# Sir Thomas Lewis

Pioneer Cardiologist and Clinical Scientist

Springer
*London*
*Berlin*
*Heidelberg*
*New York*
*Barcelona*
*Budapest*
*Hong Kong*
*Milan*
*Paris*
*Santa Clara*
*Singapore*
*Tokyo*

Arthur Hollman

# Sir Thomas Lewis

## Pioneer Cardiologist and Clinical Scientist

With 145 Figures

Springer

Dr Arthur Hollman, M.D. F.R.C.P. F.L.S.
*Emeritus consulting cardiologist, University College Hospital, London, UK*
*Honorary Senior Lecturer, Department of Medicine, University College London Medical School*

Sea Bank, Chick Hill, Pett, East Sussex TN35 4EQ, UK

*Cover illustration:* The main photograph on the front cover shows Thomas Lewis aged 27 in 1909 (Chapter 2, Figure 10)

ISBN 3-540-76049-0 Springer-Verlag Berlin Heidelberg New York

British Library Cataloguing in Publication Data
Hollman, Arthur
Sir Thomas Lewis: pioneer cardiologist and clinical scientist
1. Lewis, Sir Thomas 2. Cardiologists - Great Britain - Biography
I. Title
616.1′2′092
ISBN 3540760490

Library of Congress Cataloging-in-Publication Data
Hollman, A. (Arthur)
Sir Thomas Lewis: pioneer cardiologist and clinical scientist / Arthur Hollman.
p. cm.
Includes index.
ISBN 3-540-76049-0 (hardback: alk. paper)
1. Lewis, Thomas, Sir, 1881-1945. 2. Cardiologists-Great Britain-Biography. 3. Electrocardiography-History. I. Title.
[DNLM: 1. Lewis, Thomas, Sir, 1881-1945. 2. Cardiology-biography
WZ 100 L676H 1996]
RC666.72.L49H65 1996
616.1′2′0092-dc20
[B]
DNLM/DLC 96-9462
for Library of Congress CIP



Typeset by EXPO Holdings, Malaysia
Printed and bound by Cambridge University Press
28/3830-543210 Printed on acid-free paper

For my wife and our daughters, and in memory
of my parents who gave me a medical education

# Foreword

It is timely that Arthur Hollman's biography of Sir Thomas Lewis, with an account of his philosophy of clinical science as well as of his personal contributions to medicine, should appear now, just over 50 years since his death. While one could have anticipated that the life of such an eminent physician would have been written sooner, we have the advantage of the detailed scrutiny of his work and of the records to which Hollman has devoted himself for some years. Indeed, as the book went to press, he was able to locate and speak to the 87 year old Dr Werner Hess, one of the two German postgraduate students who had worked with Lewis in 1931, and confirm that his portrait shows a duelling scar. This meticulous attention to detail and the depiction of Lewis' relationships with his colleagues and students underpins the biography.

British cardiologists recognise the key role played by Lewis in the establishment of their specialty. The important influence that he had on American cardiology and on electrocardiography in particular has not been forgotten by those with a sense of history. Yet active work in cardiology, with dedication to electrocardiography, research on arrhythmias and conduction disturbances in particular, occupied no more than 15 years of his life; but he did of course continue to take a profound interest in diseases of the cardiovascular system and to teach and to write on the subject to the end of his days. A keen writer and critical journal editor, he played a key role in the genesis of the Cardiac Club, forerunner of the British Cardiac Society. Only now has the *British Heart Journal* reverted to his original journal title, *Heart*, established by Lewis in 1909.

Lewis is of course well remembered for being one of the first to describe the electrocardiographic appearances of atrial fibrillation in man, making his initial observations a few months after Rothberger and Winterberg of Vienna. He characterised virtually every other rhythm disorder save for the pre-excitation syndromes, but did not focus on cardiac infarction and ischaemia, where the electrocardiograph has played so major a role. He was not always right when it came to the distinction between left and right bundle branch block, the importance of left ventricular failure and the mechanical problems created by valve disease, but as he considered the evidence over the years, he did where necessary accept the views of others. Cardiac catheterisation was introduced towards the end of his life and he was rather negative about it. Yet, over all, he had a profound positive influence in the development of cardiology as a specialty, and in the recognition of war-induced stress, during the First World War, and Paul Wood took matters further during the Second World War.

As he completed the classical third edition of his Mechanism and Graphic Registration of the Heart Beat, Lewis turned to other aspects of medicine including cutaneous reactions, peripheral vascular disease, and pain perception. Underlying all these various interests was his quest for the physiological explanation for clinical phenomena, in other words clinical science. Careful observation of physical signs allied to their sound interpretation still forms a proper scaffold for clinical medicine at the end of this century, and the importance of linking basic research with clinical presentation is as valid today as he had demonstrated it to be from the outset of his career.

We get an absorbing picture of a man who was clearly perceived in different ways by those who worked with him; above all, a man who concentrated powerfully on what he was doing and who was an explicit and stimulating clinical teacher to his pupil who now gives us this account of his life. We are fully apprised of his family background and see the interplay of family life and friendships. In Arthur Hollman, his teacher Sir Thomas Lewis has found a fair and thorough biographer who while critical where appropriate is sympathetic to him and his cause in giving us a detailed account of a man of considerable intellect and influence.

Dennis M. Krikler

# Preface

*For your own satisfaction and for mine, please read this preface*

St. Francis of Sales: preface to *Introduction to Devout Life* (1609)

When I was a medical student at University College Hospital from 1943 to 1945 I had the good fortune to be a pupil of Sir Thomas Lewis. I was a clinical clerk on his firm for three months and attended his course of lectures. As a result I became very interested in clinical science and with Sir Thomas' help I started to investigate the mechanism of 'stitch' in his department. So it was natural for me to remember him with respect as a great medical scientist and a fine teacher. This led me on the tenth anniversary of his death to ask some of his former associates to record their reminiscences of working with him in a special issue of the *University College Hospital Magazine*. In his lectures, Lewis spoke about former great physicians and of medical discoveries and this gave me my first interest in the history of medicine. I then realised that many medical biographies were based on second and third hand accounts and I therefore resolved to obtain further information from men and women who had worked directly with Lewis. With the generous assistance of the Wellcome Trust I was able to record interviews with 24 of his research associates, house physicians or students, and I believe that these oral history recordings could also be of value to other medical historians. In addition I obtained useful information from informal interviews and from correspondence.

This is the first biography of Lewis and although originally I did not intend to write it myself, it gradually became apparent that I would be the author. An especial catalyst to that idea came from Dr Dennis Krikler when he recommended to the British Cardiac Society that I should be appointed their Thomas Lewis Lecturer in 1981 in order to speak on Lewis' work. Dr Krikler has been a tremendous source of encouragement and information ever since and I am deeply grateful to him. It has of course taken far too long and although it is now completed I do not wish to imply that it could not be usefully extended. I continue to see areas that could well be expanded or better explained, but one has to draw a line somewhere.

I decided that the book should consist mainly of accounts of Lewis' scientific work. Perhaps this sounds obvious but what I have tried to do is to concentrate on his own achievements as an electrophysiologist and clinical scientist without, as a rule, describing what other investigators were doing at the same time. To have done so would have meant diluting the essential message about Lewis' work with a rather poor history of cardiology and experimental medicine. In any case, a lot of his work was truly original. I have also attempted to summarise the main points of his research endeavours rather than give long accounts of them. Like all attempts to write briefly, this has involved much more work than writing at length, because I have had to try and understand the nature of his research. In some cases, especially the effort syndrome and pain, this was not always an easy thing to do. However I have not hesitated to quote directly, and sometimes at length, from his own writing when I felt that this would give a better picture of what he was saying, rather than paraphrase it. The other decision I made early on was that this would be a book for doctors. So there are inevitably technical aspects which I regret non-medical readers will find difficult to follow. On the whole the layout is chronological, but at times it was appropriate to deviate from this approach. For example there are separate chapters on clinical science, on his hospital, departmental and teaching work, and on his family life and hobbies.

But although Lewis' work is described quite briefly, I have gone to some trouble to give as many references as I can to all aspects of it, including even brief passages of his correspondence, in order to help other workers. I have read every reference myself. No reference has been included for the sake of completeness. Some of the references, particularly to those in the Wellcome Institute Contemporary Medical Archives Centre, are being published for the first time, for example Lewis' help to German Jewish refugee doctors.

It is a mistake to regard Lewis just as a cardiovascular specialist (he disliked the term cardiologist). His mission in life was that of experimental medicine, or clinical science as he came to call it, but his work on the heart was the first, and became the best known, of his research endeavours. In fact his investigations into pain, in my opinion, were intellectually even better than his highly praised electrocardiographic studies. And his identification of a chemical factor, the H substance, as the mechanism of injury to the skin was also a fine achievement. However many do still remember him chiefly for his seminal work on the electrophysiology of the heart and on cardiac arrhythmias, and I have not hesitated to give emphasis to these exciting discoveries. Being a cardiologist, I am not free from bias in this respect!

In some quarters there is now a strong tendency to play down the personal contributions of individuals and to emphasise instead the general events of their lifetime. In other words to demonstrate the importance of what is called social history. But I have not felt the urge to join this movement.

Quite apart from being an essential duty, it is a great pleasure to thank those who have encouraged, assisted and educated me during the writing of this book. Dr Gerald Graham, formerly my colleague at the Hospital for Sick Children, London, did the most important thing by recommending my work to Springer Verlag. Writing a book is one thing, but getting it published it quite another, and Dr Graham did this without my even asking him for help. I am deeply grateful to him for his assistance which came entirely from kindness of heart and his interest in the subject.

Professor John Pattison is the Dean of University College London Medical School and I cannot thank him enough for the continued interest he has taken in this book which has led to the School providing the essential and very generous financial support needed to ensure publication.

A draft of the manuscript was perused in detail by Dr Howard Burchell of St Paul Minnesota who gave it his approval. Because he is one of the world's leading cardiac historians his approval was important and I thank him warmly for it, and for all his help. It has been good also to have the appreciated support and advice of other historian friends in the United States, namely Drs W. Bruce Fye, Paul Kligfield and Charles F. Wooley.

Dr John Honour was Lewis' personal laboratory assistant for 18 years. He has been a friend ever since my student days and I cannot overestimate the value of the information he has given me on many occasions. I wish to thank him warmly for his unstinted help and advice.

I have been fortunate in having tremendous support and help from Sir Thomas' family. Lady Lewis, who survived her husband by 44 years, very kindly talked to me on several occasions and her assistance was invaluable. The eldest daughter Pat and her husband Sinclair Watson have been of immense help. They have answered many queries, have supplied family photographs, and have been generous with their time and hospitality. The younger daughter Pip, Mrs Phillipa Althaus, wrote a nice account of her father. The son, Dr Christopher Lewis, has written a long and valuable account of recollections of his father. I am deeply grateful to them all.

I thank the Wellcome Trust for its important help and financial support. The staff of the Wellcome Institute for the History of Medicine have been very helpful and I am grateful to Dr Christopher Lawrence for his advice.

Mrs Julie Beckwith, assistant librarian at the Royal College of Physicians London, has my warm thanks for answering an almost unending number of enquiries with precision and good humour.

Mr Stephen Paratian has taken many photographs for me and Mrs Berti Rooke-Ley has often given secretarial help. They both work in UCL Medical School and I am grateful for their assistance.

It has been a pleasure to work with Springer and I appreciate the friendly and immensely efficient help I have had from Rebecca Moore, Nick Mowat and Nicolas Wilson.

My wife, Catharine, has patiently put up with long and solitary hours when I have either been writing in my study, or visiting libraries. Luckily she too was a medical student at University College Hospital so the project was quite a personal one for her also and she has followed it with especial interest and with great benefit to myself for which I offer her my very best thanks.

The Greek physician Galen (131–201) is said to have given the following reasons why a man should write a book. 'Firstly, to satisfy his own friends; secondly to exercise his best mental powers; and thirdly to be saved from the oblivion incident to old age'. I sincerely hope that my family and friends will give their approval to this book. Should they do so then I too will be satisfied.

Arthur Hollman

## Numbering of Notes and References

Bracketed superior numbers in the text refer to Notes shown at the end of each chapter. Unbracketed superior numbers refer to the References section which starts on page 279.

# Acknowledgements

I am grateful to Mrs Patricia Watson (née Lewis) for generously lending me photographs of her family and her father's associates and allowing me to publish them. Dr Herbert J. Levine kindly gave me a photograph of his father, Dr Samuel A. Levine. I thank Dr Joel D. Howell and Dr D.W. Sonneborn for lending me photographs taken at Ann Arbor of Willem Einthoven, Frank N. Wilson and Sir Thomas and Lady Lewis. Dr A.J. Honour kindly gave me a photograph of himself, and Dr Alan Sykes supplied a picture of A.D. Waller.

Permission to reproduce pictorial and written material in their possession has been granted by the following authorities.

The Museum Boerhaave Leiden for Figures 3.1 and 7.1. The British Medical Journal Publishing Group for Figures 3.9, 11.4 and 11.5. The Gambit Press, Boston, for the quotation from reference 255. Peabody and Arnold, Boston, for Figures 13.1, 13.2, 13.3, 13.5, 17.1, 17.2 and 17.6. The Medical Research Council for quotations from their archives. The National Library of Medicine Washington DC for Figure 2.10. The Portland Press Ltd for Figures 14.1, 14.2 and 14.4. The Rockefeller Foundation for Figure 2.10. The Royal College of Physicians of London for Figures 2.2, 9.5, 10.2, 11.2, and 14.3. The Royal Society of London for Lewis' personal record. Shaw and Sons Ltd for Figures 2.7, 3.11 and 5.3. The Librarian University College London for Figures 1.8 and 2.1. The Wellcome Institute Library London for Figures 5.1, 5.4, and 9.3.

If by unintended oversight I have omitted to request permission to publish, or have failed in any way to acknowledge copyright material, I offer my sincere apologies.

# *Contents*

# Chronology

1881 Born in Cardiff, Wales.

1893 Attended Clifton College Bristol for one year. Before and after that he was educated at home.

1895 Decided at the age of 13 to become a doctor.

1898 Home tuition continued by a tutor, until aged 16.

1898 Went to University College Cardiff.

1902 B Sc (Wales) with honours. 2nd MB (London) with gold medal. Primary FRCS (England).

1902 Publishes his first scientific paper.

1902 Enters University College Hospital London (UCH).

1904 Elected to the Physiological Society. Conjoint diploma.

1905 Final MB BS (London) with University gold medal. D Sc (Wales).

1905 House surgeon and house physician at UCH, until 1906.

1906 Undertakes original research work on the pulse.

1907 Appointed to the staff of the City of London Hospital and the Seamans' Hospital. Working in the laboratory of Professor E.H. Starling at University College London (UCL). MD (London), MRCP (London). Elected Fellow of UCL.

1908 Meets Dr James Mackenzie, a pioneer of cardiac investigation, who greatly influences his career, and who encourages him to study irregular heart action.

1909 Starts private consulting practice in Wimpole Street.

1909 Founds the journal *Heart* and becomes its first editor. Now aged 27.

1909 Visits Willem Einthoven, the great pioneer of electrocardiography in Leiden, and initiates a long collaboration and friendship with him.

1909 Acquires his first electrocardiograph machine and begins an intensive study of cardiac arrhythmias. Elucidates atrial fibrillation in man.

1910 Awarded a Beit Memorial Fellowship. Appointed lecturer in cardiac pathology at UCH.

1911 Pioneer monograph *The Mechanism of the Heart Beat.*

1912 Appointed assistant physician at UCH. Elected FRCP (London). Writes a teaching book on *Clinical disorders of the heart beat*, followed in 1913 by *Clinical Electrocardiography.*

1914 Invited to the United States of America to give the Herter and the Harvey Lectures.

1914 His first communication to the Royal Society of London.

1916 Appointed physician at the Military Heart Hospital Hampstead. Appointed physician on the staff of the Medical Research Committee, the first full time post in clinical medicine in Britain. Commences research work on 'Soldier's Heart', which he re-names the Effort Syndrome. Gives up private practice.

1916 Marries Miss Lorna James of Merthyr Tydfil, Wales.

1917 Croonian Lecture at the Royal Society summarises his outstanding work in cardiac electrophysiology.

1918 Monograph *The Soldier's Heart and the Effort Syndrome.* Elected a Fellow of the Royal Society of London.

1918 First child, Patricia, is born.

1919 Appointed Physician at UCH, and establishes the Department of Clinical Research in UCH Medical School under the Medical Research Council.

1920 Appointed Commander of the British Empire. Writes an article for *British Birds* on the Little Tern.

1921 Created a Knight Bachelor. Intensive study of the mechanism of atrial flutter and fibrillation leading to his hypothesis of the circus movement.

1922 Founder member and first chairman of the Cardiac Club.

1922 Gives invited lectures in the United States.

1923 Second child, Christopher, is born.

1924 Studies the vascular reactions of the skin to injury and proposes the 'H substance' as the mechanism of the triple response to injury. Gives up research on the heart.

1925 Publishes the third and highly acclaimed edition of *The Mechanism and Graphic Registration of the Heart Beat.*

1927 Monograph, *The blood vessels of the human skin and their responses.* Has a myocardial infarction at the age of 45 and recovers well. Awarded the Royal Medal of the Royal Society.

1929 Commences a study of Raynaud's disease.

1930 He founds, with others, the Medical Research Society and becomes its first chairman.

1931 Research on pain in muscular ischaemia, with its cause identified as a chemical substance, 'factor P'.

1931 Third child, Phillipa (Pip), is born. A third lecture tour in the United States when he enjoys bird watching with Dr Frank Wilson at Ann Arbor.

1932 He has been a member of the Council of the Royal Society from 1925–26 and 1930–32.

1932 Identifies the mechanism of Raynaud's disease.

1933 Delivers the Harveian Oration on Clinical Science. He founds the journal, *Clinical Science incorporating Heart* and becomes its editor. He is appointed a member of the Medical Research Council, and serves until 1937.

1933 *Diseases of the Heart* is published and becomes very popular with students and doctors.

1933 The family moves to a new house in the country with a large garden and a trout stream.

1934 He recounts his own research work in *Clinical Science, illustrated by personal experiences.*

1935 Has a second myocardial infarction. Delivers the Huxley Lecture on clinical science.

1936 Writes an excellent teaching book, *Vascular disorders of the limbs.*

1937 He proposes that cutaneous hyperalgesia is due to a hitherto undescribed 'nocifensor system' of nerves in the skin. His hypothesis is attacked but is validated 50 years later.

1938 Makes a teaching film on heart failure called 'The signs of venous congestion'.

1939 Concludes three years work on the double pain response in the skin, and on the experimental production of referred pain.

1939 The outbreak of World War 2 terminates the work in his department, never to be re-established. The hospital and medical school are evacuated from London.

1940 Takes charge of teaching UCH students at Llandough Hospital near Cardiff Wales.

1941 Is awarded the Copley Medal of the Royal Society which is its most prestigious award.

1942 His monograph *Pain* is published in the United States.

1944 Articles on reform in medical education.

1945 His book *Exercises in Human Physiology* is designed to introduce physiology students to clinical medicine.

1945 Dies at his home with a third myocardial infarction on March 17 at the age of 63.

# Chapter 1

## Early life • Family • Education • Medical School at University College Cardiff and University College London

THOMAS LEWIS was born in Cardiff, Wales, on December 26 1881 at *Teigel House* in Roath, a district in the centre of the city. A few years later his parents moved into the countryside a few miles north of Cardiff to a house called *Tynant* at Taff's Well, which remained his home until he was a young man. He was the third of five children and his only sister died in infancy. His father, Henry Lewis (1850–1916) was one of ten children of Thomas Lewis (1819–1881) and Mary Lester (1822–1902) both of Abersychan, Monmouthshire. Henry's forbears were Monmouthshire yeomen, belonging to an old Welsh family whose origin could be traced back to 1000 A.D. His pedigree is in the College of Heralds, and his armorial bearings[(1)] were those of 1) Rhys Goch; 2) Howell of Caerleon; 3) Caradwg Greich Fras; and 4) Howell Dola.[41] His mother, Katherine Hannah Davies was the daughter of Owen Davies of Cardiff who owned slate quarries in North Wales, and Hannah Davis who came from a Somerset family.

Henry Lewis (Fig. 1.1) was a mining engineer, a pioneer in the South Wales coal trade, who became president of the Coal Owners Association. Like two of his relatives before him he owned a colliery, and he won the Albert Medal for bravery during rescue work underground. Lewis said, "My father was a man of exceptionally strong upright and lovable character. He was widely read, unusually clear minded, and ambitious for his sons. I attribute my success as a student very largely to his constant stimulus and encouragement. The interest and guidance of my parents was constant".[223]

The family was Methodist but their upbringing was not narrow for the works of Darwin, Huxley, Lyell, Mill and Tyndal, together with many books on natural history and chemistry were in the library of several thousand volumes. His mother (Fig. 1.2), who was an only child, was described as an interesting person who gave the children all their early lessons.[377] She, too, was ambitious for them and taught herself Latin in order that they might learn it from her.

### Home and family

The family home *Tynant* at Taff's Well (Fig. 1.3) had been made from a row of cottages at the end of which was a public house. The boys (Fig. 1.4) used to spend

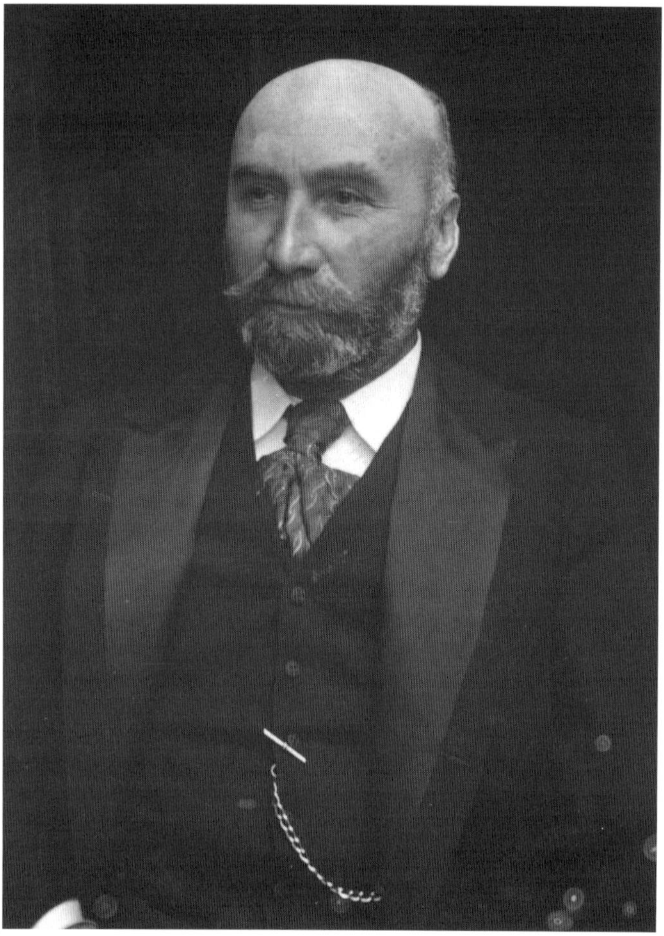

*Figure 1.1* *Henry Lewis, aged 40. 'A man of exceptionally strong character', a trait which was reflected in his son.*

all their spare time in the fields and woods and on the mountains. The eldest was Lester who became an engineer in the British Army. He went on an army expedition to Tibet, and later served in the 1914–1918 War winning the Distinguished Service Order and Bar. He had two sons neither of whom had children and he died in 1960. After Tom the next was Clifford, considered by his father to have the best brain of all his sons. He trained to be a barrister but had a nervous breakdown and on medical advice his parents took him on a holiday to California, where they visited Yosemite National Park; but he never worked and later he lived with his mother in Bath until her death in 1938. He died in 1947. The youngest was Trevor, who followed the family tradition and became a mining engineer in Bilbao, Spain. He was tragically killed in the 1914–1918 War, whilst bravely trying to clear away an unexploded grenade.

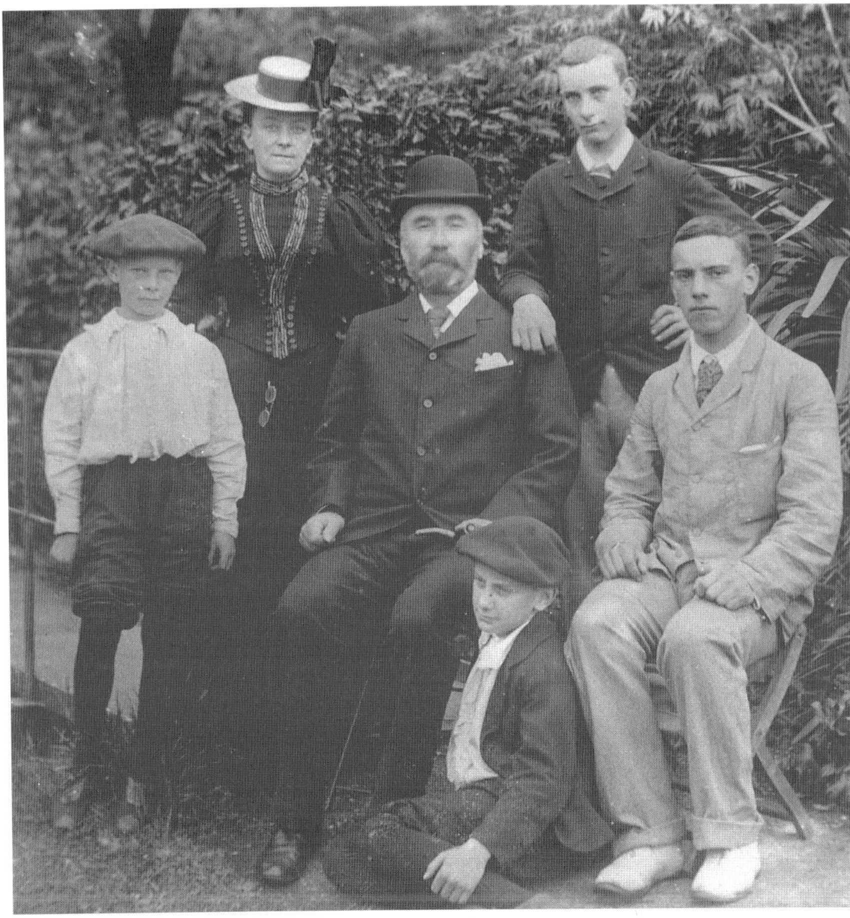

*Figure 1.2 The Lewis family in about 1896. Tom is behind his father, with Lester, Clifford and Trevor from right to left.*

## Early education

Tom was educated at home until he was ten years old and then went to Clifton College, Bristol as a boarder to join his brother Lester. Judging by the letters he sent home, one written in French, he enjoyed being at school. "The boys in my bedroom are very nice", "I am getting on well with my music", – a reference to his learning to play the violin, and interestingly, "I find my work is much easier with the other boys than at home".[378] However he was considered to be a delicate child and after one year Mrs Lewis decided to have him home again, where he stayed until he was aged 16½. In fact he seems to have been a normal, healthy lad, so maybe Mrs Lewis, who had a strong personality, just wanted to have him back with her. For the last two years he had a Cardiff graduate, Mr Morgan, as his tutor and got on well with him, but he lacked the stimulus of a busy classroom and had no practical work in, for example, physics and chemistry. This may have been why he failed the University of London matriculation examination at the age of

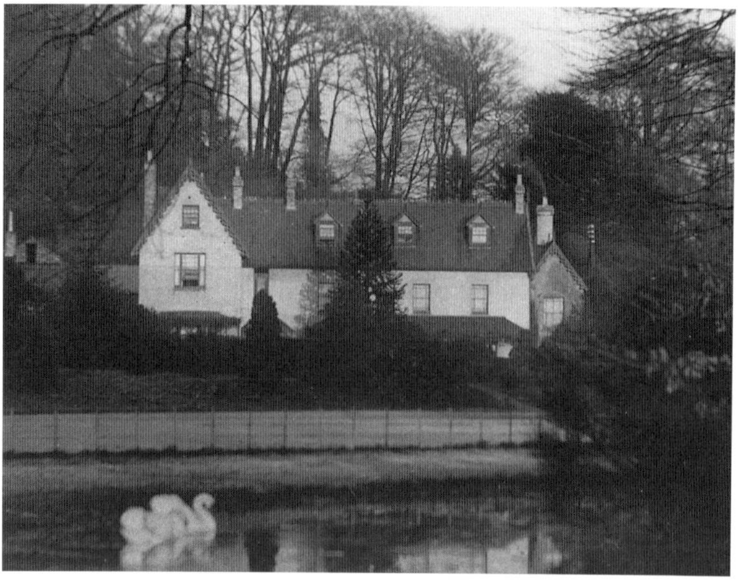

*Figure 1.3 The family home* Tynant *at Taff's Well near Cardiff Wales.*

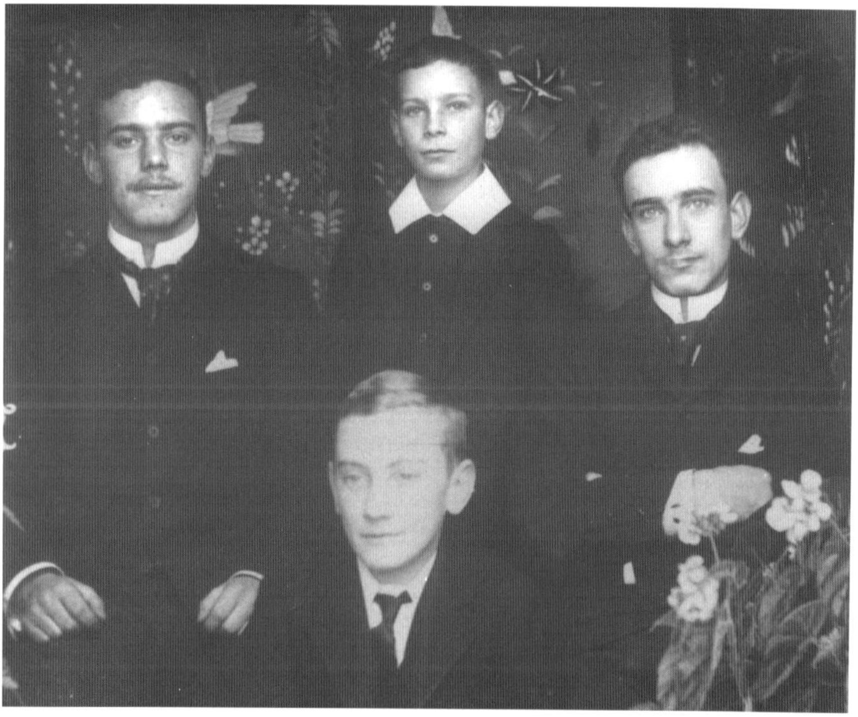

*Figure 1.4 The four sons in about 1900. Clifford in front with Lester, Trevor and Tom from left to right. Tom would be aged about 18.*

15.[(2)] "My failure to matriculate goaded me to apply myself to my books. I failed in no subsequent examinations".[223]

Nevertheless his own explanation of the failure was that he did not really start to work until after that episode, his chief interests up to then, he said, being in natural history, hunting and shooting. He took these interests seriously, possessing the two volume *A History of British Birds* by William Yarrell, 1836, and the four volume *A History of British Fishes* by the same author, 1884. Both of these books were illustrated field guides. At some stage he also commenced his life-long interest in photography, developing and printing the pictures himself.

## College and medical school in Cardiff • First scientific papers

Having matriculated in the first division in June 1898 at age 16, he entered the Science Department at University College, Cardiff, going there each day on his bicycle. His college studies were directed towards a career in medicine and luckily we know from his own writing the very unusual reason that led him in that direction:

> I decided to become a doctor before entering my teens, for the curious reason that conjuring fascinated me, and because two family doctors both conjured I fancied that doctoring was a prerequisite to sleight of hand. Very fortunately a certain manual dexterity and a persistent curiosity in respect of natural objects and phenomena made his career suitable.[223]

The subjects he took were chemistry, physics and biology. He said that he worked hard, but was surprised when he gained scholarships which paid his fees while at College. He passed the first part of the London MB examination (the 1st MB) in July 1899 and then went to the medical school in Cardiff.[(3)] Incidentally, he became a second lieutenant in the volunteer forces of the Welsh Regiment in 1901. During his three years of preclinical studies there were two teachers who especially influenced him. They were Francis Dixon, Professor of Anatomy and Swale Vincent,[(4)] Lecturer in Physiology, and he became a student demonstrator in anatomy and then in histology. His potential was recognized by Vincent who asked him – and Lewis was still only 18 – to undertake research with him on the proteins of unstriped muscle. "The request came as a complete surprise to me. I have always been grateful to Vincent for giving me my first introduction to scientific work".[189] His first two scientific papers, written with Vincent, were published in 1901 in the *Journal of Physiology.* They were on the proteins of unstriped muscle and on the chemistry and heat rigor curves of muscle.[322,323] Then he wrote, by himself, a 54-page paper on the structure and function of the haemolymph glands and spleen (Fig. 1.5) which was published in an important international journal.[110] It was a full, detailed and professionally written account which was to become a standard work on the subject. It had two full page colour plates of the microscopical appearances, each reproducing several of his own excellent water colour drawings (Fig. 1.6). To be sole author of this scholarly work at the age of 19 was a notable achievement.

(Aus der Internationalen Monatsschrift f. Anatomie u. Physiologie. 1902. Bd. XX. Heft 1/2.)

(From the Physiological Laboratory, Cardiff, December 20th, 1901.)

**The Structure and Functions of the hæmolymph Glands and Spleen.**

By

**Thomas Lewis, B. Sc.,**
University of Wales.

(With Plates I, II.)

Contents.



1

*Figure 1.5 Title page of his first scientific article written at age 19 (From reference 110).*

His diligence and natural grasp of method is well demonstrated in the collection of reprints of papers which he made at this time, and had bound up in a volume labelled *Ductless Glands chiefly histological.*[521] There are 44 papers of which 25 were written by Vincent who probably also gave him some of the others, though it is quite likely that this was the time when he first learnt to write to authors for their reprints. Seven were from the journal *Anatomischer Anzeiger* so he may even then have had some knowledge of German. At the back of the volume there were indices with detailed lists of the articles, journals and authors.

He became a Bachelor of Science, Wales, taking a pass degree in June 1901 and proceeding to a double honours degree a year later. In July 1902 at the age of 20, Lewis (Fig. 1.7) passed the 2nd MB (London) examination with first class honours

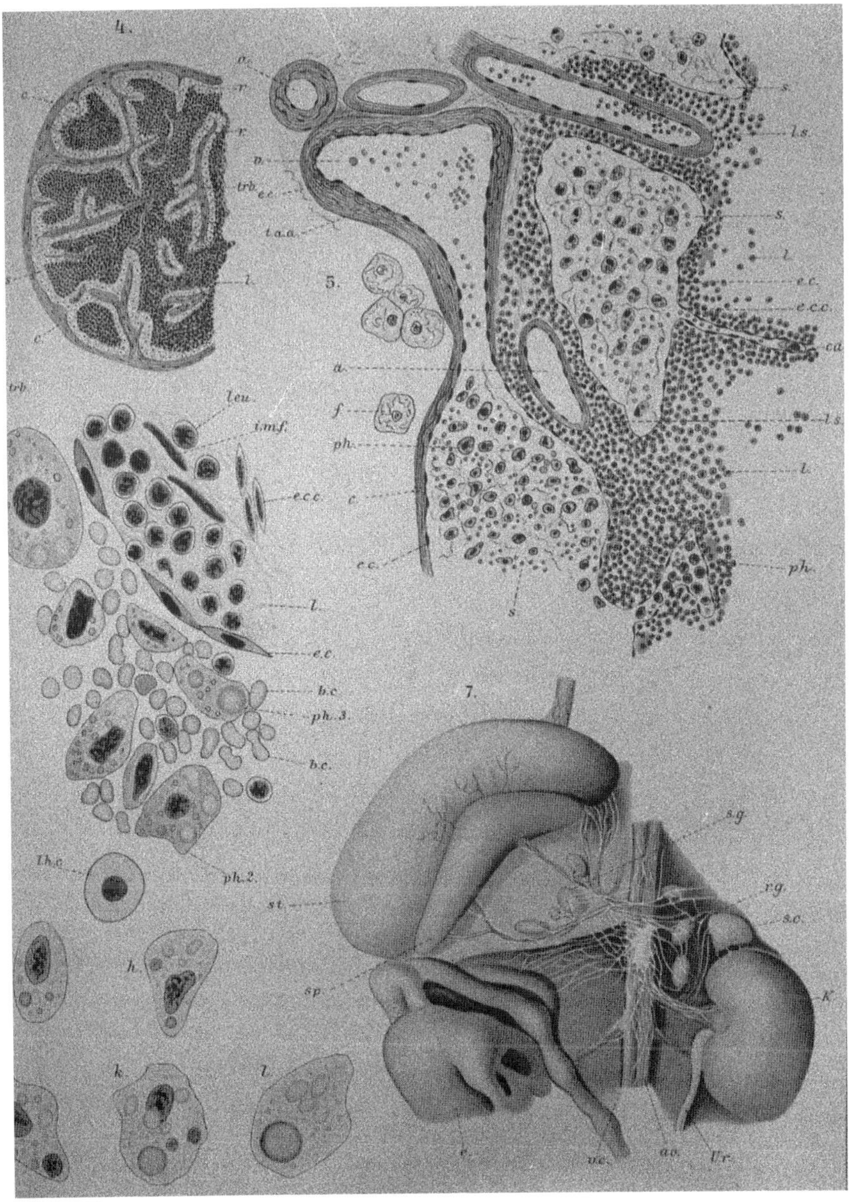


*Figure 1.6 Plate 1 of the article, drawn and coloured by himself, showing a dissection of the haemal glands of the rat (bottom right) with microscopic sections of a gland shown top right × 250, and middle left × 1000. (From reference 110).*

in anatomy and physiology and was awarded the gold medal. A group of seven papers, four being written during these student days, gained him, at the age of 22, the degree of Doctor of Science, Wales. It was a remarkable beginning to what was to be a remarkable career.

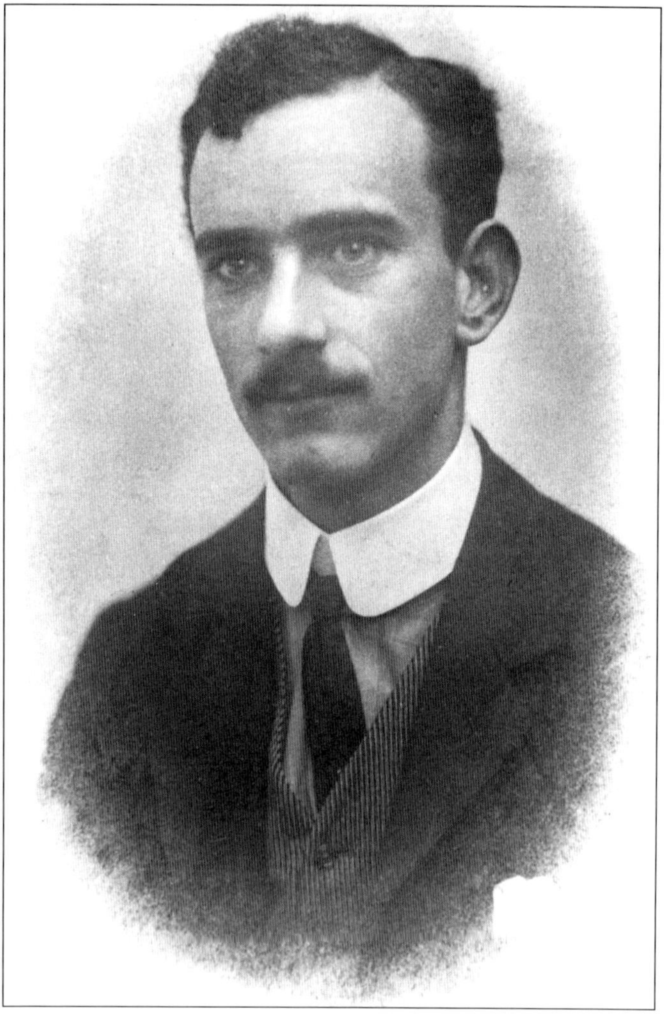

*Figure 1.7 Thomas Lewis, the young Cardiff undergraduate, aged 20, sporting a moustache for the first time.*

## Enters University College Hospital and meets the leading physiologists at University College London

In October 1902 he enrolled in the medical school at University College Hospital, London, (UCH) with an Entrance Exhibition. At that time the School, which became independent in 1907, was still part of the Faculty of Medicine of University College London (UCL).[5] Soon afterwards he passed the primary FRCS[6] examination. The hospital had several doctors of academic distinction on its staff and it naturally had close links with the College, but in spite of this Lewis found the transition from the scientific discipline of his Cardiff work and studies to the atmosphere of hospital routine a difficult one. He used to say that to go to hospital after a training in science was like working in a market garden after being in a botanical laboratory.[50] In another comment he wrote, "There is an abrupt passage to a foreign atmosphere where opportunism reigns with the voice of authority, (and) where memory is more extolled than reason...".[236]

However his aptitude for scientific work stood him in good stead because it was no doubt through Swale Vincent, a former lecturer at UCL, that he gained an introduction at the College (Fig. 1.8) to the leading physiologists of the day, namely Ernest H Starling[(7)] and William M Bayliss,[(8)] and to the pharmacologist Arthur R Cushny.[(9)] In fact he used to lunch regularly with these three, all Fellows of the Royal Society, at the ABC restaurant in Tottenham Court Road though still a student and their junior by 15 or more years, and he learnt, he said, much from them.[50]

This was a time when UCL was exceptionally strong in cardiovascular research. Starling and Bayliss had done pioneer studies on the electrical activity of the heart and on pressures in the heart and blood vessels. Starling (Fig. 1.9) went on to design his famous heart–lung preparation and Bayliss to investigate the vasomotor system. Cushny had worked on experimental and human arrhythmias and had been first to suggest that atrial fibrillation in the dog had a counterpart in humans. In addition the neurosurgeon Sir Victor Horsley[(10)] had a laboratory in the College in which junior hospital staff were often invited to work. Lewis greatly admired Starling and Horsley saying that "both were inspiring men of outstanding intellect and originality". He was elected to the Physiological Society at the age of 22 and it was there that he first met the pharmacologist H H Dale,[(11)] later Sir Henry, and President of the Royal Society, who became a close friend. Dale said that:

> Lewis indeed had a precocious maturity of outlook and scientific judgement which made it natural for him to associate with older men: though he was my junior by 6

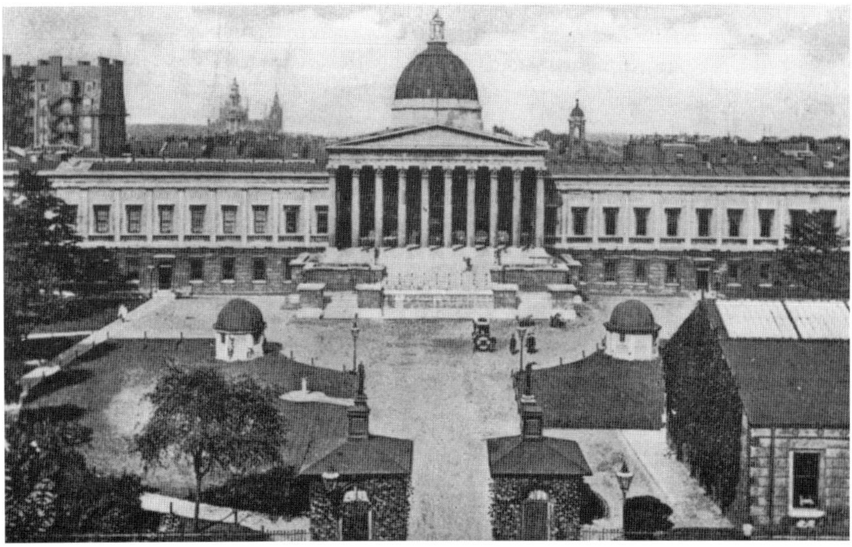

*Figure 1.8 University College London at the time when he worked there as a medical student in 1904.*

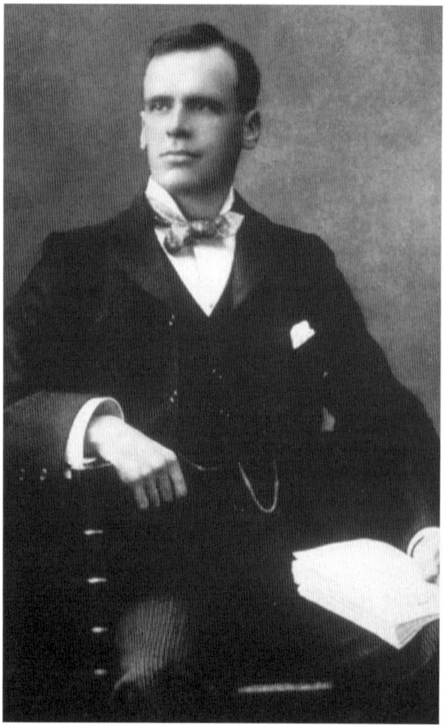

*Figure 1.9 Ernest Henry Starling at the time he became professor of physiology at UCL in 1899.*

> years, it never occurred to me to think of him as other than a contemporary in scientific development and experience. I remember the impression of assured scientific competence and judgement produced by his first serious piece of research, on sphygmograph records, when he described it to the Physiological Society.[46]

Whilst an undergraduate he won the Fellowes silver medal in clinical medicine on two occasions, a silver medal in surgery, the Tuke medal in morbid anatomy, and the Bruce medal in surgery and bacteriology and he became the Atkinson Scholar, but "his individualism and intentness in his work kept him apart from his fellow students".[50] Lewis wrote, "During the whole of my student career at UCH I was dabbling in research in spare time, but produced nothing of consequence".[223]

## Letters to his mother and a hunting trip in Norway with his father and brothers

He wrote several letters to his mother at this time.[378] The first, in October 1902, relates that, "I saw Victor Horsley do two of his famous brain operations last week, he is exceedingly smart using both hands equally well. Please ask Dobbins to see that he has eased the springs of our guns put by for the winter". Another tells us that he had at some time taken up photography as a hobby: "I have no toning solution so I am afraid I cannot do prints". It was addressed to "My dear mother" and signed, "With love to all, believe me, your affectionate son Tom". The next has a good sketch in ink of a consultant physician, Dr Vivian Poore, who "is exceedingly witty but teaches us very little medicine". A further letter has good drawings done at the Zoo with sketches of birds and a tortoise which reveal his artistic ability, ending with the comment "there is a surprising want of elegance in the foot of a tortoise". At the end of the first term he says that he is playing "soccer" for UCH adding, "You need have no anxiety of my talking about colliery matters". There is no clue as to what these matters were, possibly they were financial, for as we shall see later, he certainly relied to some extent at least on an income from his family's coal mines. In September 1904 he wrote from Norway where he was on a hunting expedition with his father, Clifford and Trevor. They were hunting elk and he made careful notes, which have been kept, of the day-to-day events during this time.[520] One of them, for example, reads:

> Monday. Found bull 9.45, winded us and ran, picked up trail and dog winded. Sighted crossing a glade at 180 yards. Tom – miss. Cliff – shot traversing body from right perinaeum to left lung. "Coup de grace" 11.30 Home 12.50 ? 12 miles. Old bull 18 hands. 4+6 = 10 points.

And what was striking were the several statistical analyses he made of the expedition. He recorded the average days, miles and hours per elk and the average miles per day with a table showing how they applied to each member of the party. Altogether in 17 days they killed 6 elk, and walked 332 miles in 135 hours. This holiday, and the visit his parents and Clifford made to California, show that his family had ample means.

## Notes to Chapter 1

(1) Armorial bearings, which are an essential part of heraldry, originated in the 12th century as a symbol on armour. A coat-of-arms referred to a person with distinctive clothing who was entitled to carry weapons and to bear arms, armorial bearings, became the mark of a gentleman. They were awarded to important members of a community, and could be inherited by their family, such as the Howells of Caerleon, a town in Wales. The College of Heralds in London is the reference centre for all aspects of heraldry.

(2) To matriculate means literally to be placed on a register. It was the essential first step to gaining entry to a university.

(3) The degree in the University of London which enabled one to be placed on the Medical Register and practice as a doctor was that of Bachelor of Medicine and Bachelor of Surgery, abbreviated to MB BS but often just called the MB. The 1st MB was in scientific subjects such as physics. The 2nd MB comprised anatomy, physiology, pharmacology and biochemistry, whilst the 3rd or final MB was the examination in clinical subjects.

(4) Thomas Swale Vincent, FRS Ed, 1868–1934, worked under Professor E A Schafer and then under Professor E H Starling at UCL until he was appointed lecturer in physiology at Cardiff in 1900. He was a pioneer of the then recently discovered functions of the endocrine glands, especially of the suprarenal glands, and was valued for his critical and sceptical mind. From 1920 to 1930 he was professor of physiology at the Middlesex Hospital, London. He was described as an essentially shy man which gave

an impression of brusqueness, and interestingly this was later to be a description of the young man, Thomas Lewis, whom he selected to be his assistant.

(5) University College London was founded in 1826, and opened in 1828, as the University of London, with the express aim of being free of all religious constraints, in contrast to Oxford and Cambridge. In order to provide clinical experience for the students in its faculty of medicine, a hospital was built opposite the College in Gower Street. University College Hospital, at first named the North London Hospital, opened in 1834. A fine new hospital with 300 beds, built on a cruciform plan, was opened in November 1906. In 1907 the clinical, as opposed to the basic sciences, portion of the faculty of medicine of UCL separated from the College and became University College Hospital Medical School.

(6) The first part, "the Primary", of the examination for Fellowship of the Royal College of Surgeons of England. The primary FRCS was a difficult test of advanced knowledge in anatomy.

(7) Ernest Henry Starling, FRS, 1866–1927, was the professor, and head of the department, of physiology at UCL from 1899 to 1922. He was known as the "arch-experimentalist" to his friends in Europe, and as "the clinician's physiologist" in Britain. His famous heart–lung preparation enabled him to define the factors governing cardiac output which he summarized in his Law of the Heart. Together with Bayliss he discovered secretin, and did early electrocardiographic work. He had a dynamic personality and was an inspiring teacher who was always keen on helping young people.

(8) William Maddock Bayliss, FRS, (later Sir William), 1860–1924, was a physiologist who worked closely with Starling at UCL. In 1891 they did pioneer work on the electrophysiology of the mammalian heart, and in 1902 they discovered the hormone secretin. Bayliss wrote a monograph on *The Vasomotor System* and gained the Copley Medal, the highest award of the Royal Society of London.

(9) Arthur Cushny, FRS, 1866–1926, was a Scotsman who worked at Ann Arbor USA until 1905 when he became professor of pharmacology at UCL. He did early work on digitalis and arrhythmias, and on the pharmacology of optical isomers, and was especially known for his authoritative monograph, *The Secretion of Urine*.

(10) Victor Horsley, FRS, (later Sir Victor), 1857–1916, was named after Queen Victoria at her command. He was a pioneer neurosurgeon noted for his work on the localization of function in the brain. Every working day he went from the hospital to UCL to undertake research on the brain and any keen medical resident at UCH was certain of an invitation to his laboratory. He was a strong opponent of the anti-vivisection movement and of the use of alcohol. He was awarded the Royal Medal of the Royal Society.

(11) Henry Hallett Dale, FRS, (later Sir Henry), 1875–1968, was an experimental pharmacologist of great distinction who was a joint recipient in 1936 of the Nobel Prize for his work on the chemical transmission of nerve impulses. He became the first director of the National Institute for Medical Research in 1928, and was later the chairman of The Wellcome Trust. He was president of the Royal Society from 1940–1945 and was awarded its Copley Medal.

# Chapter 2

## Graduates • House appointments at University College Hospital • Research on pulse and blood pressure • Meets Dr James Mackenzie in 1908 • Becomes editor of *Heart*

THOMAS LEWIS qualified as a doctor with the Conjoint diploma[(1)] in July 1904 at the age of 22 and then proceeded in 1905 to gain a triple distinction in the final MB BS examination, with the University gold medal. His first appointment at University College Hospital (Fig. 2.1) was as house surgeon to Sir Victor Horsley in 1904. (Fig. 2.2, *overleaf*) He had initially thought of being a surgeon but during this job he found that work in the operating theatre was too physically exhausting.[362] In later years he often spoke about Horsley, and always with admiration, 'he bore himself like a prince and behaved like one', but he did say that Horsley left him to do operations on his own that nobody with his inexperience should have been allowed to do.[515] He worked also in Horsley's laboratory and wrote a paper, under his own name, in *Brain* about the case of a dog with defective cerebellar lobes.[111] Horsley would not permit his own name to appear jointly on a paper because he knew it would detract the credit from a junior's work.[293]

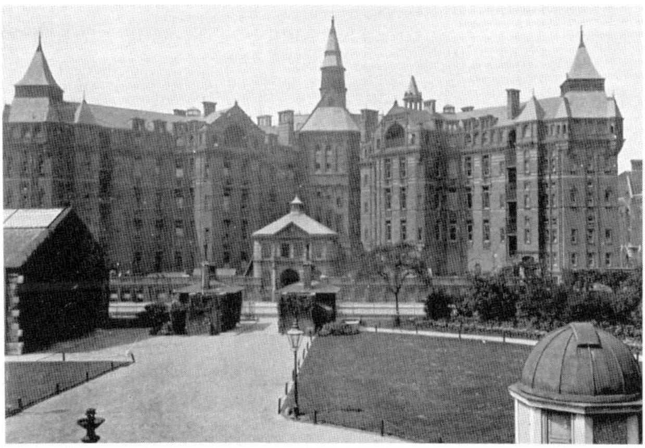

*Figure 2.1 University College Hospital, when completed, in 1906. Two wings and the central block were in use when Lewis became a medical student in 1902.*

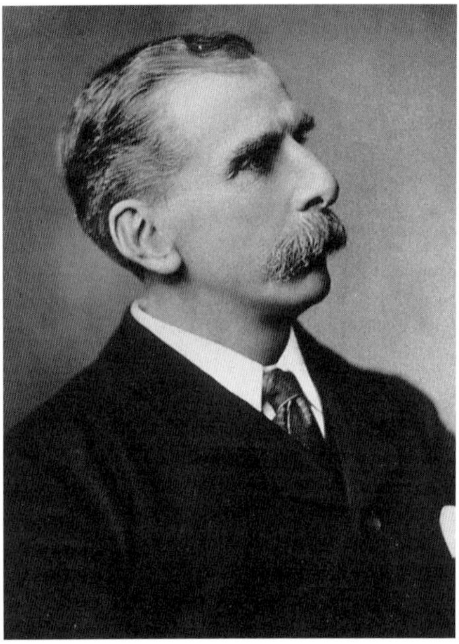

*Figure 2.2* *Sir Victor Horsley. Pioneer neurosurgeon and Lewis' first chief, 'a man of outstanding intellect and ability'.*

## His first cardiological work

Then came an important, perhaps a decisive, point in his career when he first started to study the cardiovascular system, by undertaking research on the pulse whilst he was house physician to Sir Thomas Barlow(2) in 1905–6. He started off by making a detailed analysis of the clinical features of 20 patients with aortic regurgitation, including on each a pulse tracing done with the Dudgeon sphygmograph(3) and a measurement of the systolic blood pressure. These findings were written up in *The Lancet* of 15 September 1906 with the title, The pulse in aortic disease; the relation of pulse curves to blood pressure (Fig. 2.3) and this was Lewis's first cardiological paper.[112] It was followed during the next twelve months with no less than seven other articles on either the pulse or the blood pressure, utilising both clinical and experimental observations. In one of them he again used the Dudgeon sphygmograph which he cleverly modified to make it a sensitive way of measuring the systolic blood pressure.[80] At this time in 1906 it was only the systolic blood pressure that was measured, by palpating the radial artery and using the newly introduced pneumatic cuff of S Riva-Rocci.[104] The discovery in 1905 of the auscultatory method by N S Korotkoff took a long time to be recognized and introduced into practice, and indeed even 20 years later some doctors were still not using it. The Dudgeon sphygmograph (Fig. 2.4) was a compact instrument which fastened onto the wrist and enabled one to record the arterial pulse on a short strip of smoked paper. It was very convenient for clinical use and it was even possible to add a second tracing using a tambour and stylus. Lewis used such a method to show the changes in the pulse with the alterations in

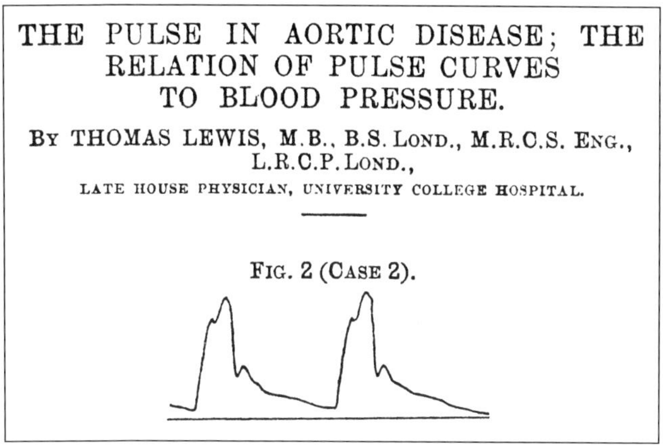

THE PULSE IN AORTIC DISEASE; THE RELATION OF PULSE CURVES TO BLOOD PRESSURE.

BY THOMAS LEWIS, M.B., B.S. LOND., M.R.C.S. ENG., L.R.C.P. LOND.,

LATE HOUSE PHYSICIAN, UNIVERSITY COLLEGE HOSPITAL.

FIG. 2 (CASE 2).

*Figure 2.3 The title, and one figure, in Lewis' first article on heart disease in 1906. (From reference 112.)*

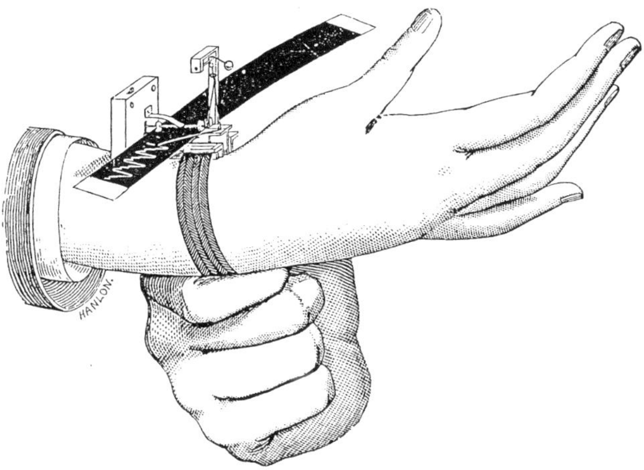


*Figure 2.4 Dudgeon's sphygmograph showing a recording of the radial arterial pulse. From Bramwell B. (1884) Diseases of the Heart. Young J. Pentland, Edinburgh*

intrathoracic pressure that occurred with the manoeuvres of Valsalva and Müller. He also made a careful study of the bisferiens type of pulse.[80] Later he wrote, 'My first really original work was done on the pulse and respiration while a house physician. It was a repetition of earlier work by Leonard Hill and I was greatly stimulated by his generous acknowledgment of its correctness'.[223] Leonard E Hill[(4)] had done original work on the pulse[48] and Lewis went on to write a chapter on the pulse for Hill's *Further Advances in Physiology.*[120] His research continued both in the hospital and also in Starling's laboratory. He was clearly fascinated by the various waves in arterial pulse curves and by inserting artificial waves into the tracing he was able to prove that the first wave was not an artefact. A paper on 'The factors influencing the prominence of the dicrotic wave' is notable for having experimental studies at the bedside together with good studies in the laboratory.[113] By observing patients who required a venesection he was able to show that blood loss produced a dicrotic pulse. In order to study the dicrotic wave under controlled conditions he devised a reservoir system with an artificial 'pulse' made from a silk tambour with a sphygmograph mounted above it. These papers show his early ability to devise good experimental methods and to link clinical and laboratory investigations, – a combination which became his personal hallmark in the discipline of clinical science.[80] At that time he had to publish some of his papers in physiological journals, for there was no other suitable English one available. They are impressive papers, with up to 33 pages and 28 figures each and for a young and busy doctor this was a huge research output which presaged the tremendous volume of his later work. Clearly the cardiovascular system had gripped his imagination, and Hill's introduction may have catalysed an interest in the subject which he had gained from Starling's outstanding work, and from his friendship with him and his associates. Maybe the dynamic nature of circulatory work had a personal appeal to him too, which would have been lacking in research on one of Starling's other interests such as the endocrine system. He then went to Berlin for a few months in the autumn of 1906 to study German and 25 years later he still urged his assistants to learn that language. On returning to Britain he took the MD London degree[(5)] and he passed the Membership examination (MRCP) of the Royal College of Physicians.[(6)]

## Obtains his first hospital consultant posts

In 1907 he was appointed Assistant Physician to the Seamen's Hospital Greenwich, and Physician to Out Patients at the City of London Hospital. He had glowing testimonials from his former chiefs on applying for these posts. Sir Thomas Barlow wrote, 'I cannot speak too highly of his efficiency. I found him remarkably quick and at the same time dependable…he was enthusiastic in new enquiries and investigations'.[344] Sir Victor Horsley wrote, 'Few men have a more intelligent appreciation of the needs of a patient or are more skilled in meeting them. It is difficult to express adequately the high character of Dr T. Lewis's claim for this appointment'.[370] But these posts left him enough time to continue with work in Starling's laboratory at UCL where he undertook very thorough and technically demanding animal work. In one study he recorded simultaneously the pericardial, tracheal and arterial pressures in 44 cats, and described the relationship of respiration to blood pressure in a 42-page paper.[115] This paper, published in 1908, also contained clinical work showing that the blood pressure fell in normal subjects on inspiration and hence that pulsus paradoxus was a misnomer. It is a token of the high regard that his seniors must have had of him that he was now elected a Fellow of UCL at the age of only 25.

## Meets T.R. Elliott, a lifelong friend

By now Thomas Renton Elliott[(7)] had come to UCH as a medical student at the late age of 29 after brilliant physiological work at Cambridge. He was the first, from his work on adrenaline, to advance the concept of a chemical neurotransmitter.

He met Lewis at a meeting of the Physiological Society in London early in 1906 and soon afterwards, when Lewis left the residence at UCH, they took rooms together in Camden Town, a mile or so north of the hospital. He became one of Lewis' closest and certainly most important friends giving him constant and invaluable support during his whole career and becoming his physician. When Elliott retired in 1939 Lewis wrote a charming account of their early days together:

> I went to live with him in noisy ill-kept rooms in Mornington Place where all the passing trains of the Midland Railway vomited smoke and spat ashes at us. There we worked together in our common sitting-room in the evenings, and dined in it monotonously on what passed for boiled mutton and parsley sauce. From there we took a never forgotten holiday in the Channel Islands, going to Sark to explore its under-water caves and natural aquaria, to lie on its sunlit rocks and to swim in its surfbroken channels. We hauled up great skate from the depths and on a grassy slope we exposed their still beating hearts and watched in these before they died, the forward blocks and reversed rhythms which Gaskell had described. He was the same Elliott then that he has since been, a frequent change in his thoughtful and ruddy countenance coming first at the corners of his mouth, soon to move in whimsical smile or to break in genial and hearty laughter; he was always vigourous physically and mentally; eager and enthusiastic but scrupulously exacting and critical in his work; downright in his mature thought and clear speech; full of kindliness and help for others. He was a fascinating and stimulating companion for these reasons and for his enjoyment of life through his keen perception of things best worth while.[215]

Lewis still had time to pursue his boyhood enthusiasm for bird watching, going to the Norfolk Broads for this in June 1908. He wrote to his mother saying that he saw bearded tits which he described as perhaps the most beautiful English species, and also many reed warblers' nests, which he photographed.[378]

## The electrocardiogram and Einthoven's string galvanometer

The year 1908 is a landmark in Lewis' career because it saw the beginning of his work on cardiac arrhythmias. This original, truly pioneering work led him to elucidate nearly every presently known cardiac irregularity and rightly made him world famous. It was also an important time in the development of methods to analyse cardiac arrhythmias. Mechanical recordings of the heart beat had been in use for over 50 years and their clinical application was greatly facilitated by Dr James Mackenzie[(8)] in the late 1890's.[272] Mackenzie modified the Dudgeon syphygmograph by using an attached tambour (Fig. 2.5, *overleaf*) so that a simultaneous recording could be made of the venous pulse. Therefore the arterial and venous pulses of a patient could be readily recorded in a patient's home with this easily portable apparatus.[264] But there remained the drawback that the recording had to be made on smoked paper. Mackenzie overcame this problem by inventing an ink-writing polygraph in 1906 and this apparatus, which he published in 1908 (Fig. 2.6), became widely used for the analysis of arrhythmias.[265] But these mechanical recordings could yield only indirect evidence of impulse formation in the heart. Direct evidence had to come from electrical recordings and at first these could only be made by placing electrodes directly onto an

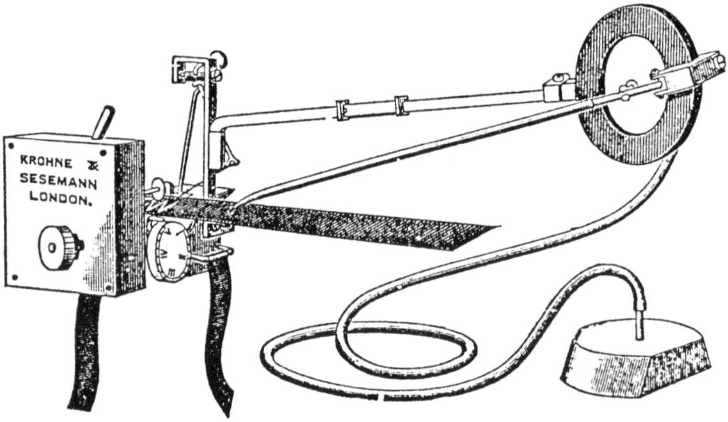


*Figure 2.5 The clinical polygraph of Dr James Mackenzie. Venous and hepatic pulses and the apex beat could be recorded by using the cup receiver linked to the tambour. (From reference 264.)*

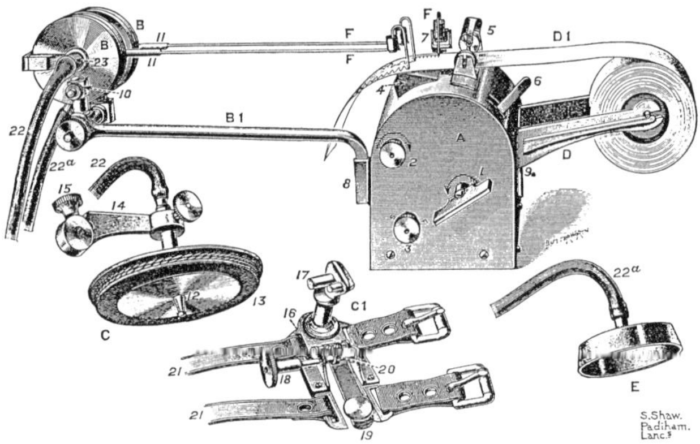


*Figure 2.6 The ink polygraph of Dr James Mackenzie, with arterial contact on the left, and a cup receiver on the right. (From reference 265.)*

animal's heart and recording the potentials with Lippmann's capillary electrometer in which a mercury column was moved by the current. However, in 1887 Augustus D. Waller(9) demonstrated for the first time that the electrometer could pick up the electrical activity of the human heart, in fact on himself, from contacts on the body. It was his idea to call the recording an electrocardiogram.[27] But although the apparatus was sensitive the recordings were flawed by a slow response time due to inertia of the mercury column.

This drawback was overcome by Willem Einthoven,(10) the professor of physiology in Leiden, Holland, who solved the problem by means of a mathematical correction. Using this method he was the first to discover that tracings taken from patients with heart disease were markedly different from normal subjects and he made the stimulating suggestion that the electrocardiogram might have value in cardiac diagnosis. But this technique was laborious because it involved redrawing each tracing and he set out to develop a better instrument than the electrometer. The technical and theoretical problems involved were very considerable, especially the requirement for high sensitivity, and it is a tribute to Einthoven's genius that he overcame them with his invention of an extremely sensitive string galvanometer capable of recording cardiac potentials. It consisted essentially of a fine silver-plated quartz fibre which was suspended between the poles of a powerful electromagnet. Changes in the current flowing through the fibre caused it to move in the magnetic field and the movement was magnified and then recorded photographically. The fibre was always referred to as 'the string'. He published a preliminary report of his invention in 1901, when he was aged 41, and then gave a detailed description of the galvanometer and the records obtained with it in his classic paper of 1903.[315] Einthoven's string galvanometer gave highly accurate recordings of changes in electrical potential and even his early electrocardiograms have hardly been surpassed for their quality. Naturally this invention aroused great interest but Einthoven was unable to provide models of his apparatus. In any case it was a massive affair, weighing over 600 pounds (300 kg), occupying two rooms and requiring five men to operate it. Einthoven approached Max Edelmann in Munich and Horace Darwin in Cambridge with the suggestion that they should produce, under a royalty agreement, a commercial electrocardiograph.[63] The Edelmann Company brought out their redesigned, much smaller, model in 1906. The Cambridge Scientific Instrument Company, of which Darwin (later Sir Horace) was the director and cofounder, also proceeded with a new design.[15] It was made to a very high standard in the company's workshops and the first model, a galvanometer only, was sold to the physiological laboratory in Sheffield, whilst the first electrocardiograph went to Professor Edward A Schafer's[(11)] laboratory in Edinburgh in 1908. Edelmann soon stopped paying royalties on the grounds that the invention was not new[28] and thereafter Einthoven dealt only with the Cambridge Company who honoured their agreement even though, as Darwin pointed out to him, the invention had not been patented.[29]

## Research work on arrhythmias

Lewis's first arrhythmia paper was published in the *Journal of Physiology*[245] in 1908 in collaboration with Arthur S Macnalty. It described a patient with heart block and was entitled 'A note on the simultaneous occurrence of sinus and ventricular rhythm in man'; although it was illustrated chiefly with Mackenzie polygraph curves, it did have one electrocardiogram taken on November 12 1908 which was recorded in Waller's physiological laboratory at the Imperial Institute in South Kensington, where he had the first Einthoven string galvanometer in London. A unique feature is the appearance for the first time of Lewis' famous 'ladder' diagram for arrhythmia analysis, in this instance being constructed from the polygraph tracings. (Fig. 2.7, *overleaf*) By showing the relationship to each other of atrial and ventricular contractions the diagram illustrates the way the electrical impulse is transmitted through the heart. Unknown to him it had been described in 1895 by Theodor W. Engelmann.[(12),80,99] There are two unusual features to this paper by Lewis. Firstly, it is difficult to read and one gets the

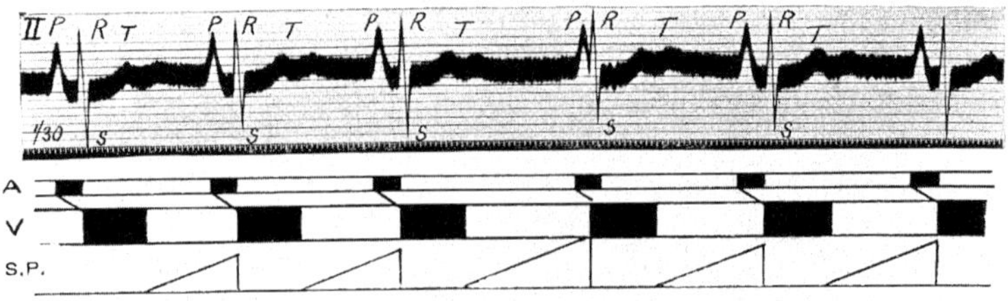


*Figure 2.7* *The ladder diagram of Lewis showing conduction from auricle (A) to ventricle (V), and stimulus production (S.P.) in the ventricle. On the electrocardiogram the fourth RS complex is a ventricular escape beat due to slowing of the sinus rhythm. 'The zig-zag line (S-P) represents the building-up of impulses which from time to time are responsible for ventricular escape'. (From reference 168.)*

impression that Lewis was fumbling with a subject he did not fully understand. Secondly, it is almost the only time that he expresses thanks to a technical assistant, in this case, 'Gratitude to Mr Symes for the trouble he has taken in rendering me conversant with the management of the apparatus'. Waller's apparatus was used again for a paper in 1909 entitled 'Single and successive extrasystoles'.[116] The three electrocardiograms in it, like the one in his first paper, look odd because they are recorded unconventionally from right to left. Furthermore Lewis has used Waller's nomenclature of **a** and **v** in labelling them and not the PQRST of Einthoven. (Fig. 2.8) Heart block was also the subject for a lecture he gave at the London Hospital in which he carefully analysed all the evidence, clinical and experimental, for its causation and concluded that it is usually due in man to a lesion of the bundle of His.[114] We now know that the lesions are more often to be found in the bundle branches, rather than the His bundle itself.

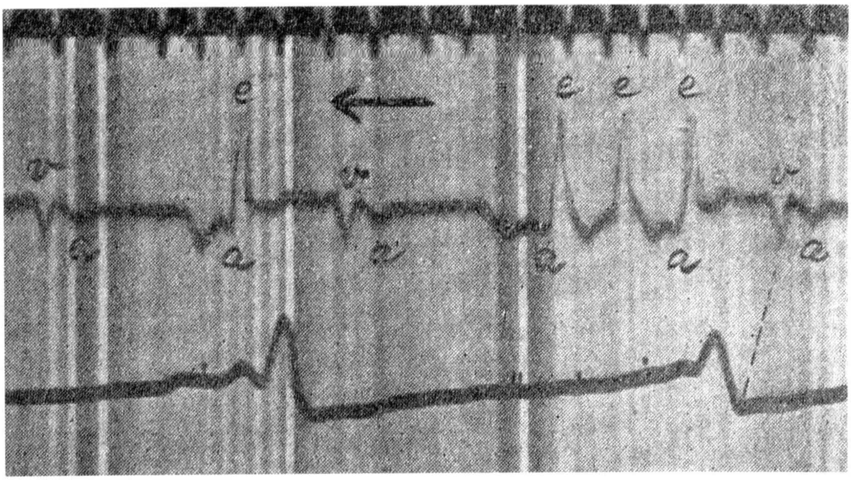

*Figure 2.8* *An electrocardiogram taken in Professor A. Waller's laboratory in 1909. It is unconventionally recorded from right to left and deflections are labelled a and v. Ventricular extrasystoles are e. Radial pulse below. (From reference 116.)*

Henry Lewis, now aged 58, clearly thought this an opportune time to give some fatherly advice to his son on the conduct of his coming career. In a warmly written letter he says that:

> ...the attitude you should adopt generally towards your comrades in the profession should be one of consideration...let them down as lightly as you possibly can (if they are in error)...when I was your age I went wrong in this way and did myself no good.[374]

But it seems that father and son were alike in their reaction to criticism. Dr Edward M. Brockbank wrote an article in the *Quarterly Journal of Medicine* saying that Lewis and others had given wrong interpretations of polygraph curves. In reply Lewis wrote that Brockbank had done no original work himself on the subject and said, 'His criticisms are totally invalid'.[126] In fact Lewis was to become well known for his trenchant comments on other peoples work when he thought it was wrong, though he never resented well informed criticism.[50]

## An article on genetics

In 1908, with his colleague Dennis Embleton, who was a clinical pathologist, he wrote a long paper in *Biometrika* on a family whose 44 members had only one finger on their hands, and two toes on their feet; 'Split hand and split foot deformities'. It is illustrated with good radiographs ('skiagraphs') and there is detailed consideration of the possible genetics.[241] This paper was well outside Lewis' other interests and indeed his training. Sir Cyril Clarke[(13)] has kindly reviewed it and says that the authors made three important errors in their contention that Mendelian inheritance could not explain the inheritance of the condition and that their conclusions were entirely wrong. Sir Cyril adds:

> In 1917 my father was invalided out of the Army with what I suspect were extrasystoles. He was seen by Tommy Lewis who gave a very bad prognosis 'About six months to live'. My father proceeded to survive and live a very active life for another 31 years. My opinion of Tommy Lewis as a geneticist is much the same as my view of him as a clinician.[508]

## Meets Dr James Mackenzie in 1908

A major event in Lewis's life came in 1908 when he met Dr James Mackenzie (Fig. 2.9, *overleaf*) for the first time. Mackenzie was well known in Europe and North America, though much less so in Britain, for his work on the venous and arterial pulses on which he had written a notable monograph in 1902 entitled, *The Study of the Pulse, Arterial, Venous and Hepatic and of the Movements of the Heart.*[264] He had an especial interest in cardiac arrhythmias which he shared with the Dutch cardiologist Karel Wenckebach,[(14)] who had written an acclaimed book on the subject which Mackenzie had had translated into English.[61] It was remarkable that the whole of Mackenzie's research, which also included important studies on pain, had been done during his 28 years as a general practitioner in the industrial Lancashire town of Burnley. Now, at the age of 54, he had made the challenging decision to move to London to further his research and to promote interest in

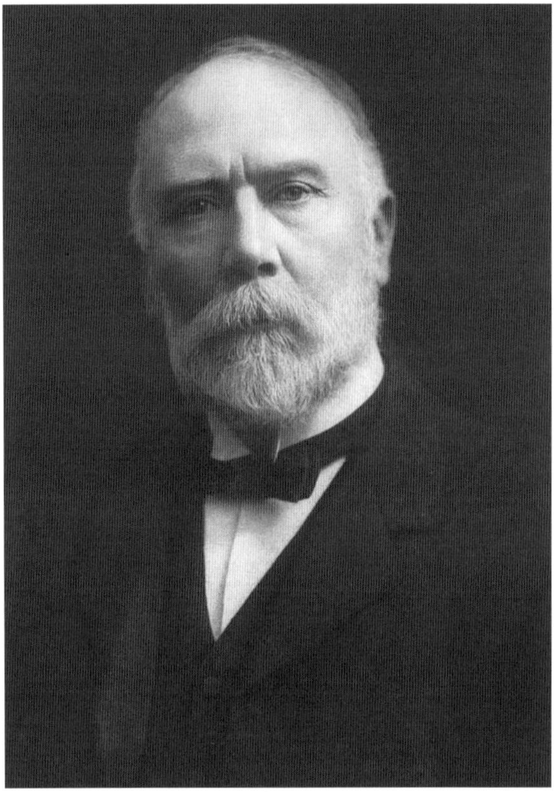

*Figure 2.9 Sir James Mackenzie in about 1910.*

his work, and he became a consultant physician at Mount Vernon Hospital.[74] Although Lewis was well acquainted with Mackenzie's work, the personal contact was very important to him. Lewis was 28 years his junior, 'yet he extended to me a friendship which soon became intimate and highly prized ... we were in almost daily and personal communication'.[166] This friendship was obviously a stimulus to Lewis for his work on arrhythmias, but even more important was: 'Mackenzie's critical approach to Medicine and his independence of authority, under the spell of which I fell at UCH, came as a revelation to me'.[223] 'He was the first authority in clinical medicine on whose lips I frequently heard the words "I don't know" and he taught Lewis to see, "where clinical knowledge ends and ignorance begins"'.[166]

## The journal *Heart* is founded in 1909

It was now becoming increasingly obvious that a journal was needed exclusively for work on cardiovascular problems and in the summer of 1908 Lewis suggested to Mackenzie that a journal should be founded for the study of the circulation.[380]

They would have known that the French journal, *Archives des Maladies du Coeur et des Vaisseaux et du Sang* had just been started, in 1907. Mackenzie arranged in January 1909 for the new journal to be published by Shaw and Sons and in March 1909 he asked Lewis to be its editor. Lewis who was now 27, (Fig. 2.10), had no editorial experience but Mackenzie's reputation gained support for the journal in North America as well as in Britain. Invitations to collaborators were sent out in the last weeks of April and during May final arrangements were made with the publishers. Lewis wrote that, 'One of the chief reasons for accelerating publication was the fact that several articles were ready'.[380] To give an example of efficient work by both editor and publisher one can refer to the article by A.R. Cushny on aconitine. It was received on May 24 and sent to the publisher on May 27, with a proof going to the author on June 7. The four papers of Part 1 of Volume 1 went to press on June 9 and the first issue appeared on July 1st. The title page (Fig. 2.11) was headed: 'HEART. A journal for the study of the circulation. Edited by Thomas Lewis, M.D., aided in the selection of papers by Dr W.H. Gaskell, Prof A.R. Cushny, Dr Leonard Hill, Dr J. Mackenzie, Prof. A W Hewlett (Ann Arbor) and Prof. G.N. Stewart (Cleveland).' There were 44

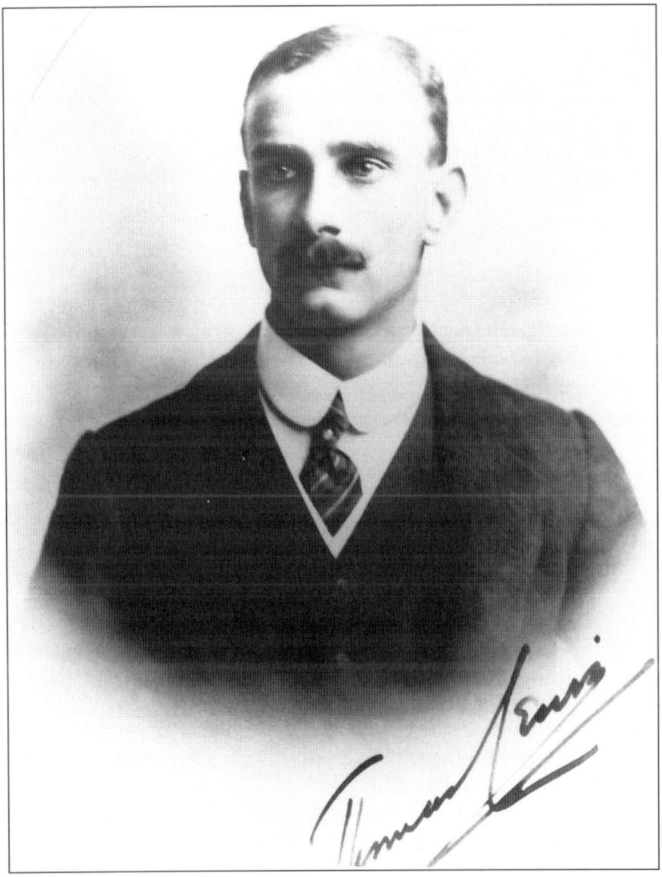

*Figure 2.10 Thomas Lewis aged 27 in 1909.*

HEART.

A JOURNAL FOR THE STUDY OF THE CIRCULATION.

EDITED BY

THOMAS LEWIS, M.D.,

AIDED IN THE SELECTION OF PAPERS BY

Dr. W. H. Gaskell.

Prof. A. R. Cushny (London).
Dr. Leonard Hill (London).
Dr. J. Mackenzie (London).
Prof. A. W. Hewlett (Ann Arbor).
Prof. G. N. Stewart (Cleveland).

WITH THE COLLABORATION OF

Prof. J. G. Adami (Montreal).
Sir T. Clifford Allbutt (Cambridge).
Prof. W. M. Bayliss (London).
Dr. C. Bolton (London).
Prof. J. R. Bradford (London).
Dr. W. Langdon Brown (London).
Sir Lauder Brunton, Bt. (London).
Dr. W. J. Calvert (Dallas).
Prof. A. J. Carlson (Chicago).
Dr. Alexis Carrel (New York).
Dr. A. E. Cohn (New York).
Dr. C. M. Cooper (San Francisco).
Dr. John Cowan (Glasgow).
Prof. George W. Crile (Cleveland).
Prof. Harvey Cushing (Baltimore).
Dr. George Dock (New Orleans).
Prof. W. Einthoven (Leyden).
Prof. J. Erlanger (Madison).
Dr. A. G. Gibson (Oxford).
Dr. G. A. Gibson (Edinburgh).
Dr. A. M. Gossage (London).
Prof F. Gotch (Oxford).
Prof. T. Wardrop Griffith (Leeds).
Prof. Ch. C. Guthrie (St. Louis).
Dr. J. Hay (Liverpool).
Prof. Y. Henderson (New Haven).
Dr. W. P. Herringham (London).
Dr. A. D. Hirschfelder (Baltimore).
Prof. Ch. F. Hoover (Cleveland).
Prof. Wm. H. Howell (Baltimore).
Prof. T. C. Janeway (New York).
Prof. A. Keith (London).
Prof. J. A. MacWilliam (Aberdeen).
Dr. S. J. Meltzer (New York).
Prof. Joseph L. Miller (Chicago).
Sir R. Douglas Powell, Bt. (London).
Dr. W. T. Ritchie (Edinburgh).
Prof. Torald Sollmann (Cleveland).
Prof. E. H. Starling (London).
Prof. Graham Steell (Manchester).
Prof. W. S. Thayer (Baltimore).
Prof. A. D. Waller (London).
Prof. G. S. Woodhead (Cambridge).
Sir Almroth E. Wright (London).

VOL. I.
1909-1910

London:
Shaw & Sons, Fetter Lane, Fleet Street, E.C.

1910

*Figure 2.11 Title page of the first volume of* Heart, *1910.*

collaborators of whom 21 were from the U.S.A, one from Canada and only one, Professor W. Einthoven from Europe.

The Prefatory Note was written by Walter H. Gaskell, FRS[15] the Cambridge physiologist whose work on the rhythmical contraction of cardiac muscle was much admired by Lewis. Gaskell said in his note that medicine was losing its empiric character and was founding itself more and more on facts derived from the experimental sciences of physiology, pathology and pharmacology. The results of animal experiments were now being applied to man and laboratory methods were being used for diagnosis. It was 'of vital importance for the medical man to keep in touch with the workers in the laboratories, and to apply the most recent knowledge gained by them directly to man'. The journal, he said, would be of great value to the clinician because it would focus together work in the laboratory and in the hospital, and also to the physiologist who would be reminded of 'the nature of the problems which, in the opinion of the medical man, are pressing urgently for solution'.

Lewis' preface was a notably mature and authoritative statement from the young editor:

Editorial Preface

It has been decided that it is now essential that those specially seeking new facts and new conclusions relating to haemodynamic problems should reap the advantages of a special Journal, in which such facts and the conclusions drawn from them may be placed on record.

This resolve comes from the conviction that students of the circulation are now seriously hampered in their work by the difficulty of keeping in touch with the papers that appear, so widely scattered, in the various publications of more general scope.

The Journal affirms a single object, the progress of knowledge of the mechanism by which the blood circulates in health and disease. A closer union of thought amongst workers in the separate branches of medical science must contribute to the attainment of this end.

To know the pump, which Harvey revealed to us, more intimately; to understand more definitely the forces which regulate its action, and the mechanism by which it distributes the constant stream of blood, bathing and feeding the tissues of the body; to determine the causes which impair the circulatory functions; to see more clearly the means of prevention and the remedies which palliate where injury to the heart or vessels is concerned; such is the scope of this Journal. The field is sufficient for many workers.

The Journal requires communications, containing, above all, original and carefully ascertained facts, and conclusions consonant with such facts and previous observations. By the record of fact and the statement of new principles progress will be ensured.

The advances of recent years are largely indebted to Gaskell and his work for their initiation, and this Journal heartily appreciates the message he sends it as it takes the first step on its course.

Lewis' own paper in the first number was on paroxysmal tachycardia, Mackenzie's was on nodal bradycardia, whilst Cushny wrote on aconitine arrhythmias and Hill on measurement of systolic blood pressure. It was a good start to what became under Lewis' critical editing one of the finest medical journals of the century. Of the 326 articles in the 16 volumes of *Heart* issued between 1909 and 1933 he was author or part author of one quarter.

## Notes to Chapter 2

(1) The Conjoint was a diploma which enabled one to qualify as a doctor. With it one became a licentiate of the Royal College of Physicians of London (LRCP) and also a member of the Royal College of Surgeons of England (MRCS), hence the name conjoint.

(2) Thomas Barlow Bt, KCVO, FRS, (later Sir Thomas) 1845–1945, was a physician of great distinction. He was on the staff of the Hospital for Sick Children London as well as UCH. He described infantile scurvy (Barlow's disease) and was President of the Royal College of Physicians of London from 1910–1914.

(3) The Dudgeon syphygmograph recorded the radial arterial pulse onto a strip of smoked paper 18 cm by 3 cm. It was a small device, driven by clockwork, which was fastened onto to the wrist by a cloth strap. Being portable and easy to use it became widely employed by clinicians, and replaced the rather cumbersome Marey syphyg-

mograph. Dr James Mackenzie modified it by adding a tambour which could be used to record a second tracing from the venous pulse, or apex beat or liver.

(4) Sir Leonard Erskine Hill, FRS, 1866–1962, knighted in 1930, was a graduate of UCH who became a lecturer in physiology firstly at UCL and then at the London Hospital. From 1914 to 1930 he was Director of Applied Physiology at the National Institute for Medical Research, London.

(5) The degree of Doctor of Medicine (MD) was a post-graduate degree in Britain, unlike other countries where it was the qualifying or graduating degree in medicine.

(6) To enter on a career as a hospital consultant it was essential to become a Member of the Royal College of Physicians of London (MRCP). This was obtained by taking the difficult Membership examination. There was a searching clinical part, and the written papers included translations from Greek and Latin.

(7) Thomas Renton Elliott, FRS, 1877–1961, was a brilliant experimental physiologist who was the first to suggest chemical neurotransmission with his work on adrenaline in Cambridge, when aged 23 to 28. He entered UCH as a medical student at the late age of 29, when he formed his life-long friendship with Thomas Lewis. In 1920 he occupied the first full time chair of clinical medicine in London at UCH Medical School, and also became director of the Medical Unit. He was an influential member of the Medical Research Council and did much to promote academic medicine in Britain, giving wise guidance in the establishment of whole time professorial units in medical schools, and becoming secretary to the Beit Fellowship.

(8) James Mackenzie, FRS, (later Sir James), 1853–1925, had worldwide eminence as a clinical investigator of the cardiovascular system. For over 25 years he worked as a general practitioner in the industrial town of Burnley in Lancashire and it was then that he made his pioneer studies, unaided, of the venous and arterial pulses. His work on arrhythmias was of great importance, and he also did seminal work on the mechanism of pain. He became a consultant at the London Hospital at the age of 54 and in 1918 he founded an institute at St Andrews in Scotland to pursue his life's ambition of attempting to understand the significance and prognosis of symptoms. He can be identified as the first pure cardiologist in Britain, and he also was a wise and thoughtful physician with a philosophical interest in the principles of medicine.

(9) Augustus Désiré Waller, FRS, 1856–1922, was a pioneer electrophysiologist who summarized his work in 1903 in a book entitled *Signs of life from their electrical aspect*. He was lecturer in physiology at St Mary's Hospital Medical School London for 20 years, during which time he recorded the first human electrocardiogram. He then founded the University of London Physiological Laboratory in South Kensington and was director there from 1902–1922. It was his father who described Wallerian degeneration.

(10) Willem Einthoven, FRS, 1860–1927, became the professor of physiology in Leiden Holland at the age of 25. He had an early interest in recording electrical action currents from exposed animal hearts using Lippmann's electrometer and saw Waller demonstrate this apparatus. It was Einthoven who, in 1895, labelled the deflections P Q R S and T. In 1906 he discovered the U wave. His invention of the string galvanometer in 1901 made it possible for the first time to record the electrical events in the cardiac cycle faithfully, and revolutionized the diagnosis of cardiac disease. Einthoven has rightly been hailed as the father of electrocardiography, and he was the sole recipient in 1924 of the Nobel Prize for physiology or medicine.

(11) Edward Albert Schafer, later Sir Edward Sharpey–Schafer, FRS, 1850–1935, was professor of physiology firstly at University College London and then, from 1899, in Edinburgh. He devised a method of artificial respiration and was a noted for his work on cerebral localization.

(12) Theodor Wilhelm Engelmann, (1843–1909), was a pioneer electrophysiologist who worked in Utrecht and later at the Physiological Institute in Berlin. He was the first to represent graphically, in 1878, the diphasic time course of cardiac potentials, the

'Doppelschwankung'. He recognized experimental extrasystoles prior to electrocardiography.

(13) Cyril Clarke, FRS, (later Sir Cyril) 1907–, is a renowned medical geneticist who devised Rhesus immunization to prevent haemolytic disease of the new-born. He was President of the Royal College of Physicians of London from 1972–1976.

(14) Karel Frederik Wenckebach, 1864–1940, was a notable Dutch physician, who had studied under T.W. Engelmann. His chief interest was in cardiac arrhythmias and he was the first to identify extrasystoles in man. In 1900 he became professor of medicine at Groningen in Holland and later held the chairs of medicine in Strasbourg and Vienna. He recognized the importance of James Mackenzie's work, for which he had great admiration, well before it was accepted in Britain and they became close friends. He is known eponymously for the type of heart block called the Wenckebach phenomenon.

(15) Walter Holbrook Gaskell, FRS, 1847–1914, was a noted physiologist who studied first under Carl Ludwig in Leipzig and then under Michael Foster in Cambridge. He did fundamental work on the sympathetic nervous system, especially on the cardiac nerves. He showed for the first time that the cardiac muscle fibre was endowed with the property of rhythmical contraction and was not, as supposed, a passive agent of the nerve cell. He gave great encouragement to the younger men in his department at Cambridge.

# Chapter 3

## The electrocardiograph • Elucidates atrial fibrillation and other arrhythmias • Gets his own department • Writes a much acclaimed monograph • Meets Willem Einthoven

AFTER WILLEM EINTHOVEN had published the full description of his string galvanometer in 1903, he started to make a systematic study of its clinical applications and also to make advances in electrocardiographic theory.[315] He introduced the standard method of recording using three leads connected to the limbs, which led to the important concept of the electrical axis of the heart.[63] In the next few years Einthoven described the patterns of right and left ventricular hypertrophy, left atrial hypertrophy, and several arrhythmias including extrasystoles and complete heart block. In order to get these recordings, he arranged for the University Hospital in Leiden to be connected to his physiological laboratory by one mile of special telephone cable. He described this method and the electrocardiograms obtained with it in a paper published in 1906 in the *Archives Internationales de Physiologie* entitled 'Le Telecardiogramme'.[51] Lewis wrote for a reprint of it in May 1908 and this signalled the start of a close and fruitful friendship which lasted for 18 years. Their correspondence has been published by Herman A Snellen[(1)] in his excellent book *Two Pioneers of Electrocardiography*.[317] It has been said that it was Mackenzie who initiated this approach to Einthoven, and certainly his link with Holland through his friendship with Wenckebach could support this. On the other hand Lewis was well up in the physiological literature. Lewis visited Leiden in September 1909 and wrote to thank Einthoven (Fig. 3.1) for the 'delightful and instructive day' which he spent there. He was shown round by George Fahr,[(2)] an American assistant who became Professor of Medicine at the University of Minnesota. Fahr asked Lewis what he would like to see and got the reply, 'Everything'; One wonders why he thought one day was sufficient. But he made time to write to his parents and his mother replied thanking him for 'the nice long letter written at Leiden. It gladdened us to learn you had such a lovely time there'.[375]

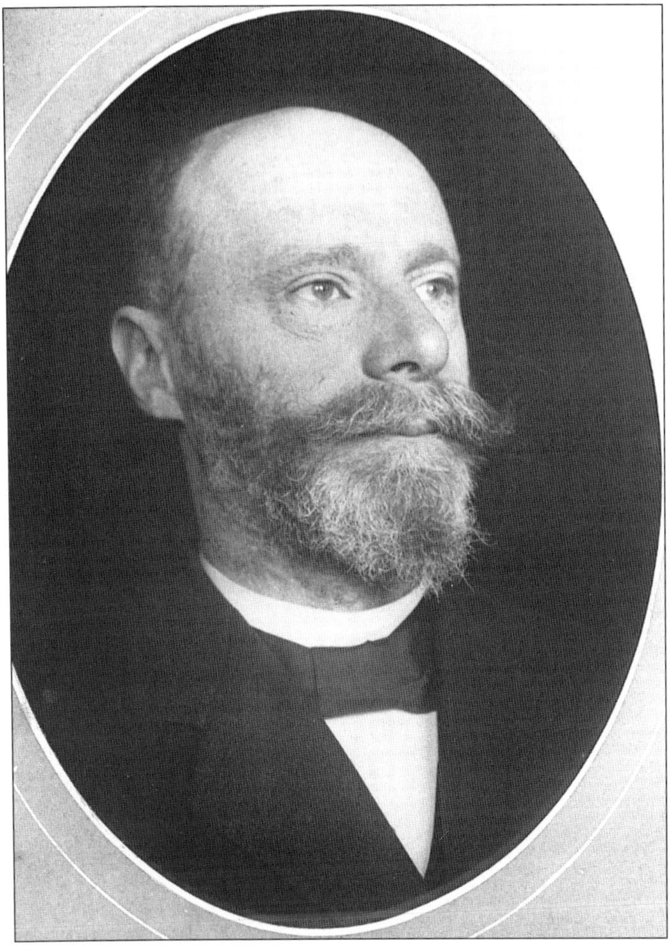

*Figure 3.1 Willem Einthoven aged 46 in 1906 the year of his very influential paper 'Le Télécardiogramme'.*

## Obtains his first electrocardiograph apparatus in 1909

At this time the only electrocardiograph suitable for clinical use was the model made by Edelmann and Sons of Munich under licence from Einthoven and early in 1909 Lewis purchased what was known as the large pattern of it. This was installed in a basement room in the medical school just behind the lift shaft. That position was not an indication that the school thought the apparatus to be unimportant. It was considered at the time, wrongly as it turned out, that the galvanometer was so sensitive to vibration that it could not be placed on the floor of a building, but had to be put on concrete in a basement. Dr Strickland Goodall's electrocardiograph in Harley Street was likewise installed inconveniently in the basement of his house.

## Dr A.E. Cohn, his first American research assistant

Lewis' research assistant at this time, his first, was Alfred E. Cohn,[(3)] aged 30, of New York who had been studying for two years in Freiburg and Vienna. (Fig. 3.2) He wrote an account of his time in London:

> When I arrived in London in the Spring of 1909 Thomas Lewis had just acquired one of these instruments. Dr James Mackenzie – not yet Sir James – beside working with E H Starling took me off to work with Lewis...I did, as I say, begin to work with Lewis in the basement of University College Hospital just behind the elevator shaft. Could you imagine a worse place? At that time Lewis had not yet acquired Edelmann's resistance box for compensation of the skin current. Neither he nor I knew much, if anything, about galvanometers. We tried to manage Lewis' machine without the necessary compensating apparatus and did not know when we came in the morning where, or whether, we would find the string. But we went on merrily this way the whole of the summer.[25]

The problem of 'finding the string' was always a problem with the Einthoven galvanometer when the operator was not an expert. In his article on the development of the electrocardiograph, S.L. Barron recollected that finding the string after it disappeared required patience and practice and that although an experienced technician, such as himself, could perform the task in a matter of minutes 'the distracted physician often spent fruitless hours'.[14] Lewis may have continued to get help from Mr Symes, and although it has never been established

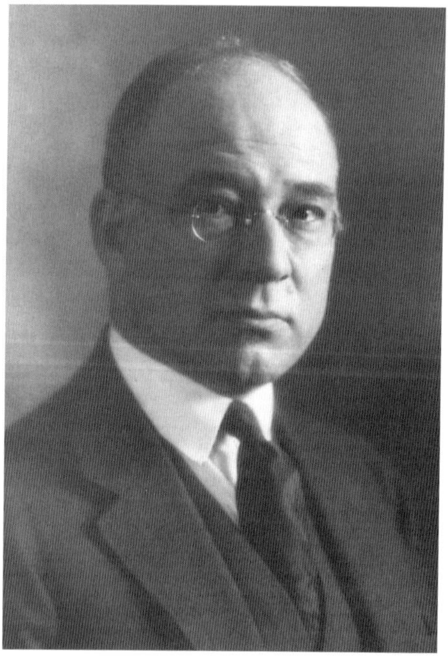

*Figure 3.2 Alfred E. Cohn of New York, Lewis' first research assistant in 1909.*

which apparatus Waller originally had it is quite likely that it was an Edelmann model.

When Cohn returned home he took an Edelmann apparatus with him and this, together with one at Johns Hopkins Hospital, became in 1909 the first electrocardiographs in the United States. He set it up at Mount Sinai Hospital, New York and Dr Horatio B. Williams,[(4)] a physiologist at Cornell, who had been trained in both engineering and medicine, made the essential compensating device for him. Williams had visited Einthoven in 1911 and by 1915 he was able, with the mechanical assistance of Charles F. Hindle,[(5)] to construct the first American electrocardiograph and deliver it to Cohn, then at the Rockefeller Institute. Cohn continued to collaborate with Lewis for four years after he left London and in particular gave expert help with the pathology of the conducting system. In July he wrote to acknowledge the receipt of three hearts which Lewis had sent him. Two were cases of complete heart block, one from an adult and the other from a child with diphtheria. The third, of nodal bradycardia, was from a Mr Macdonald and Cohn said, 'Macdonald's heart is beautiful. There is an aneurysm behind the aortic flap of the mitral valve which has destroyed the AV junction'.[352] Cohn initiated what was to be a long and distinguished line of American research workers in Lewis' department which went on for the next 28 years. The next to come were Adele and Bernard S. Oppenheimer,[(6)] also from the Mount Sinai Hospital, who wrote a paper in *Heart* with Lewis in 1910 on the site of origin of the heart beat in the dog heart.[255]

The outstanding problem that the electrocardiograph was likely to solve was that of complete irregularity of the heart. This common condition had puzzled physicians for over a century and had been known by a variety of descriptive terms such as 'rebellious palpitations', 'delirium cordis' and 'pulsus irregularis perpetuus'.[100,121] Using Ludwig's kymographic method it had been studied by several workers such as Marey and Potain from 1863 onwards,[316] but it was Mackenzie who had done most to elucidate its mechanism. By using his own simple and portable modification of the Dudgeon sphygmograph he was able to record venous and arterial pulses during his visits to patients in their homes. He discovered that with the commencement of an irregular pulse beat, the wave of atrial contraction disappeared from the venous pulse, as did the presystolic murmur of mitral stenosis, and he concluded therefore that the atria must have become paralysed. Haemodynamically this was correct. But he then changed his mind and decided that the pacemaker had moved to the atrioventricular (AV) node, and that atrial contraction was masked by the simultaneous ventricular contraction. The condition, he declared, was due to nodal rhythm.[96] So the stage was well set for further investigation when Lewis tackled the subject in 1909. He later wrote as to how this had come about.[194] The stimulus had come from Mackenzie for 'like all those who then met him (I) was forced to an interest in his great problem...the puzzle of this form of disorderly heart action and its peculiar responsiveness to digitalis, which he himself had already discovered, dominated Mackenzie's thoughts'. One can imagine his excitement at using his newly acquired electrocardiograph, 'at a time when the need to explain the irregularity of the heart in the patient was urgent' – and, as far as he knew, being the first to do this. The Edelmann electrocardiograph was ideal for arrhythmia analysis because it used a continuous roll of photographic paper (Fig. 3.3, *overleaf*) thus allowing long recordings to be made.

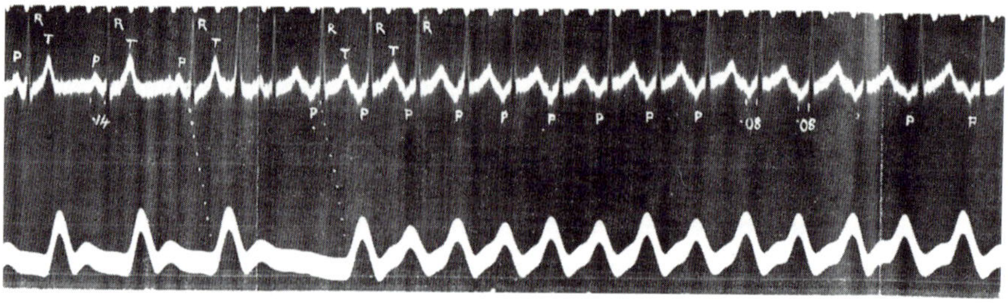

*Figure 3.3* *A long strip of electrocardiogram (10 seconds), with a pulse tracing, taken with the Edelmann apparatus. It shows a paroxysm of junctional tachycardia. (From reference 121.)*

## Nodal rhythm is identified

As it happened, the first step towards elucidating the problem came from studying a different arrhythmia, and Lewis' account of that step is worth quoting at some length:

> And then as chance directed there came an observation that changed fundamentally our direction of thought. It was in the earliest days of electrocardiography in this country, when a man came to my department suffering from paroxysmal tachycardia. I won from him what in that year was unique, namely, a complete series of venous and electrocardiographic curves, in and out of his attacks. These records gave a startlingly plain record of true nodal rhythm...producing high pointed venous waves..and inverted P waves. (They) were altogether different from those of the disorder that had been under intensive study, and showed that this could not in fact be due to nodal rhythm...they drew the focus of attention away from the intricacies of jugular curves where it had rested too long.[195]

These recordings, (Fig. 3.4) which were made in October 1909, also served to emphasise the weak point in Mackenzie's hypothesis of nodal rhythm, namely its inability to explain the irregularity of the ventricle. Having proved that nodal rhythm was not the basis of the disorder, Lewis' next move came from his recollection of a paper by A.R. Cushny and C.W. Edmunds on 'Paroxysmal irregularity of the heart and auricular fibrillation', published in 1907, in which they had shown that pulse tracings in patients resembled those in the dog with fibrilla-

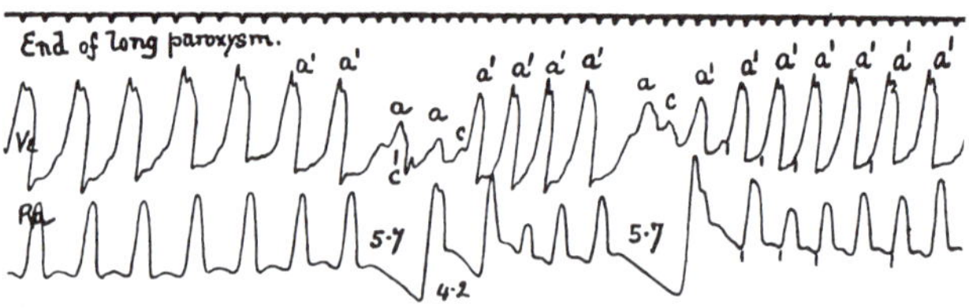


*Figure 3.4* *An ink polygraph recording of the jugular venous, and arterial, pulses showing the giant 'a' waves of nodal rhythm during three paroxysms of nodal tachycardia. (From* Heart *1910:2;134.)*

tion[43]. 'I believe,' he said, 'that it was a remembrance of this paper, read some time before and forgotten, which finally led me to examine the irregularity of auricular fibrillation more closely'.[130] Cushny had in fact shown earlier, in 1899, that the cardiac rhythm in dogs with experimental atrial fibrillation, 'physiological delirium auriculae', was similar to that of patients with 'delirium cordis'.[63] Regarding Cushny's work Lewis said that it had been discussed many times by Mackenzie and himself 'and both of us had talked of it with Cushny; but the evidence seemed so slight that the evidence had not been entertained seriously, I think, by any one of us'.[196] Cushny however, referring to his paper with Edmunds, told a different tale saying, 'Their diagnosis was received with doubt by the various schools of investigators of heart disease, and efforts to arouse interest in the diagnosis and to extend it to the large group of cases previously described by Mackenzie proved fruitless'.[42] Lewis started his series of investigations by taking a large number of venous and electrocardiographic records from a dog with fibrillation, 'My conviction on this subject dates from the experiment performed on this animal on November 11th 1909'. He employed the clinical polygraph to record venous and arterial pulses from the dog so that they had the appearance of being taken from a patient. He then showed these curves, without comment, to Mackenzie who said they were from a patient with nodal rhythm. 'From this moment my task was easy, for the electric curves which I had obtained were equally convincing'. He acknowledged that 'the auricular fibrillation theory won Dr Mackenzie's support – support so generously given and so valuable, for it was withdrawn from the rival hypothesis, 'nodal rhythm'.[130]

## Mechanism of atrial fibrillation; the final proof

Lewis then proceeded to record electrocardiograms in no less than 30 patients with the disorder and showed the presence of rapid irregular oscillations and an absence of the normal atrial beats, the P waves. He ascribed the oscillations, which he labelled 'f' waves, to fibrillation of the atria, and was careful to show that the ventricles were stimulated in the usual way by impulses arriving at the A–V node. But he was not content just with assuming that the 'f' waves come from the atria. He put two electrodes on the chest wall near the right atrium, the first time that chest leads had ever been used, and got a tracing dominated by 'f' waves. (See Fig. 6.5) Furthermore in a patient with paroxysmal irregularity these same leads showed obvious P waves when in regular rhythm. This was as far as proof could go in the human, but his animal work gave valuable supporting evidence. When the dog atria were faradized, the electrocardiogram showed 'f' waves very like the human, and of course the fibrillating muscle could be actually seen. (Fig. 3.5, *overleaf*) But Lewis warned that, 'It would be a very simple and serious fallacy to imagine that the human disease has been reproduced in the animal; it will be appreciated that it was merely an end product...which had been provoked'. However he felt reassured that no serious error had arisen, 'because the argument in proof was not confined to mere comparison, but consisted largely of direct reasoning from observations on man himself.' But he still wanted to see the atria fibrillating when this occurred naturally from disease, not from experiment, and 'it occurred to me that if I could find a similar pathological affection in any of the lower animals, it might finally settle the nature of the irregular-

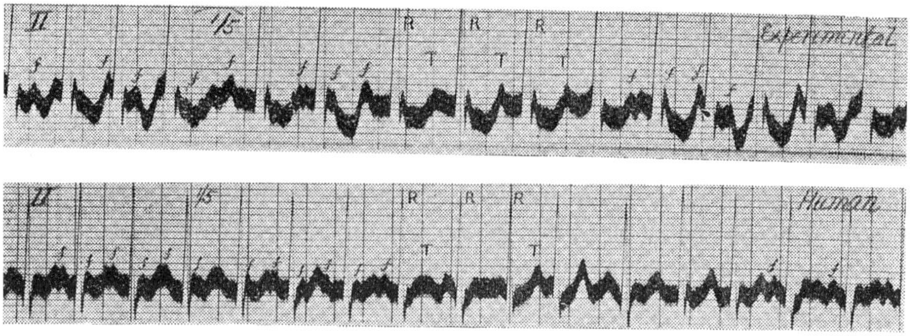


*Figure 3.5 Electrocardiograms to show the similarity of atrial fibrillation produced experimentally in the dog (upper) and the naturally occurring arrhythmia in the human (lower). (From reference 157.)*

ity with which I had to deal'.[127] He discovered that there was a rare condition in horses called 'tumultuous action of the heart' and with the help of veterinary surgeons he was able to examine five horses with this condition. In one, a polygraph record showed complete irregularity of the heart and a characteristic plateau form of the venous pulse with fine oscillations on it. Another animal was taken to the mews behind the medical school and connected by long wires to the galvanometer. The tracing was 'characteristic of experimental fibrillation and complete irregularity of the human heart...the oscillation...which is due to the fibrillating auricle...is obscurely seen in several places in these curves' and resembled that of the human condition. The horse was then killed and when the heart was exposed '...the auricle seemed to be standing still. A closer inspection of the right auricle now revealed the presence of a fine fibrillary movement in its walls'.[127] The hearts of three horses were sent to Cohn in New York who reported that the sino-auricular node was normal, as was the conducting system.[33]

It was a great achievement to delineate atrial fibrillation in man but Lewis generously acknowledged that 'this final conclusion is the outcome of the studies of a large body of workers'. Ironically Mackenzie had noted rapid oscillations in venous pulse records but had disregarded them, and Einthoven had recorded electrocardiograms showing 'f' waves, but they were not alone in overlooking their findings. Lewis confessed his own failure in this direction:

> A curious illustration of how obtuse the mind can remain in failing to correlate facts within its knowledge is that for some time I had already possessed a series of electrocardiograms from patients exhibiting the disordered heart action and a second series from dogs in which the auricles had been thrown into disorderly action by faradization. These then were ready, but had not been looked at side by side.[196]

## Publishes his classic paper on atrial fibrillation and just misses priority

Lewis's 66-page paper in the March 1910 issue of *Heart* (Fig. 3.6) is a masterly and comprehensive account and review entitled 'Auricular fibrillation and its relationship to clinical irregularity of the heart'.[121] It was illustrated with 36 electro-

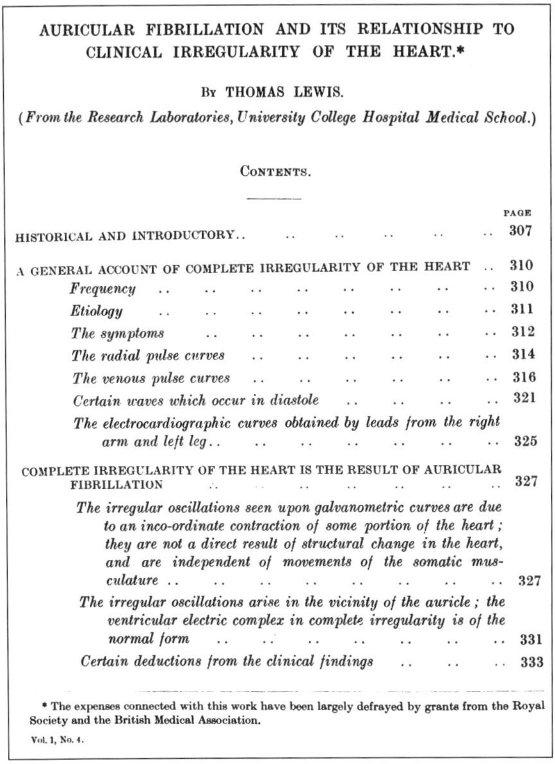

AURICULAR FIBRILLATION AND ITS RELATIONSHIP TO CLINICAL IRREGULARITY OF THE HEART.*

By THOMAS LEWIS.

(*From the Research Laboratories, University College Hospital Medical School.*)

CONTENTS.



* The expenses connected with this work have been largely defrayed by grants from the Royal Society and the British Medical Association.

Vol. 1, No. 4.

*Figure 3.6 Title page of Lewis' seminal paper on the identity of atrial fibrillation. (From reference 121.)*

cardiograms. An especially fine one from the technical point of view is a recording which shows the mechanical events in the atrium and ventricle of a dog taken simultaneously with the electrocardiogram. The Edelmann machine had certainly been mastered, but surprisingly there is no mention of it in the paper, nor is there any reference to Cohn. Prior to this major article Lewis had given a preliminary account of the conclusions in a half page article – the shortest he ever wrote – in the *British Medical Journal* of November 27 1909, entitled 'Auricular fibrillation: a common clinical condition', in which he said that, 'the facts point clearly to the conclusion that the irregularity in question is the result of auricular fibrillation...'.[118] Shortly after this article appeared he first saw a paper in the June 17 1909 issue of *Wiener klinische Wochenschrift*, in which Carl J. Rothberger[(7)] and Heinrich Winterberg from Vienna gave a convincing account of the mechanism of the condition, with electrocardiograms from dog experiments and patients, thus achieving definite priority.[310] They too referred to the papers of Mackenzie and Cushny. Lewis acknowledged their priority, albeit with reservations:

> While these investigations were in progress this conclusion has been partially and independently arrived at by Rothberger and Winterberg, working in Vienna. In their preliminary communication they conclude that certain cases of *pulsus irregularis perpetuus* are due to fibrillation. A large clinical experience of such cases exempts me from the necessity of restricting my conclusions, and permits me to assert that all such cases belong to a single group, and that the mechanism is the same in all.[121]

Mackenzie was quick to acknowledge the validity of Lewis' work as is shown by a letter he wrote to Dr William E. Hume[(8)] on March 6 1910, 'Recent observations have shown that the disappearance of all signs of the auricle is not due to 'paralysis of the auricle' or both **a** and **v** contracting together as I had inferred, but to the passing into fibrillary contractions'.[527] Further papers on arrhythmias, which were clearly intended for the general reader, followed in the *British Medical Journal* and in *The Lancet*, but papers with detailed discussion went naturally into his own journal *Heart*, though some were also published in the *Quarterly Journal of Medicine*. He wrote one paper each in French[123] and German,[124] the first and last ones written by himself in a foreign language– and it does seems likely that they came from his own pen and not via a translator. Certainly he was well-acquainted with the German and French literature as evidenced by the frequent references to them in his articles.

## Intensive studies of arrhythmias

Altogether in the first three years after getting his own electrocardiograph he published 29 papers on arrhythmias. Whilst some were only descriptive such as those on extrasystoles, others were based on experimental animal work. They included early work on the pacemaker of the heart, the production of heart block by asphyxia and the induction of paroxysmal tachycardia by ligation of the coronary arteries. His research assistants during this time were Bernard and Adele Oppenheimer from New York, Gordon C Mathison from UCL, M.D. Silberberg from Australia, E.G. Mack from the medical school, and Gordon M. Holmes, later a famous London neurologist. In delineating the sino-atrial node as the pacemaker of the heart he showed his mastery of experimental technique.[122] Stimulating electrodes were attached to various points on the atria or the venae cavae, and also remarkably to the internal surface of the right atrium with the electrodes protruding beyond a glass tube which had been introduced via the internal jugular vein. The electrodes terminated in tiny trout hooks – shades of his happy boyhood days fishing in Wales! It was therefore at an early stage in his career that he began to combine laboratory experiment with clinical observation as a deliberate pattern of research work which was to become almost a personal hallmark. This was the time when his later important concept of Clinical Science started to take shape. Two articles in the *British Medical Journal* appeared as reports of the Science Committee of the British Medical Association and his work, which he described as being from the research department of University College Hospital Medical School, was supported by grants from the Association and from the Royal Society. He got private consulting rooms at 58a Wimpole Street in 1909, but having put up his plate there, did not often use them.

## Obtains a research fellowship • Gets his own cardiographic department

However financial security came soon, and it came unexpectedly, when he was appointed in March 1910 as the first holder of a Beit Memorial Fellowship for Medical Research.[(9)] It was a remarkably fine and original idea to establish these

Fellowships which were to be of such value to young medical scientists. He held this for the full period of three years from 1910–1912 and nine others were also appointed for this period. One of them, Edward Mellanby,[(10)] was to become secretary of the Medical Research Council. The Fellowship freed him from private practice and he resigned from the Seamen's Hospital. As evidence of the continuing close relationship he had with his parents, and for its own interest, it is worth reproducing a letter he wrote on February 12 1910:

> Dear Mother,
>
> Please thank Father for his letter. I don't think there will be any harm in taking down the plate for 3 years. And for the following reasons. 1. I am seeing no patients and do not anticipate many for several years. 2. I shall be only 31 when it goes up again. 3. I can't hope to do much practice until Mackenzie retires and that will be in from 3–5 years time. 4. A run of patients would seriously interfere with my research work. 5. In 3 years I shall make a reputation which will be lasting if things go as they are going. I shall have leisure to teach and interview medical men, for the scheme includes one hospital less. If I am not in practice I shall be listened to more attentively and shall meet with more support from competitors. 6. The Beit brings £250 a year, or a total of £750 which is more than I am likely to make in 7 years practice. Apart from monetary considerations I feel that by devoting my time more exclusively to heart work (hospital & laboratory) practice will come quicker in the end. 7. ... the holding of the Beit will increase my chances at UCH. If they take me they know that I do not compete with them for 3 years ... On Thursday I had the horse up to the galvanometer and it shows that I have the right animal ... I lunched with the Evan Jones at the Carlton, another swell affair. The 4th number of *Heart* is nearly ready. Its early publication will leave me very free as there will be 4 months interval before the 1st number of Vol.2.
>
> With love
> from
> Tom[381]

The journal *Heart* was already proving a success for as Lewis had pointed out in his preface 'the field is sufficient for many workers'. The first number of volume two contained eight papers, whilst the second issued in November was larger with nine papers in 95 pages, four of them from the United States. An interesting one came from Charles C. Guthrie in Pittsburgh who described the changes in vein grafts which had been used to join up divided arteries.[70]

The year 1910 closed with the momentous news that he had gained his own department. On December 16, 10 days before his 29th birthday he learnt that approval had been given to establish a cardiographic department in the hospital and that he would be the Honorary Officer in charge with an annually renewable appointment.[349] Although it was situated in the medical school, this was a hospital department, one which served the clinical needs of the patients, and the title remained in being until 1930.

## *The Mechanism of the Heart Beat* establishes his reputation

In 1910 he certainly had the need of free time because he was writing his monograph (Fig. 3.7, *overleaf*) to be published by Shaw and Sons in 1911, entitled *The*

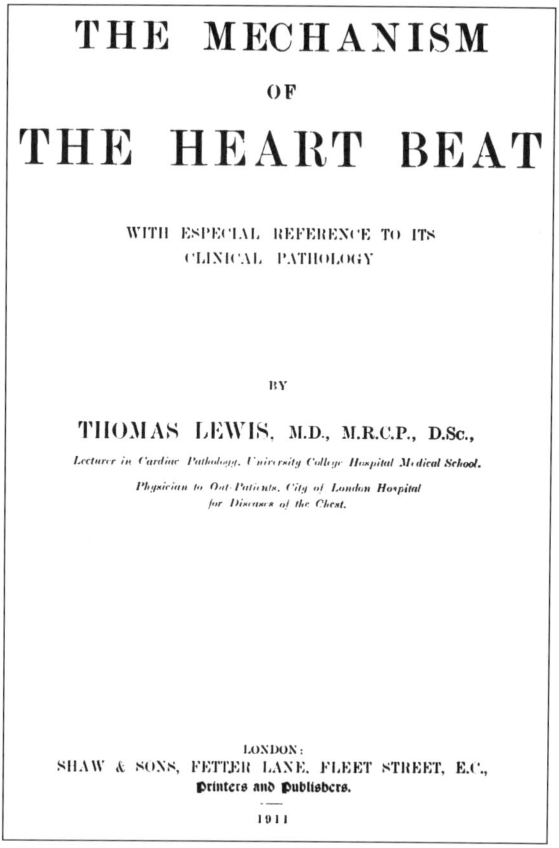

THE MECHANISM

OF

THE HEART BEAT

WITH ESPECIAL REFERENCE TO ITS
CLINICAL PATHOLOGY

BY

THOMAS LEWIS, M.D., M.R.C.P., D.Sc.,

*Lecturer in Cardiac Pathology, University College Hospital Medical School.*

*Physician to Out-Patients, City of London Hospital for Diseases of the Chest.*

LONDON:
SHAW & SONS, FETTER LANE, FLEET STREET, E.C.,
**Printers and Publishers.**

1911

*Figure 3.7 Title page of the monograph which was hailed as the bible of electrocardiography.*

*Mechanism of the Heart Beat* with the subtitle *with especial reference to its clinical pathology.*[128] It is a remarkable book that deals with every aspect of the investigation and analysis, or as he liked to call it, the clinical pathology, of the heart beat. Having shown how the normal cardiac rhythm, the 'cardiac mechanism', may be analysed from the point of view of the arterial pulse, the venous pulse and the electrocardiogram, he then goes on to describe individual arrhythmias using these methods of investigation. When a rhythm is physiological he employs the term homogenetic, whilst a pathological one is called heterogenetic and extrasystoles for example are described under this heading. The pacemaker of the heart, and the transmission of the impulse to the ventricle are carefully described. There are full accounts of paroxysmal tachycardia and heart block, with separate chapters on the vagus and the Adams–Stokes syndrome. The chapters on atrial fibrillation, naturally, are comprehensive. Every arrhythmia has an account of its experimental production in the dog, as well as the clinical features. The contributions of previous workers are well acknowledged. Mechanical recordings of the pulse, apex beat and venous pulse are often described and illustrated, but the important emphasis of the book was on electrocardiography. This, after all was what everyone wanted to learn about, and Lewis was the person best qualified to teach it. The 23 chapters cover 295 pages and contain detailed discussions on the literature in addition to recounting his own work, some of it unpublished. There are as many references to foreign language papers as there are to those in English. For example, he quotes from ten journals and several monographs written in German. The work is liberally illustrated with 227 figures, some of them being composite ones containing up to five separate recordings of the electrocardiogram. One can only guess at the amount of work required to produce this book, in which he had to prepare all the figures as well as the text and the over 300 references himself. There had been two previous books on electrocardiography. The first was by Alexander F. Samojloff from Russia in 1909[102] and the second by Friedrich Kraus and Georg F. Nicolai from Germany in 1910.[99] Although his book was not the first on the subject it soon came to be described as the bible of electrocardiography. The preface is dated December 1910 and acknowledges his indebtedness to the Beit Memorial Research Fund for the 'leisure in which to write' and records, 'my appreciation of the unfailing kindness of my friend Dr. James Mackenzie'. It is dedicated to James Mackenzie and Willem Einthoven. He sent a copy to Einthoven saying that the credit for the work on which it was based belonged to him and Mackenzie. Einthoven modestly replied[317] that, 'your discoveries in the field of the pathology of the heart increase the value of the string galvanometer greatly'.

Papers on clinical arrhythmias continued to appear in rapid succession. There were 18 from 1911 to 1912 and they included observations on atrial flutter which had awaited the electrocardiogram for its recognition,[131] and on other forms of atrial and nodal tachycardias as well as extrasystoles, complete heart block and further work on atrial fibrillation.

## Ventricular fibrillation

Of particular interest was his study with Dr Alfred Goodman Levy[(11),95] in 1911 on arrhythmias due to chloroform which critically examined the decades-old contention that this anaesthetic agent was associated with sudden death during induction especially if the patient was apprehensive. Using cats they showed that a low concentration of chloroform produced multifocal extrasystoles and that the addition of adrenaline led to ventricular fibrillation.[108] This arrhythmia had been postulated by John A. MacWilliam in 1889[58] as the cause of sudden death, and as Lewis pointed out, 'If fibrillation of the auricles is so frequent in the human subject, it is natural to ask why a similarly disturbed ventricle is so rare. Its rarity is more apparent than real for fibrillation of the ventricles spells death'.[170] When MacWilliam died in 1937 Lewis said, 'He was a most lovable man of very unusual innate modesty. I have long had a strong admiration for his early work; he was one of the chief pioneers of cardiac physiology in this country. In 1889 he suggested that this ventricular fibrillation of his is probably a frequent cause of sudden death in man...this suggestion was for its time brilliant and has been abundantly justified since'.[414] Although Lewis was now deeply involved with research he still retained his interest in natural history as is shown by the fact that in 1911 he obtained a large textbook on fungi, *A Monograph of the*

*Mycetazoa,* by Arthur Lister. He purchased this from the well known medical and scientific bookshop in Gower Street, H.K. Lewis and Sons, which was used by generations of students at the college and hospital, and who became the publishers of one of his books. This firm was not related to his own family.

## The heart spa at Bad Nauheim

It is surprising to find in the *University College Hospital Magazine* for 1911 a paper on the spa at Bad Nauheim.[125] This spa had gained a considerable reputation in the treatment of heart disease, especially with a regime of brine baths and resistive exercises devised by Drs August and Theodor Schott. Osler had described their results as striking and Arthur D. Hirschfelder, the cardiologist at Johns Hopkins, praised them in his textbook.[302] But James Mackenzie, who had visited the spa, wrote at length in 1908 about 'the unmerited reputation of the Nauheim baths...Of wonderful cures I saw none'.[266] With typical thoroughness Lewis objectively analysed all the features of treatment there such as the chemical composition of the springs and the types of baths, and also of the cost for five weeks of £100. He found little evidence that cardiac size was reduced or that pulse irregularities were diminished, both of these being claimed as benefits of the regime. A fall of blood pressure was stated to occur, but he added that it was an open secret that occasionally patients died of apoplexy in the baths. He had the firm impression that the great majority of the visitors did not have heart disease. The official guide gave a list of the diseases in which the Nauheim treatment was indicated and there was, he said, 'a most unfortunate similarity between the list and that found on the wrappers of many proprietary remedies'. It was a fault he said to crowd together many patients, largely of the neurotic type, and intent upon their ailments. Presumably he wrote this article as a result of going there during his stay in Germany.

## Appointed lecturer in cardiac pathology

In 1911 he obtained his first academic post in UCH Medical School, which had become independent of UCL in 1907. He was appointed lecturer in cardiac pathology in the department of pathology and morbid anatomy and it should be explained that there was then a close association between pathology and clinical medicine. The director of the department was Dr Charles Bolton[(12)] who was a physician to the hospital, as well as giving the lectures in general pathology in the medical school. His department had facilities for clinical research in addition to laboratories for bacteriology, chemistry and histology. Pathology demonstrations were given by clinicians, for example, in surgery by Mr Wilfred Trotter.[(13)] The medical school prospectus for its 84th session in 1911–1912 states that, 'Dr T. Lewis will give six lectures on the graphic methods of investigating heart disease'. It also has an entry for the cardiographic department, the rooms of which 'are fitted with a string galvanometer...and other instruments used in the analysis of cardiac mechanisms' and notes that patients will be examined there on Wednesdays and Saturdays at 11 a.m.

## Willem Einthoven visits London in 1912

The year 1912 was a very significant one for Lewis. It opened with a visit to London by Einthoven who had been invited to address the Chelsea Clinical Society.[52] On learning of this Lewis and Sir William Osler[(14)] arranged a special meeting for him of the clinical section of the Royal Society of Medicine. This took place in UCH Medical School on March 20 and it gave Einthoven his first opportunity to meet Mackenzie whose books he admired. Lewis gave a fluent welcome:

> The School was proud to entertain such a man, a worker whose name was for ever stamped in the annals of clinical medicine. The advances in our knowledge came, as a rule, through the invention and introduction of new methods. It was given to few men to make these discoveries; it had been given to Einthoven. Such men were incalculable benefactors of the human race. The Professor had given the profession a perfected instrument, and a method of unrivalled precision.[132]

In his own paper Lewis pointed out that the electrocardiogram enabled nearly all arrhythmias to be analysed with precision and that as a result 'The chapter of the analysis of cardiac irregularities was fast closing'.[132] After only four years work with a new technique this sounds like a rather over-confident, even a rash, statement to make but in retrospect one can see that it was factual and largely correct.

## He installs a Cambridge electrocardiograph apparatus

The next important event came soon afterwards when he was able to start using the Cambridge electrocardiograph. The Cambridge Scientific Instrument Company[(15)] was directed by Horace Darwin, FRS, who entered into a royalty agreement with Einthoven in 1904 to make a new version of the string galvanometer. Darwin invited W.D. Duddell, FRS, known for his exceptional ability in designing new instruments, to create an entirely new design for the string galvanometer and the first instrument was made in 1905.[29] It was a great success, having a very compact electromagnet and a new type of string carrier. The early models were of the galvanometer only, and used just for physiological work, because it took a few years for the full significance of its diagnostic value to be appreciated. By 1908 Cambridge had manufactured a complete electrocardiograph but it was not until 1911 that the first complete apparatus, or 'outfit' as it was called, was available for clinical use, and Lewis was supplied with the first one, on hire, in that year. (Fig. 3.8, *overleaf*) The electrocardiograms were recorded on a glass photographic plate and an ingenious, oil-damped, falling-plate camera enabled a variety of recording speeds to be used, either slow for arrhythmias or fast for detailed analysis of the complexes.

## His technical assistant, Mr B.A. Robinson

Horace Darwin sent his assistant Bernard A. Robinson (Fig. 3.9, *overleaf*) to work with Lewis every week in order to facilitate development of the apparatus. Robinson had previously worked with a company which used the string

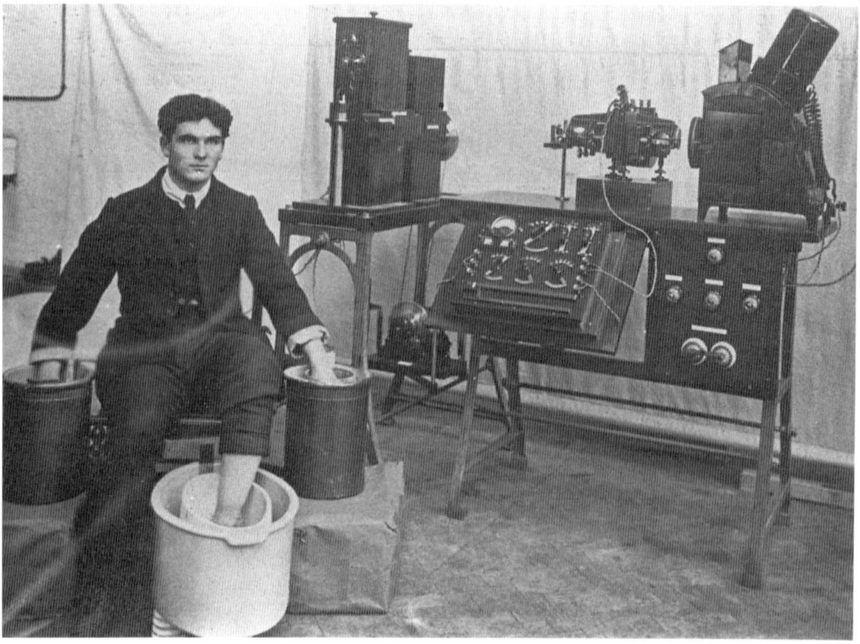

*Figure 3.8* *The first complete Cambridge electrocardiograph apparatus in 1911. From right to left, arc lamp, string galvanometer and two cameras. The camera on the left has an oil-damped falling plate, and the one on the right is a continuous paper camera.*

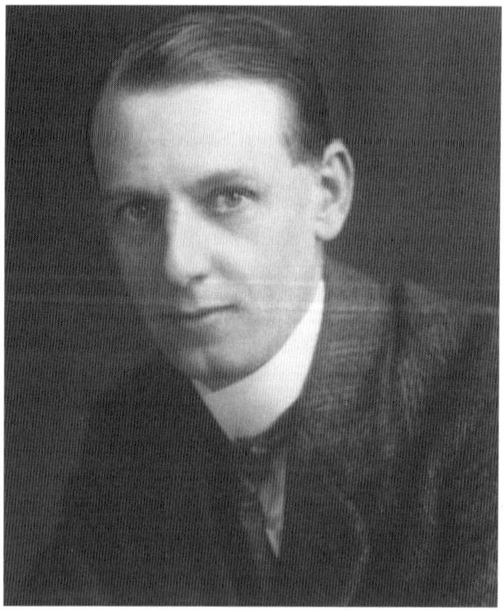

*Figure 3.9* *Bernard A. Robinson, Lewis' indispensable technical assistant from 1912 to 1914.*

galvanometer to send high speed radio-telegraph messages across the North Sea, and he had visited Einthoven in 1907. Robinson later wrote:

> I was introduced to Dr Lewis in July 1912. At that time he was working with the Edelmann string galvanometer and had not got the Cambridge machine working. Thursday was his research day in each week and it was arranged that as much as possible I would spend Thursdays with him. This co-operation was the main factor in the very rapid development of the cardiograph between 1912 and 1915. It relieved Lewis of all responsibility for the operation of the instruments so that he could concentrate on the physiological side. At the same time I was on the spot to counter any difficulties and immediately report to Cambridge suggested modifications for regular hospital and clinical use. As each new type of equipment was produced it was submitted to him for criticism, and we used prototypes together before being put into production. From then onwards Lewis used only Cambridge equipment. Thus the Cardiograph became a unified Outfit and each one supplied strictly up to date.
>
> Lewis was 31 and I was 24 when I started working with him and that was an education in itself. During the three years I was associated with him so closely I never once saw him ruffled. He had a most equable temperament. Slim in figure, those penetrating eyes under heavy eyelashes were very expressive. Always quietly speaking, when anything went wrong we would look at each other and instinctively felt 'Come on let's try again'. He had infinite patience and there was much affection between us. He once told some visitors, 'When 'BAR' is here the instruments always behave, so when he is away his photo hangs up'. Most of the work at that time was done on anaesthetized dogs and Lewis was most careful that they were tenderly treated before being 'put under', and never under any circumstances allowed to recover consciousness.
>
> One always had to have a plentiful supply of experimental electrodes ready. Often half a dozen or more electrodes were in use at one time and the greatest care had to be taken in the positioning, and the right connection maintained for the recording. There was obvious pleasure in producing some irregular function of the heart; of taking the record, and then restoring normal rhythm without altering the position of the electrodes. When we met a week later sometimes he would say 'I'm puzzled by such and such a record last week so we must repeat and check each step'. It really was a joy to work with him.[83]

It is clear that it was only with Robinson's invaluable assistance that he was able to do some of his finest experimental work. A little known invention of Robinson's was his introduction of silver-plated glass fibres or 'strings' for the galvanometer which were easier to make than the quartz fibres used by Einthoven. Another innovation came after he noticed that Lewis, like Waller and Einthoven, sometimes placed a pulse tracing on the electrocardiograph recording. This was done by placing the writing arm of the Mackenzie polygraph in the beam of light, and Robinson saw that its pneumatic system lacked sensitivity. Lewis took him to Harley Street to discuss the matter with Mackenzie who agreed with him. Robinson redesigned the instrument and the first model was tested out and approved by Lewis in July 1914.[83] It was called the Mackenzie–Lewis polygraph. (Fig. 3.10, *overleaf*)

One of the first clinical studies Lewis did with the Cambridge apparatus was a remarkable one in which, with the help of the obstetric registrar Mr Clifford White, he took electrocardiograms on new-born babies to show their physiological right ventricular hypertrophy.[141] The tracings were repeated every two weeks to demonstrate regression of the hypertrophy, and there is a splendid illustration (Fig. 3.11, *overleaf*) of this in *Clinical Electrocardiography.*[136] Technical problems

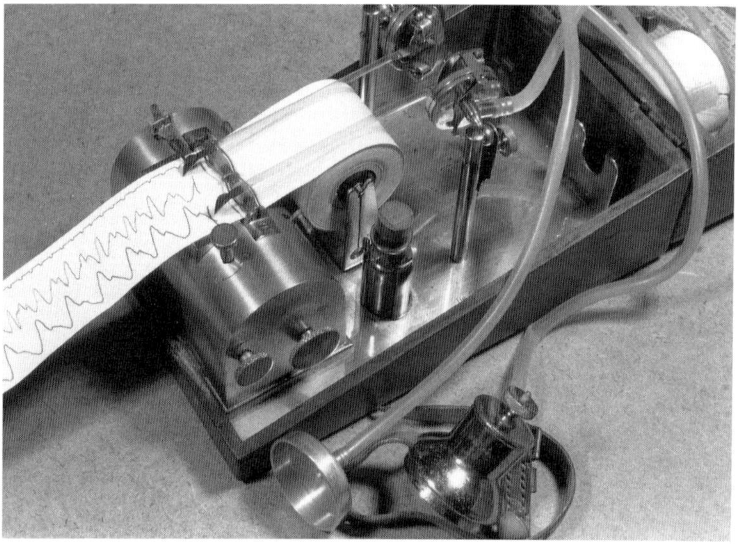

*Figure 3.10 The Mackenzie–Lewis ink polygraph with venous and arterial tracings. The tubing is modern.*

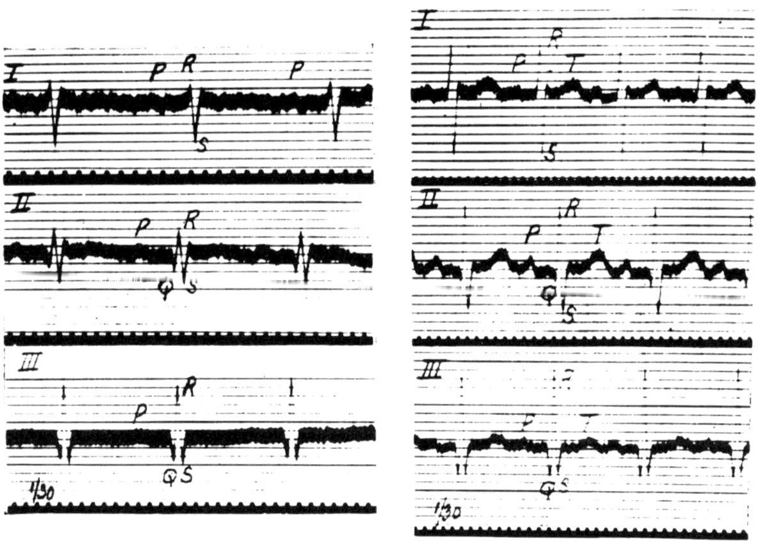

*Figure 3.11 Electrocardiograms from a child two hours after birth (left) and at age six weeks (right) which show the resolution of physiological right ventricular preponderance. This was a technically remarkable achievement for its time in 1913. (From reference 136.)*

with this study called for one of his frequent requests for help to Einthoven who sent him some zinc–iron wire and recommended using 20% salt solution to moisten the cotton wool electrodes.[317]

# Study of heart murmurs, and phonocardiograms

The new apparatus also gave him the opportunity to make recordings of the heart sounds and murmurs, with a carbon microphone made by Cambridge to a design of Einthoven. Initially he used two string galvanometers side by side in order to record the phonocardiogram and electrocardiogram simultaneously, a method first used in 1911 by L. Bull in Boulogne.[23] However in 1913 an ingenious double string carrier was designed at Cambridge by A.P. Apthorpe and this enabled two tracings to be made simultaneously with only one galvanometer.[308] The phonocardiograms in his two papers are of high quality and demonstrate well the murmurs of aortic regurgitation (Fig. 3.12) and patent ductus arteriosus, which are difficult to record.[134,135] He made especial studies of mitral stenosis and his recordings (Fig. 3.13) clearly show the opening snap of the mitral valve. But this distinctive feature was not recognized by him, and even in later years he called it a reduplicated second sound. This is a surprising omission because it had been described in France 30 years beforehand. However, in an earlier paper he made a

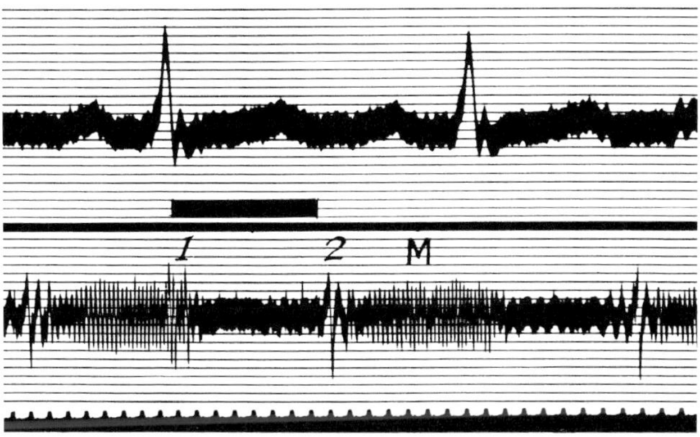


*Figure 3.12 Phonocardiogram of an aortic diastolic murmur M from a patient with a ruptured aortic susp. (From reference 188.)*

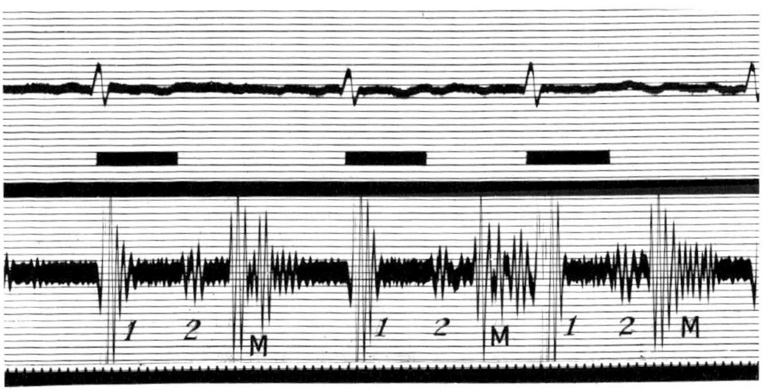


*Figure 3.13 Phonocardiogram in mitral stenosis showing the diastolic murmur, M. Note the loud opening snap of the mitral valve just before M. (From reference 134.)*

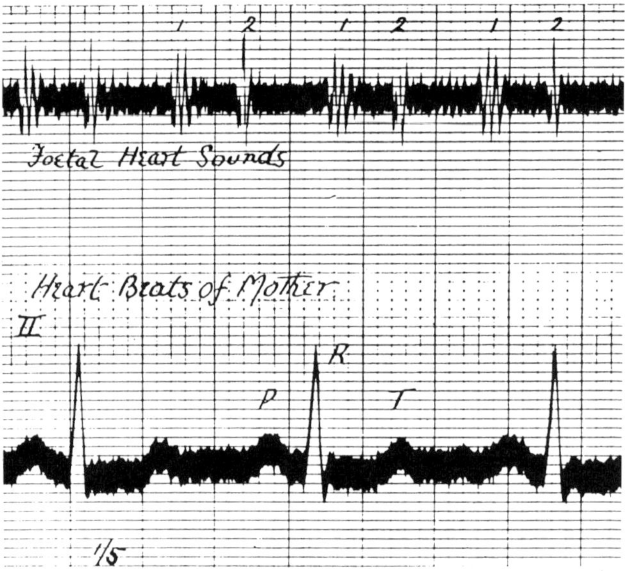


*Figure 3.14 Simultaneous recordings, using the twin string galvanometer, of the heart sounds of the foetus and the electrocardiogram of the mother. A fine technical achievement.*

very astute observation at the bedside in a man with mitral stenosis. He noted that a previously heard presystolic murmur had disappeared and that there was no atrial wave in the apex beat tracing though there was definitely an atrial wave in the jugular venous pulse. He decided that the left atrium had become paralysed whilst the right atrium continued to beat normally.[117] This situation seems so unlikely that it was a bold conclusion to reach, but typically for him he stuck to the facts. This remarkable and distinctive syndrome does in fact occur in severe mitral stenosis but it was overlooked by all subsequent observers until 1980 when modern studies showed that Lewis' interpretation was the correct one.[71] Naturally for Lewis, the experimental physiologist, these studies had to include animal work. In dogs he perforated an aortic cusp and recorded not only the immediate diastolic murmur but also a presystolic murmur which he likened to that described in man by Dr Austin Flint of New York in 1862, and named after him.[135] Austin Flint had noted a mitral presystolic murmur, apparently indicating mitral stenosis, in two patients with aortic regurgitation who had normal mitral valves.

## Notes to Chapter 3

(1) Herman Adrianus Snellen, 1905– , is a distinguished cardiologist, formerly professor of medicine at Leiden University and a noted medical historian. Author of three books about Willem Einthoven and also one on the history of cardiology.

(2) George Edmeston Fahr, 1882–1968, was an American physician, a pioneer of electrocardiography, who became professor of medicine at Minneapolis General Hospital. He was an assistant to Willem Einthoven from 1909 to 1913 when he collaborated in important work on the electrical axis of the heart.

(3) Alfred Einstein Cohn, 1879–1957, was a cardiologist at Mount Sinai Hospital, New York. He studied first under Ludwig Aschoff in Vienna and then went to London where he did some of the earliest research work in electrocardiography with Thomas Lewis in 1909.

(4) Horatio Burt Williams, 1877–1955, was an American physician who also graduated in engineering, and who became professor of physiology at Columbia University. After visiting Einthoven's laboratory in 1911 he designed the first electrocardiograph to be manufactured outside Europe.

(5) Charles F Hindle was a gifted mechanic in the College of Physicians and Surgeons New York. He constructed an electrocardiograph to Williams' design and then formed the Hindle Instrument Company. His excellent portable machine of 1921 was well ahead of the model made in Cambridge, England.

(6) Bernard Sutro Oppenheimer, 1876–1958, graduated MD in 1901 and developed an early interest in cardiology. He became Lewis' second American research worker in 1910 and was one of the first physicians to use the electrocardiograph in the United States. He was Chief of the Medical Service at the Mount Sinai Hospital in New York. He was a strong advocate of postgraduate medical training and for many years he was chairman of the committee on medical education of the New York Academy of Medicine. Whilst in London he married Enid Tribe who was a distinguished physiologist.

Adele Oppenheimer, 1874–1960, worked with Lewis being co-author of a paper in 1910, and later she collaborated with Bernard in a paper in 1912 on the nerve fibrils in the sino-auricular node.

(7) Carl J Rothberger was an outstanding exponent of cardiac electrophysiology who worked in the Institute for General and Experimental Pathology in Vienna. He wrote extensively on arrhythmias and also on experimental bundle branch block. The 1925, 3rd, edition of Lewis' book on *The Mechanism and Graphic Registration of the Heart Beat* refers to 36 papers written by Rothberger in collaboration chiefly with H Winterberg, and also with H Eppinger, A F Hecht, R Kaufmann, Y Miki and E Nobel between 1909 and 1923.

(8) William Errington Hume, (later Sir William), 1879–1960, was a consultant physician at Newcastle-upon-Tyne and an early specialist in cardiology, writing on cardiac arrhythmias. He did good work on The Soldiers' Heart in 1916–1918 and gave the Harveian Oration in 1943 on 'The Physician in War'. Cardinal Hume is his son.

(9) Otto Beit, (later Sir Otto), 1865–1930, was a South African millionaire who made his fortune from diamonds. In December 1909 he founded and endowed the Beit Memorial Fellowships for Medical Research in memory of his late brother Mr Alfred Beit, 'to promote the advancement by Research of Medicine and the allied Sciences in their relation to medicine'. A fellowship was for a period of three years, and this far-sighted enterprise made it possible for talented young research workers to pursue a career which otherwise would have been closed to them. A woman, Dr Ida Smedley, was among the first ten to be elected.

(10) Edward Mellanby, FRS, (later Sir Edward), 1884–1955, became professor of pharmacology in Sheffield in 1920. He showed that rickets was due to deficiency of vitamin D. From 1933 to 1940 he was secretary of the Medical Research Council. He was a forceful secretary who initiated the National Institute for Medical Research.

(11) Alfred Goodman Levy, 1866–1954, qualified from University College Hospital in 1892 and then became a pioneer doctor in Rhodesia. He then became an anaesthetist at Guy's Hospital London and undertook research work with Thomas Lewis on chloroform. Later he was on the staff of the London Jewish Hospital and the London Chest Hospital.

(12) Charles Bolton, FRS, 1870–1947, was a consulting physician at University College Hospital. When the new medical school opened in 1907 he was made Director of Research. This was an unusual post at that time for a physician in a London hospital and it emphasizes the scientific eminence of the clinical staff at UCH, some of whom

like Bolton were Fellows of the Royal Society. Lewis worked originally in Bolton's laboratories.

(13) Wilfred Batten Trotter, FRS, 1872–1939, was a consulting surgeon at University College Hospital from 1906–1938. He was a fine surgeon but is best known for his book *Instincts of the Herd in Peace and War* and also for other essays on the philosophy of medicine, such as 'Has the intellect a function?'

(14) William Osler, FRS, (later Sir William), 1849–1919, was one of the greatest physicians of the late 19th and early 20th centuries. He worked first in Canada, and then in the United States where he was the originator of combining scientific work in the laboratory with clinical work. He wrote original articles on endocarditis and angina pectoris. From 1904 was Regius Professor of Medicine in Oxford. He was an inspiring leader of the medical profession, and a great medical historian.

(15) The Cambridge Scientific Instrument Company was founded in 1881 to manufacture physiological apparatus, initially for Trinity College Cambridge. H Darwin, later Sir Horace, the seventh child of Charles Darwin was at first in control of instrument making. The company later manufactured many types of laboratory apparatus and was very highly regarded for the fine quality of its designs and workmanship.

# Chapter 4

## Appointed to the staff of UCH • Studies on the excitatory wave, bundle branch block, and ventricular hypertrophy • Research in medicine • Visit to Canada and the United States of America

IN NOVEMBER 1912 he achieved his ambition by being promoted to the clinical staff of UCH as an assistant physician, with charge of four beds. The full physicians were Sir John Rose Bradford, Dr Sidney Martin, Dr J. Risien Russell, Dr H. Batty Shaw, Dr Frederick J Poynton and Dr Charles Bolton. It was Batty Shaw who at some stage advised Lewis to give up his research and do some proper clinical work! The other assistant physician was T.R. Elliott, four years his senior, who had been appointed only a year after qualifying in 1910. The London Hospital had also wanted to appoint Lewis, and the Dean of their medical college wrote a letter of congratulation saying 'I am more than sorry that we shall not have the distinction of having you as a member of our Staff...'[484] There is an interesting background to this comment. Two years previously Mackenzie had been appointed lecturer in cardiac research in the London Hospital Medical College but he did not have clinical duties and the medical staff were reluctant to give him a consultant appointment without competition. As a result he was thinking of resigning and was looking for a successor, and Lewis' growing reputation made him an obvious choice. Later Mackenzie did get a consultant post at the London Hospital where he established an excellent Cardiac Department which attracted visiting physicians from all over the world. But as his Resident Medical Officer at Mount Vernon who had trained at the London Hospital, had predicted, he was never, according to Linnell, completely happy at the London Hospital.[272] Lewis had given his usual serious and careful attention to the prospect of going to the London Hospital and it is worth quoting at some length from a letter which he wrote to his father from his new consulting room at 27 Queen Anne Street on November 14 1912.[520] It gives one a very clear idea, not just of that appointment, but more importantly of his considered views of what he wanted to do with his career:

> In regard to UCH and the London I do not propose deciding until I see the offers of both. There are very many things to consider and the question of title is one of the least. The first thing is *opportunity for observation*, and that naturally includes personal comfort. There are three strong arguments in favour of UCH 1) it is within easy reach 2) it is closely associated with the best laboratories and staff of scientific

> men in London 3) I know the ropes there. I should add that it is in favour with the Board of Education and that big changes are impending all round. I am prepared in view of these considerations and also from motives of sentiment (you will remember that the basis of my work has been laid at UCH and that my name is associated with the place; my friends are there; and my department is already running) to take less at UCH than at the London. It is largely a question, not of the actual position allotted, but of the prospects of quickly establishing a sound branch of special study and I am confident that I can do this at UCH with far less labour than at the London.
>
> Secondly I have no fear with regard to practice, it is a certainty within the next 10 years, and will probably come on a larger scale than is desired. A large practice means morning till midnight slavery at what is quite often anything but a congenial task. My heart is set primarily upon the study of disease, and upon the attempt to organize and control a small and efficient school to this end. What I want at UCH is the facility provided by an acknowledgment of the principle that such study can only be provided by the *special* worker. As a matter of fact they have already appointed me assistant physician (not yet official) giving me 4 beds and outpatients. What they have not done is to clearly state that *I am exempt from the general duties.* I am appointed because *they want the special work to continue at UCH* The fact remains and they know it perfectly well, *that the two together are too much for any one man.*But they have made the appointment and the exemptions are, I think, pretty certain to follow.

In the event Lewis did persuade his senior colleagues of the strength of his argument and his future at UCH as a specialist in cardiovascular work was assured. Furthermore, in a year which was so full of important events the Royal College of Physicians of London awarded him their Fellowship.[(1)] In 1912 he wrote to Einthoven saying 'I am trying to establish a postgraduate class at the school. Quite a lot of men are coming'.[317] The school prospectus for 1912–13 indicates that all the clinical and experimental work of the Cardiographic Department was available for study by qualified men, that Lewis would work with them each day from 11 to 1 o'clock and that the fee was two guineas per month or seven guineas for six months.

This postgraduate class is a good and clear example of Lewis' determination that he must always make the results of his research work available to general physicians and to the general medical practitioner. This of course meant a great deal of extra work when he was involved in time consuming and difficult experimental studies, but he conscientiously undertook this self-imposed task. He realized that his monograph on *The Mechanism of the Heart Beat* was too detailed for the general physician with an interest in the heart and he therefore set about writing two teaching books which presented the information in a shorter and more readable form.

## Books for the general physician

The first of these teaching books which came out in 1912 was *Clinical Disorders of the Heart Beat. A handbook for practitioners and students.* (Fig. 4.1) It was intended to present a modern view of cardiac irregularities as they could be detected by simple bedside signs. He did not believe it to be necessary for the practitioner to either record or interpret graphic records, because 'most of those disturbances of the heart's mechanism which are met with in everyday practice

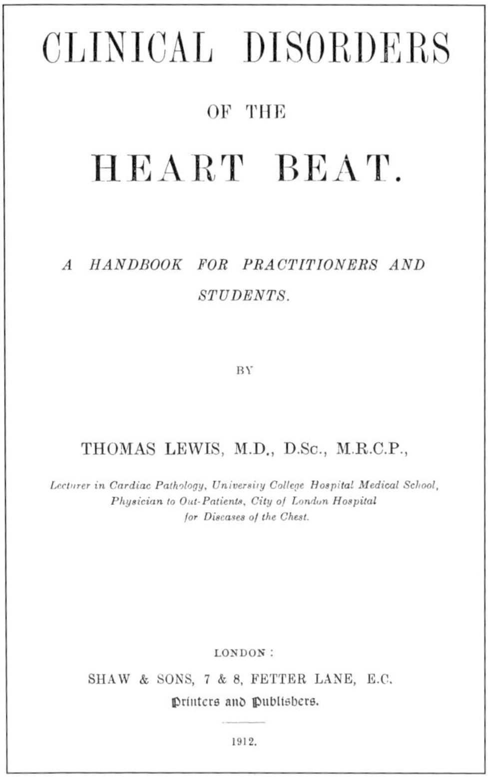

CLINICAL DISORDERS

OF THE

HEART BEAT.

*A HANDBOOK FOR PRACTITIONERS AND STUDENTS.*

BY

THOMAS LEWIS, M.D., D.Sc., M.R.C.P.,

*Lecturer in Cardiac Pathology, University College Hospital Medical School, Physician to Out-Patients, City of London Hospital for Diseases of the Chest.*

LONDON:

SHAW & SONS, 7 & 8, FETTER LANE, E.C.

Printers and Publishers.

1912.

*Figure 4.1 Title page of Lewis' first teaching book, which went through seven editions. (From reference 133.)*

can be identified by simpler means'.[133] There were chapters on sinus irregularities, heart block, extrasystoles, paroxysmal tachycardia, auricular flutter, and auricular fibrillation. The final one was on alternation of the heart which he described in a fine piece of writing, 'It is the faint cry of an anguished and fast failing muscle, which, when it comes, all should strain to hear, for it is not long repeated. A few months, a few years at most, and the end comes'. It was illustrated with polygraph curves because many doctors could take these at the bedside and their interpretation was assisted by his 'ladder' diagrams. The value that clinicians placed on this book was emphasized by the appearance of a French edition only a year later. (Fig. 4.2, *overleaf*) *Clinical Electrocardiography* (Fig. 4.3, *overleaf*) came out a year later in 1913 and it must have been a godsend to those who were trying to learn about this new subject.[136] It was intended for use in hospital work, as a supplement, he said, to *Clinical Disorders*, and significantly the title did not say it was for practitioners and students. Lewis wrote in the preface that '...this new method of examination has become essential to the modern diagnosis and treatment of cardiac patients. Those cardiac patients are few, in whom an electric examination is superfluous, and in a large and increasing percentage of cases the records profoundly modify our conception of the conditions with which we deal'. It was mostly concerned, as one might expect, with arrhythmias whilst ventricular hypertrophy and bundle branch block were dealt

LES DÉSORDRES CLINIQUES

DU

BATTEMENT DU CŒUR

PAR

TH. LEWIS

Professeur à l'École de Médecine de Londres.

TRADUIT DE L'ANGLAIS

PAR LE D[r] C. CHAUVET

Médecin consultant à Royat.

PRÉFACE DE M. LE PROF. TEISSIER, DE LYON

AVEC 47 GRAPHIQUES DANS LE TEXTE

PARIS

LIBRAIRIE FÉLIX ALCAN

108, BOULEVARD SAINT-GERMAIN, 108

1913

Tous droits de reproduction et d'adaptation réservés pour tous pays.

*Figure 4.2 The first of several translations of Lewis' books.*

CLINICAL

ELECTROCARDIOGRAPHY

BY

THOMAS LEWIS, M.D., D.Sc., F.R.C.P.,

*Assistant Physician and Lecturer on Cardiac Pathology, University College Hospital, Physician to Out-Patients, City of London Hospital.*

LONDON:

SHAW & SONS, 7 & 8, FETTER LANE, E.C.

Printers and Publishers.

1913.

*Figure 4.3 Title page of his book which was eagerly read by doctors wishing to learn about the new discipline of electrocardiography in 1913. (From reference 136.)*

with under the heading of 'rhythmic but anomalous electrocardiograms'. The book was illustrated with several dozen high quality electrocardiograms. (Fig. 4.4) These books went through six and seven editions respectively, indicating the value placed on them by generations of students as well as physicians. Lewis eventually fused them into a single volume which he completed in 1945 just before he died.[238] Another valuable account, written for the general practitioner, was a long paper in the *British Medical Journal* on 'Electrocardiography and its importance in the clinical examination of heart affections'.[129] It was well illustrated and it gave the general reader a full account of the subject written in clear English. In addition to arrhythmias, the use of the electrocardiogram in diagnosing ventricular hypertrophy was also emphasized.

The year ended with an invitation from his father to join in a trip to St Moritz, for two weeks over Christmas, which Lewis said he would be very glad to join. He seems to have been well acquainted with skiing because, in accepting, he warned his father that it was rather early in the winter adding, 'I believe the place was a dismal failure last year'.[520]

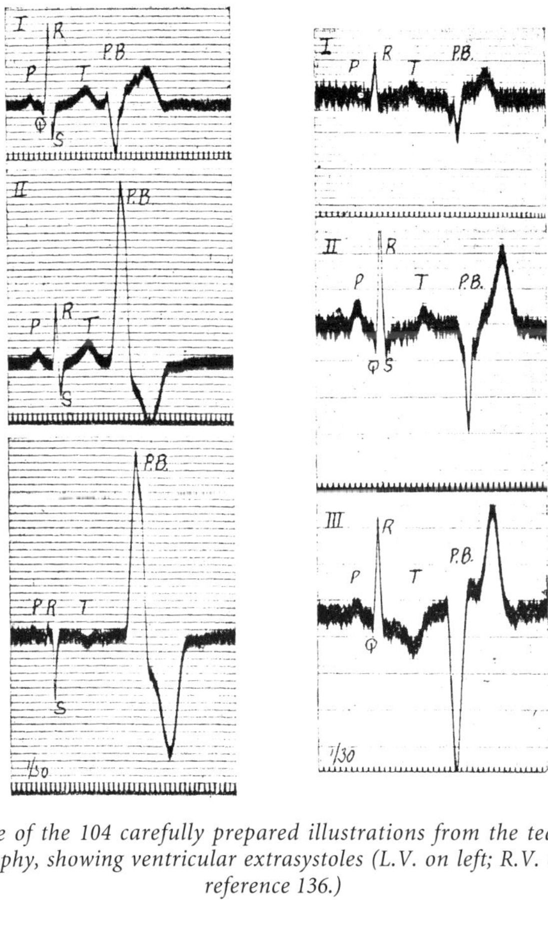


*Figure 4.4 One of the 104 carefully prepared illustrations from the teaching book on electrocardiography, showing ventricular extrasystoles (L.V. on left; R.V. on right. (From reference 136.)*

## The end of work on clinical arrhythmias

In 1913 he published a paper which appeared in the *American Journal of Medical Sciences* on premature nodal beats in a child.[239] This was his second paper in an American journal. His co-author was Herbert W. Allen from San Francisco, his fourth American associate, who wrote, 'I look back with much pleasure and satisfaction to my stay and work with you'.[342] These were to be the last purely clinical papers he ever wrote on arrhythmias; all future ones were detailed investigations of atrial fibrillation and flutter. This confirmed his remark at the Royal Society of Medicine meeting that the analysis of irregularities was nearly complete and it revealed his considerable ability, shown throughout his career, to judge when a line of enquiry was becoming worked out.

## A study of heart failure with Professor J. Barcroft

Although his experimental work remained with the electrocardiogram his clinical research then changed to a study of heart failure, a subject which remained a life long interest. He had observed that cardiac and renal patients who were very breathless usually had slight or no cyanosis in contrast to the lack of dyspnoea in deeply cyanosed patients with congenital heart disease. He decided that a factor other than deficient oxygenation of the blood was causing the dyspnoea, and enlisted the help of Joseph Barcroft,[(2)] a Cambridge physiologist. Barcroft was an expert in the analysis of alveolar air and blood gases, and author of the book *The Respiratory Function of the Blood*. They showed that the patients with dyspnoea had acidosis due to retention of acids in excess of base such as occurs at high altitude, calling it 'acid intoxication'.[240,256] In these papers Lewis describes patients with classical paroxysmal dyspnoea, either during the day or more often at night, who had aortic regurgitation or severe hypertension but in whom he ascribes the dyspnoea 'chiefly to sudden flooding of the system with acid products'. He does not even discuss the possibility of acute left ventricular failure, and it was to take him over 20 years before he would admit that such a syndrome could be the cause. Nevertheless, this was a pioneer investigation into the biochemistry of heart failure and a good example of Lewis' mission to bring laboratory studies to the bedside.

## Family matters and letters • His father has a serious illness

A letter from home in 1913 signed 'with love, your affectionate father, H. L.' is important because it shows that from 1912 he was getting a substantial allowance, namely £200 a year, from his father.[374] This was nearly as much as his Beit Fellowship which had ended in 1912. His brothers had the same allowance too. It confirms the remark 'that poverty never dictated his career',[299] though it was also correct to point out that, 'Although the son of a well-to-do father, he was not the man to subsist on parental wealth'.[50] His father's letter continued:

> So please do yourself accordingly and in as comfortable way as possible-do not put up with poor feeding on any account. I hope you are pleased with your Barry dividend which I am told is likely to continue. P.S. It is a good investment for you to give your patients the impression that you are most prosperous.

Lewis kept well over 30 letters[520] from his parents and they show the warm feelings that existed between him and his mother and father, who were keenly interested in all aspects of his professional life. He, too, often wrote to them, and in 1913 he must have mentioned that T.R. Elliott had been made a Fellow of the Royal Society because his father replied, 'When you get it I intend making a very large bonfire here and I am hoping someday to set it on fire'.[374] Their close relationship was poignantly shown when his father fell ill, possibly with a myocardial infarction, at the age of 64. His mother wrote to say, 'Father is crying out for you and wants you home to have a talk with you. He keeps on saying, 'I want Tom, I want him, I want him, I want him''.[376]

## His friends in New York

In July 1913 Lewis wrote a letter to Dr A. Crehore in New York which contains the interesting comment, '...give my regards to my many friends in New York, Dr Williams in particular'.[382] As we have already seen his first three research associates, Cohn and the Oppenheimers were all from New York, but who were the others? After all, he had not yet visited the United States. It may be that they were the authors of papers published in *Heart* up to that time, namely the first four volumes. They were G. Draper, Leo Kessel, Howard H. Mason, G. Canby Robinson and T. Stuart Hart. Kessel and Mason were co-authors with Cohn, who had five other papers by himself. Williams could have met Lewis in London after visiting Einthoven in 1911 and Cohn might have mentioned the valuable help that Williams had given him. If we take the five volumes of *Heart* that appeared before the 1914–18 War we can see how important American contributions were to the success of the journal in its early years. 32 of the total of 110 papers came from the United States of America.

## A medical congress in London • Dr Paul D. White arrives

The 17th International Congress of Medicine was held in London in 1913 and the meeting gave him the opportunity to summarize his work showing that the sinoatrial node was the pacemaker of the heart.[137] A garden party for the Congress was held at University College London and Arthur D. Morris who was a student at the time was deputed to show visitors around the medical school. He was astonished, he said, to find that so many of them asked to see Thomas Lewis' laboratory and that his dark basement room was the Mecca of the foreign doctors including many from the United States.[529] At this time Lewis had the clinical arrhythmia work behind him and he now commenced a very difficult and ultimately a very fine experimental study in dogs on the spread of the excitatory process in the heart.[142] The work was in progress when Dr Paul D. White[(3)] aged 27 from Boston, who became one of the world's leading cardiologists, arrived in the autumn of 1913. (Fig. 4.5, *overleaf*) He had written in June from the

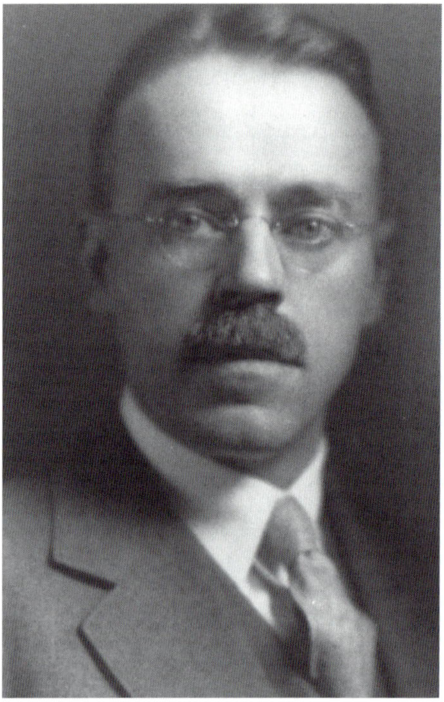

*Figure 4.5 Paul Dudley White of Boston. Photograph in 1929.*

Massachusetts General Hospital to confirm his position as a Sheldon Travelling Fellow of Harvard adding, 'my knowledge of hearts is extremely limited though I am trying to pick up a few rudiments'.[482] White recounted his immediate impressions in letters to his father, and said that although Lewis was agreeable he seemed to be naturally retiring, absent-minded and rather elusive. He soon realized that in order to learn much he had to get Lewis to give him a task to do.[254] On several occasions he went to Mackenzie's clinic at the London Hospital and gave his opinion that although Mackenzie was regarded as the foremost heart man of the time, he believed 'his day is done'. White thought there was no comparison between him and Lewis, who he considered would, before many years, be the world's greatest cardiologist, 'Even at present I think he probably is...'[295]

## Lewis' assistants give their views on working with him

Paul White's contemporary account after two months with Lewis is worth quoting:

> ...he is very taciturn and difficult to understand at first. He frightens lots of men away undoubtedly – few ever stay with him more than two, three or four weeks, which makes him all the more cynical. But we the four of us, being in earnest are hanging on like leeches and he is now just beginning to open up well. I think he

sees now that we mean business. He has certainly changed quite a bit which delights us.[295]

Nearly 60 years later when White had international fame he wrote *My Life and Medicine, an Autobiographical Memoir* in which he recounted his time at UCH with Lewis:[331]

> In October 1913, I reported to Dr Thomas Lewis for work. He stopped for a brief moment to greet me, as he stood in his cutaway morning coat at the operating table in his laboratory, massaging the heart of a dog with one hand while the other hand held his top hat and dress gloves. Impatiently he gave directions to his 'diener' (laboratory assistant) as to what to do in his absence while he was attending some official luncheon. After a short greeting my new chief paid no more attention either to me or to three others: Jonathan Meakins, a Canadian, and two other Commonwealth physicians (from India and Australia), studying in London as postgraduates with special interest in cardiovascular disease. After two weeks Meakins and I were left alone; we were obliged to remain since we had no other place to go for a year.
>
> Despite our impatience or rather our patience, while waiting to be accepted as graduate students and junior research colleagues of one of the great pioneers in electrocardiography and in the mechanism of the heart beat, I look back now with great sympathy for Dr Lewis. At the very moment of his intense preoccupation with his basic research, we were suddenly superimposed on him – ignoramuses to be trained. We were very evidently in the way and day after day Meakins and I watched on the sidelines while, with his diener, Thomas Lewis carried out experiment after experiment of great importance. Once in a while we made ward rounds with him, but this side of his job interested him little and he was always in a hurry to return to his laboratory. We admired his ability, his keenness (he had the most penetrating eyes that I have ever known), his integrity, and his complete concentration on his work, and we were anxious to join him in the excitement of the chase for knowledge – but for a long time he gave us no opportunity.
>
> Late one afternoon in December Lewis suddenly asked me if I would come back to work with him that evening and of course I accepted at once. From that moment my life in London changed completely to one of intensive research day and night. On several occasions I walked along Oxford Street with Lewis back to his lodgings (he was not yet married) and then returned to the laboratory. Night after night for weeks we measured P–R and other time intervals of the electrocardiograms of cats and dogs by the Lucas Comparator down to ten thousandths of a second under various experimental conditions. I had learned earlier how to use a slide rule, which I had brought with me, and I instructed Lewis in its use, saving countless hours of mathematical calculations. This clinched my position as a devoted slave of the master; in time this relationship changed to that of devoted friend, not only of Lewis himself but of his family. He taught me how to burn the midnight oil in London and sent me back to Boston with a basis for my cardiological career. He was one of the best teachers I have ever had, a hard taskmaster with a brain as sharp as a razor.

It is worth noting, as a comment on Lewis' dominance as a research worker, chief and teacher that White was only four years younger than him! Jonathan Meakins[(4)] (Fig. 4.6, *overleaf*) also wrote of his time at UCH and recalled that Lewis' consulting rooms in the medical school basement were distinguished chiefly by his absence because he was not keen on that type of work, and he went on to say:

> As a master Lewis was superb. He was a hard driver and did not tolerate those who did not work long and persistently. He tried you first with a subtlety of neglect which was hard to bear unless both the flesh, spirit, and determination were strong.

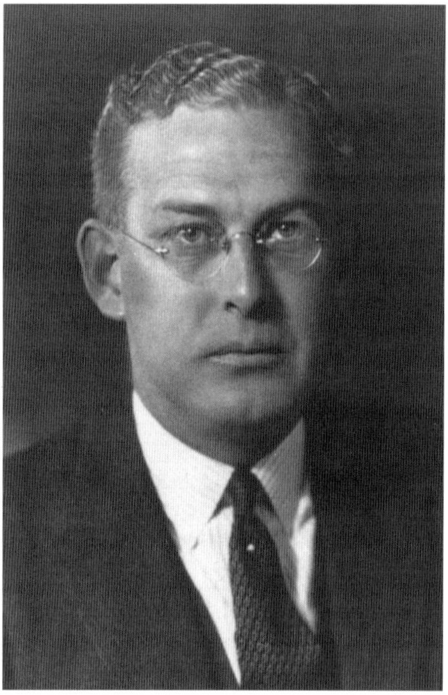

*Figure 4.6 Jonathan Campbell Meakins of Montreal. Photograph in 1929.*

> It was his way of eliminating the weak and the dilettante and withal satisfactory to everyone. He was demanding but encouraging. His smile of approbation made the sun shine even through a London fog made worse by working in a photographic dark room in a cellar. But he was also a strict scientific father who kept his children well under his eye.[281]

On one occasion Meakins and White were behindhand with their work and bribed the lab. boy for an extra key to get in at night, and Meakins said he well remembered Lewis' 'apparent wrath when he found us out of the bounds of time':[281]

> To our consternation we heard the door open and the familiar out-of-tune whistle cease. We knew we were caught! A quick question, a stern but short reprimand, a quick flashing smile and he took the centre stool and we worked till after midnight. So it was for several nights a week thereafter. He was a hard driver but appreciated an ardent worker and showed this in many subtle ways. His shyness and reticence would never permit expression by the direct approach.[281]

Only five months later, in May 1914, the first paper by Lewis, White, and Meakins was published in *Heart*,[258] and it shows how much detailed work went into this study of electrical stimulation of the dog's heart. There are 11 tables, one alone with over 300 measurements of time intervals made to 0.0001 of a second. Lewis was now at the peak of his electrophysiological studies which aimed to show the electrical events underlying cardiac contraction and his experimental work was remarkable for its scope and technical virtuosity. Electrode positions were identified with precision using drawings at the time and later by examining the whole heart embedded in paraffin wax. (Fig. 4.7) In order to follow the spread of the excitation wave he had to record the arrival of an impulse at a particular site and time it by from a reference tracing taken from a limb lead. This meant taking two electrograms simultaneously and the Cambridge double 'string' carrier containing two fibres was invaluable for this purpose, and yielded recordings of exceptional quality. (Fig. 4.8) Furthermore by using two galvanometers,

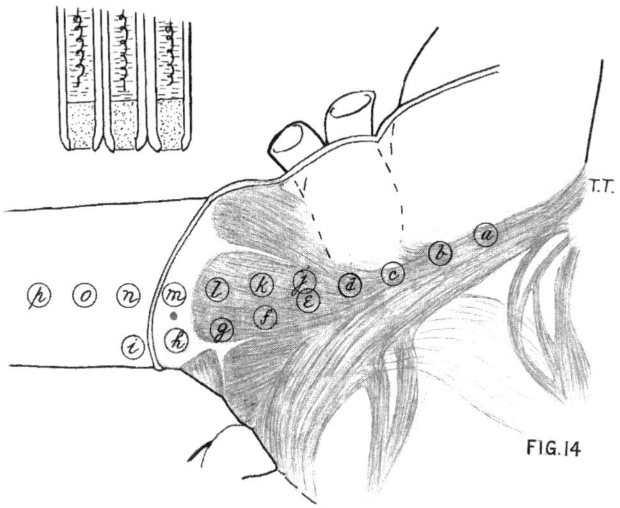


*Figure 4.7 Sketch of a dog's heart showing the 16 positions where electrodes were placed for recordings. Inferior vena cava to the left, atrium to the right. Above is shown his 'organ pipe' electrode system. (From reference 257.)*

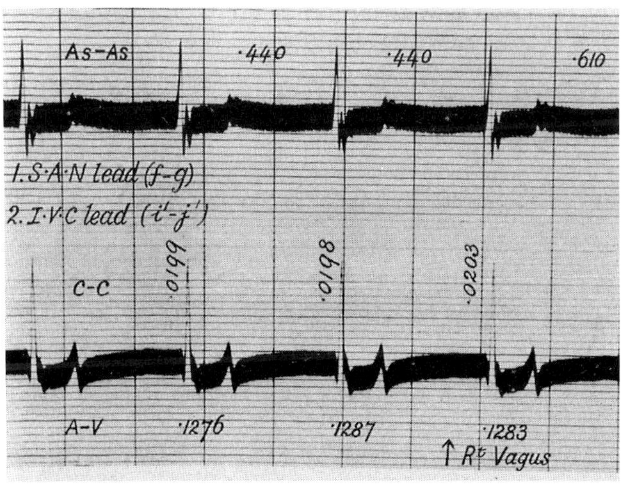


*Figure 4.8 A superb recording with the twin string galvanometer showing simultaneous electrograms from the sino-atrial node and the inferior vena cava in the dog. (From reference 257.)*

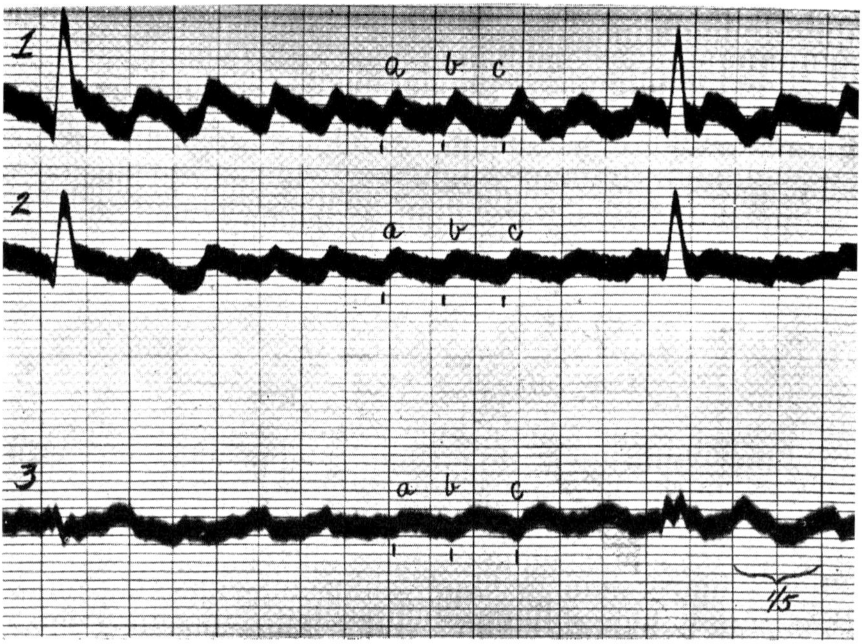


*Figure 4.9 An early example of three-channel recording. Made by using two string galvanometers, single string for the top strip and twin string for the lower two. From a patient with auricular fibrillation. (From* Heart *1921:8;359.)*

one with a double string and the other with the usual single string it was possible to record three electrograms on the same photographic plate, a remarkable achievement for 1914. (Fig. 4.9) Lewis even made recordings from inside the heart by placing glass electrodes on the interatrial septum and, via the aorta, on the outflow tract of the left ventricle. He produced nodal rhythm by devising the elegant technique of cooling the sulcus terminalis with iced water passed through a lead tube. One has to remember the small size of the dog heart to fully appreciate the excellence of his experimental work. His two classic papers entitled 'The excitatory process in the dog's heart' were presented at meetings of the Royal Society in June 1914 and February 1915.[257,251] Meakins and White were co-authors for the first, (Fig. 4.10) and Marcus A. Rothschild of New York for the second. They were read for him, because he was not a Fellow, by E.H. Starling. The final summary of this work came in 1917 with his Croonian Lecture to the Royal Society 'Upon the motion of the mammalian heart'.[145]

## Lewis's error with the interpretation of bundle branch block

Cardiac physiology had been extensively investigated in the previous few decades but demonstration of its electrical activity was limited until the electrocardiogram provided the ideal instrument for this purpose. Excellent pioneer work

PHILOSOPHICAL TRANSACTIONS

OF THE

ROYAL SOCIETY OF LONDON.

SERIES B, VOL. 205. Pp. 375–420.

[PLATES 40–43.]

---

THE EXCITATORY PROCESS IN THE DOG'S HEART.

PART I.—THE AURICLES.

BY

THOMAS LEWIS, JOHN MEAKINS, AND PAUL D. WHITE.

*Figure 4.10 Title page of the first of his papers at the Royal Society which set the seal on his scientific excellence. (From reference 257.)*

was done in Vienna by Hans Eppinger, Carl J. Rothberger, Heinrich Winterberg and Oscar Stoerk. As early as 1910 they recorded electrocardiograms after cutting either the right or left bundle branches in the dog – a delicate operation pioneered the previous year at Johns Hopkins Hospital by Lewellys F. Barker and Arthur D. Hirschfelder. This work enabled curves in the human to be identified as showing bundle branch block, an entity which Lewis was the first to recognize as being responsible for the transient widening of the QRS complex after certain atrial extrasystoles, a phenomenon he called ventricular aberration 'because they are caused by impulses which have gone astray'.

In 1915 Lewis commenced a thorough study of bundle branch block which he produced in the dog by the difficult technique of squeezing either side of the septum with a special pair of forceps, but it was his attraction to animal work that also led him, as well as the impulses, to go astray. The electrocardiographic pattern of bundle branch block in the dog is very different from that in the human, but Lewis chose to rely on the dog work to identify which bundle branch is affected in human disease. As a result he mixed up right and left bundle branch block. In the dog a lesion of the right branch gave deep negative deflections in leads II and III with left axis deviation, looking very much like left branch block in the human (though lead I was different) whilst a left branch lesion resulted in upright complexes in these leads resembling human right bundle branch block. (Fig. 4.11, *overleaf*) Taken together with a human histological study of Eppinger and Stoerk he concluded that what is really left branch block is right block, and vice versa. He ignored a histological study done by Cohn on four of his own cases which showed left branch disease in what he called right branch block, and he failed to accept Edward P. Carter's point that it was strange for patients with left heart disease to apparently have right branch block. Also he had a patient with aortic valve disease who temporarily developed bundle branch block, really left block but which he labelled right, and this led to a gentle complaint from Einthoven who wrote, 'I fear it will sometimes be difficult to decide whether the patient suffers

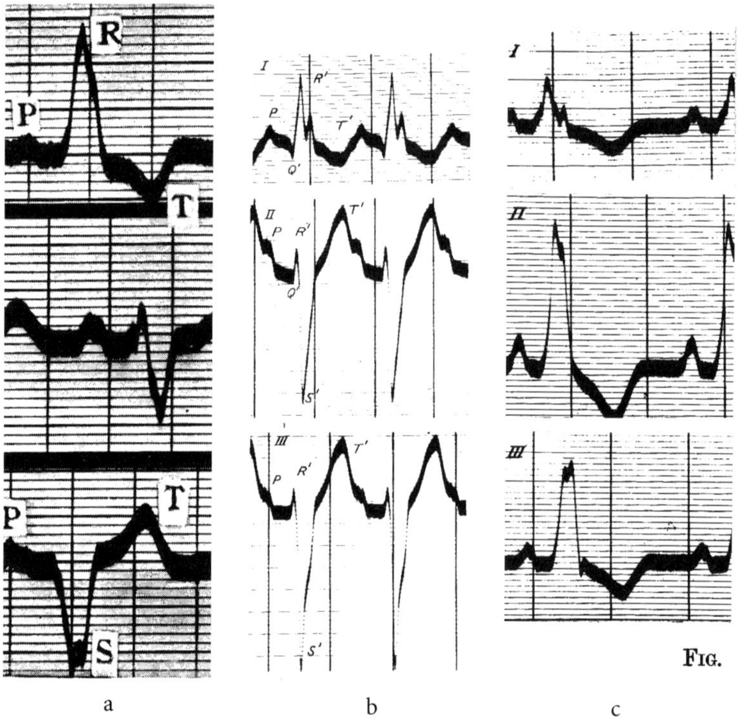

*Figure 4.11 Electrocardiograms in bundle branch block. (a) Left BBB in human (b) Right BBB in dog (c) Left BBB in dog. They show that the form of the curves produced experimentally in the dog is almost the opposite to that in the human. (From reference 81.)*

from left ventricular preponderance or from right bundle branch lesion'. The correct interpretation of human bundle branch block was given by George Fahr in 1920 by measuring the electrical axis, a piece of work which Lewis had done himself but with the opposite conclusion! But even after Frank Wilson had produced further and conclusive proof in 1932 Lewis did not hasten to correct his error. Later that year Evan Bedford(5) who was secretary to the Cardiac Club asked him to speak to the Club on this matter.[345] But Lewis declined, and replied:

> There is in fact a lot of evidence for both views. I am personally undecided as to which is true...in fact I am rather unwilling to come down on one side of the fence because I know that it influences the independent judgement of other people and I think it is desirable that they should make up their own minds.[400]

In a letter to Sir William Hume in 1935 he slightly softened his view by saying, 'Wilson's evidence is strong enough to make me feel that the old view cannot be held with confidence', but he was still reluctant to discard his original conclusion and added, 'I have come to no decision about it; have not felt it incumbent upon me to do so as I am no longer working at the subject ... I am not convinced one way or the other'.[404]

In 1937 he said that which type was which was 'a matter of debate ... (and) a matter of little practical consequence'. This last remark showed an attitude of defiance but certainly not of scientific judgment. But by 1942 he had come to label left block as 'the common type', and finally in 1944 he brought himself to use the terms 'left (1st type) and right (2nd type)'.

The full history, with references, of bundle branch block is given in my paper in *Medical History*.[81] It shows Lewis' preference for experimental compared with observational evidence, coupled with an ability on this issue to disregard other evidence and indeed common clinical sense once his mind was made up. He also had a reluctance on this and some other matters to admit that he was wrong.

## A study of ventricular hypertrophy and the cardiac impulses

The electrocardiogram's value in arrhythmias was almost self evident but Einthoven had also shown its ability to diagnose ventricular hypertrophy, and this stimulated Lewis to investigate this aspect of its use.[141] However his study soon became a more generalized enquiry into the relation of hypertrophy to physical signs and to various forms of heart disease. He devised a method of precisely separating and weighing the right and left ventricles and septum – discovering after a while that a similar method had been used by Müller in 1883. Lewis tended to work out the plan of his investigations first and read the literature later. He concluded that 'in studying hypertrophy, simple inspection of the organ is quite insufficient and that weighing the muscles of the separate chambers is alone reliable'. After weighing the heart in about 30 cases each of aortic disease and renal disease he found that isolated left ventricular hypertrophy was unusual and concluded that, especially in renal disease, general and uniform hypertrophy was common. He personally examined the precordial impulses in 80 patients who came to post mortem and found that a thrusting apex beat was usually present in left ventricular hypertrophy though the epigastric impulse (he did not examine the parasternal region) was not useful in right hypertrophy. Surprisingly he concludes that 'such physical signs ... have little or no scientific value'.

He was impressed, probably too impressed, by discrepancies in the relation of some valve lesions to hypertrophy. For example he pointed out that the left ventricle could be enlarged with mitral stenosis, and the right ventricle in aortic disease. This led him to decide 'that change in the mechanical conditions of the circulation are the sole or even chief causes of hypertrophy has not been proved'. This attitude was to be important in determining his later views on valvular disease and cardiac failure, when he played down the importance of valve lesions. In the event there were only ten cases in whom to compare the electrocardiographic and post-mortem findings, but the correlation was good. There is an interesting footnote to the paper where he gives thanks to Dr Harold S. Furness of the Lambeth Infirmary for 'his very considerable help, given to me in collecting the material upon which this paper is based; without his aid the observations would scarcely have been possible'. It has to be assumed that Lewis was unable to get enough clinical and pathological material at UCH and was glad to have the help of Furness who graduated from there 1908. The Infirmary was not a teaching hospital and probably few consultants would have thought of visiting it. In another article Lewis wrote, 'In the Poor Law infirmaries of London alone are thousands of patients upon whom no observations are made. A wealth of material goes to waste; it could be utilized without great expense; it could be utilized to the great and immediate benefit of the inmates of these institutions'.[140]

## An important statement on Research in Medicine

His days and nights must have been full to overflowing with electrophysiological and related studies, with the editing of *Heart*, writing books, and with clinical and teaching duties. Yet he found time to reflect deeply on the wider problems of medical research and presented his beliefs in a 1900 word article in the daily newspaper *The Morning Post* on April 25 1914, which was headed 'Research in Medicine. Its position and needs' and signed Junior.[140] This article is an important landmark because it is his first statement, and a very complete one at that, on the importance of clinical research and the need to provide proper support for it. He referred to this article more than once in addresses given later in life but he never reproduced it or quoted from it so it is therefore reprinted as Appendix 4. He points out that research work is usually done by the junior members of a hospital who abandon it just when they are becoming proficient because of their requirement to earn a living as a practising physician. The research worker he said must be paid, be 'independent of practice and of thoughts of practice in the future', and be provided with laboratory and hospital accommodation, adding that 'It does not follow that a man qualified for research also possesses the temperament or type of ability needful to the practising physician. Very often the reverse is true'. Because the juniors had the care of patients 'not in the wards, but as a medley in crowded outpatient and teaching departments' they had to rely on their seniors for patients to study. He attacked the consultant who whilst failing to use his own clinical material for research, restricts access to it for a junior colleague who 'is charged with pilfering if he has gathered too freely'. Lewis clearly resented the fact that, as he put it, the harvest of the research worker was culled from the fields of others who left him stubble or, by favour or oversight, a small patch of standing corn.' Let him walk ever so warily, sooner or later he is in danger of arrest for trespass'. It is interesting to find him urging the need to conduct research in wards or 'in distinct institutes' where students are not taught because the wards become 'closed classrooms during the visits of the teaching staff'. He noted that the Poor Law infirmaries contain a wealth of clinical material which goes to waste, and which could be utilized to the benefit of the patients in those institutions. The article needs to be read in full for it is cogently argued with sometimes colourful prose:

> We give the best years of our lives, we give the best work of our brains; we work for a return which if offered to a man of business he would regard as an offence … but we are aspirants who yearn to turn the few sods we can and enrich the harvest of English medicine hoping that the day may come when we may gather in the ripe corn in plenty.

The letter was written in response to the work of the Royal Commission on University Education in London chaired by Viscount Haldane which reported in 1913. Abraham Flexner, the American educationalist who had written a notable report in 1910 on North American medical schools and Sir William Osler gave evidence to it and condemned the London medical schools for their lack of laboratory facilities for clinicians, whilst Professor E.H. Starling urged that academic professorial units be established in clinical subjects. Lewis wrote, he said, because although the need for medical research had been heard, 'It seems eminently desirable that someone should speak from a different standpoint: the present position and needs of the research *worker*'.

## Visits Canada and the United States of America

Lewis' international reputation was amply confirmed in May 1914 when he received a letter from Professor William H. Welch, Dean of Johns Hopkins Hospital, Baltimore, inviting him to deliver the Herter Lectures in October, with a honorarium of $1000.[481] This invitation turned out to be only part of his first visit to North America which started in Montreal where he spoke on October 5 at the opening of the faculty of medicine of McGill University. His title was 'Observations upon cardiac syncope' but he used the occasion to emphasize that the influence of electrocardiography extended well beyond analysis of arrhythmias. Its precision, he said, had shown the value of close factual observation in the whole field of heart disease, changing our general conceptions of it, and displaying the weaknesses of the older methods:

> It has carried this branch of clinical science in one step to the level of its companion sciences in the laboratory, it has awakened a great and growing dissatisfaction with traditional cardiac philosophy. Our new philosophy is deeply rooted, it is to be trained to cover a hard and imperishable wall of fact.

This was his first use of Sir James Paget's[(6)] phrase, 'clinical science', which he later adopted to identify his campaign for the promotion of scientific medicine. By the next day he was in Baltimore where he gave the three Herter Lectures at the 25th anniversary of Johns Hopkins Hospital upon 'Clinical medicine and laboratory methods'. Lewis introduced them with a quotation from Sir Thomas Browne:[(7)]

> The fourth is a Supinity, or neglect of Enquiry, even of matters whereof we doubt; rather believing than going to see. But the mortallest enemy unto Knowledge, and that which hath done the greatest execution upon truth, hath been a peremptory adhesion unto Authority; and more especially, the establishing of our belief upon the dictates of Antiquity.

At the start of the first lecture he paid a graceful tribute to the pioneer role of Johns Hopkins University and Hospital[(8)] in 'promoting the study of Medicine upon the exacting lines of the scientific laboratory'. He would have been impressed too by the virtues of a full time system for clinical staff.[60] The lectures were on 'The method of electrocardiography exemplified', 'The relation of auricular systole to heart sounds and murmurs' and on 'Observations upon dyspnoea, with especial reference to acidosis'. The next stop was in New York where he delivered the Harvey Lecture on 'The excitation wave in the heart' on October 25. Finally he was at the Peter Bent Brigham Hospital in Boston for a week as Physician-in-Chief pro tempore leaving on November 2. His addresses were published in March 1915 in a book *Lectures on the Heart.* (Fig. 4.12, *overleaf*) In the preface, dated November 3 1914, he wrote, 'Co-operation between wards and laboratories, as my visit has clearly taught me, is nowhere more freely or widely cultivated than in the Medical Schools of America'.[143]

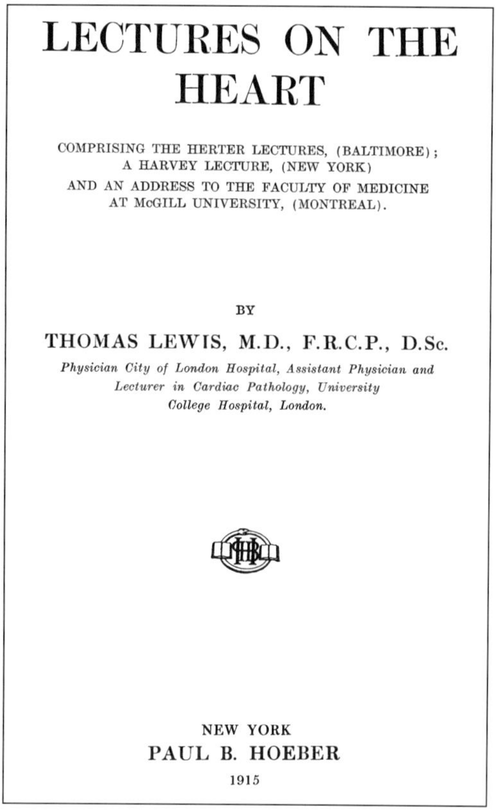
LECTURES ON THE HEART

COMPRISING THE HERTER LECTURES, (BALTIMORE);
A HARVEY LECTURE, (NEW YORK)
AND AN ADDRESS TO THE FACULTY OF MEDICINE
AT McGILL UNIVERSITY, (MONTREAL).

BY

THOMAS LEWIS, M.D., F.R.C.P., D.Sc.

*Physician City of London Hospital, Assistant Physician and Lecturer in Cardiac Pathology, University College Hospital, London.*

NEW YORK
PAUL B. HOEBER
1915

*Figure 4.12 Title page of the book containing his lectures in the United States and Canada in 1914.*

At McGill he had said that, 'While the nature of disordered heart action is a study rapidly reaching its termination, the problems which such study has opened up are manifold and far reaching'. But by the end of 1914 the World War was already into its fourth month and Lewis' efforts were soon to be diverted into a quite unanticipated study, namely that of 'Soldier's Heart'.

## Notes to Chapter 4

(1) The Fellowship of the Royal College of Physicians of London (FRCP) was awarded only by election, to Members of the College. It was an honour which indicated that the person had gained the esteem of his peers who at that time were nearly always in university teaching hospitals.

(2) Joseph Barcroft, FRS, (later Sir Joseph), 1872–1947, was a physiologist who did important work on respiration and who devised a blood gas manometer. He became professor of physiology in Cambridge where he wrote his acclaimed book, *Features in the Architecture of Physiological Function*. His expertise in blood gas work was invaluable for Lewis' research.

(3) Paul Dudley White, 1886–1973, who was on the staff of the Massachusetts General Hospital, devoted his entire career to the study of heart disease, and his textbook,

*Heart Disease* written in 1931 became a standard work. He was a pioneer in the prevention of heart disease and in furthering world wide friendship among cardiologists. He is known also for the Wolff–Parkinson–White syndrome.

(4) Jonathan Campbell Meakins, 1882–1959, was a Canadian physician who was Director of Experimental Medicine in Montreal before working with Lewis. He worked on Soldier's Heart in the Canadian Army and became professor of therapeutics in Edinburgh in 1920. From 1924 onwards he was professor of medicine at McGill University Montreal where he wrote a well-known textbook of medicine.

(5) David Evan Bedford, 1898–1978, was a consultant cardiologist at the Middlesex Hospital, London, having trained at the London Hospital under Sir John Parkinson. He was a dominant figure in British cardiology, being secretary and later president of the British Cardiac Society and the first editor, jointly with Dr Maurice Campbell, in 1939, of the *British Heart Journal.*

(6) James Paget, (later Sir James), 1814–1899, was a surgeon at St Bartholomew's Hospital who was an authority on surgical pathology. Several diseases carry his name. He had a very strong belief in the power of clinical research and urged doctors to put their faith in clinical studies and not to reject them in favour of deductions from physiology or pathology.

(7) Sir Thomas Browne, 1605–1682, was a physician in Norwich who was renowned for the richness and variety of his literary work. His most famous book, *Religio Medici*, was very influential with its wise counsels as to the conduct of life.

(8) Johns Hopkins Hospital opened in 1889 and, with its university medical school, was unique in the United States at that time in its dedication to scientific medicine, combining laboratory with clinical work. One of the first two electrocardiographs in the States was installed there by Dr Lewellys F Barker in 1909 and later Dr Edward P Carter and Dr E Cowles Andrus did early work in cardiac electrophysiology. The Hospital and University were founded under the will of a wealthy Quaker merchant, Mr Johns Hopkins.

# Chapter 5

## The Medical Research Committee • The World War • The Soldier's Heart and the Effort Syndrome

THE MEDICAL Research Committee (MRC)(1) was formed in August 1913 to administer the Medical Research Fund which had been established under a provision of the National Health Insurance Act of 1911. The original idea of the Fund was to sponsor research into tuberculosis, but fortunately the remit was later widened to include other fields of medicine.[21] The MRC was chaired by Lord Moulton FRS and its secretary was Dr Walter Morley Fletcher, FRS,(2) a medically qualified physiologist.[13] In March 1914 the Committee purchased the former North London Hospital for Consumption at Mount Vernon, Hampstead, for their Central Research Institute.[283] They established four departments in it and planned to have a total of 20 beds, but the outbreak of war on August 4 1914 abruptly altered these plans. Mount Vernon Hospital was offered to the Army Council and in November it became the Hampstead Military Hospital with 200 beds. (Fig. 5.1)

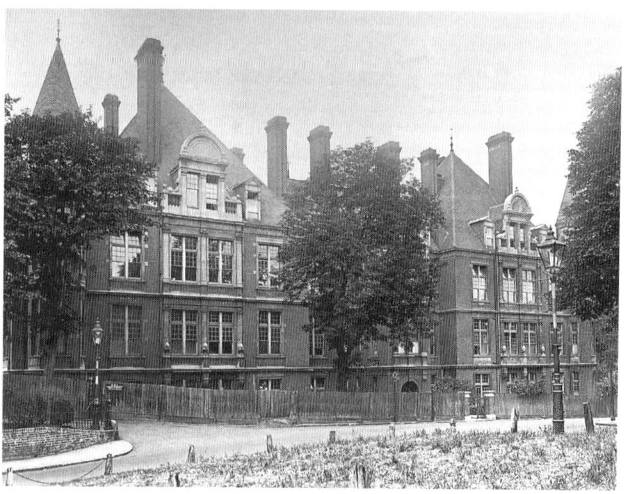

*Figure 5.1 The Mount Vernon hospital at Hampstead, which became the Military Heart Hospital in 1916.*

# Soldier's Heart • Irritable heart of soldiers • 'D.A.H and V.D.H'

Soon after the war began an important medical problem, apparently due to heart disease, declared itself. Soldiers on active service, especially after the traumatic retreat from Mons, were reporting sick with what seemed to be cardiac symptoms and were being invalided with the army medical terms of Disordered action of the heart (D.A.H.) or, if there was a heart murmur, of Valvular disease of the heart (V.D.H.). Sir James Mackenzie soon appreciated the problem and by January 1916, after only 16 months, he was able to report a study of 400 such men, of whom over 90% had a normal heart on physical examination.[269] They were suffering from what was often called 'the soldier's heart' or 'the irritable heart of soldiers', a condition which had been identified in the British Army in 1867 and especially well investigated by Dr John C. Da Costa during the American Civil War.[57] The men complained of 'feeling rotten' and only slight exertion would bring on fatigue, exhaustion, palpitation, breathlessness, giddiness and pain over the heart. Mackenzie was quick to point out that those symptoms were also 'common in civil life ... in people recovering from an exhausting illness as typhoid or influenza ... or in people who have suffered a long mental or physical strain'. He recognised that the mental and physical strain of life in the trenches was an important cause of the syndrome, but he also emphasised the role of 'bacterial and toxic influences' from febrile illnesses.

## The Military Heart Hospital founded at Hampstead

It was at the insistence of Mackenzie that a reluctant Army Medical Service accepted a proposal from the Medical Research Committee in February 1916 that the Hampstead Military Hospital should become the Military Heart Hospital to deal with this large and mounting problem.[272] Sir Clifford Allbutt[(3)] and Sir William Osler joined him as consultants whilst Lewis, Dr John Parkinson,[(4)] Dr Jonathan C. Meakins and Dr William E. Hume each had charge of 50 beds. By this time Lewis had already started to investigate the condition in soldiers admitted for special study to the military wards at UCH and, having found streptococci in the urine of 10 out of 11 patients, he concluded that 'we are dealing with an infection of the blood with organisms that are filtered out in the urine'.[37] Probably they were contaminants.

The decision to found the hospital was soon justified because in only the first three months 251 patients were admitted and discharged.[146] Lewis' scientific prestige and seniority made him the natural leader of the medical group at Hampstead, even though he was not designated as such, and the work there was directed and carried forward almost entirely by his own efforts with occasional advice from the consultants. His colleagues were all in the army: Jonathan C. Meakins and Thomas F. Cotton[(5)] were in the Canadian army, whilst John Parkinson, Francis R. Fraser,[(6)] Edward B. Gunson, John G. Slade and Alan N. Drury[(7)] were in the Royal Army Medical Corps (RAMC) as was William E. Hume who was soon posted to France – 'a serious blow'. Lewis was worried about his own status as a civilian. In a letter to Fletcher he said:

> I don't ask for khaki or anything of that sort ... but all single men under 40 should present themselves ... it makes one a little jumpy. It comes to mind because I have been asked to go as a Physician to an overseas hospital and think that I certainly ought not to accept.[490]

This was a Welsh military hospital in Mesopotamia – a country where his former chief Colonel Sir Victor Horsley was to die a few months later. Lewis was formally exempted from military service.

## Appointed to the MRC staff • Marries Miss Lorna James

Then came the most important event in Lewis' professional life. The Medical Research Committee appointed him to their permanent scientific staff, for clinical research work, on February 16 1916. (Fig. 5.2) 'This appointment' he said

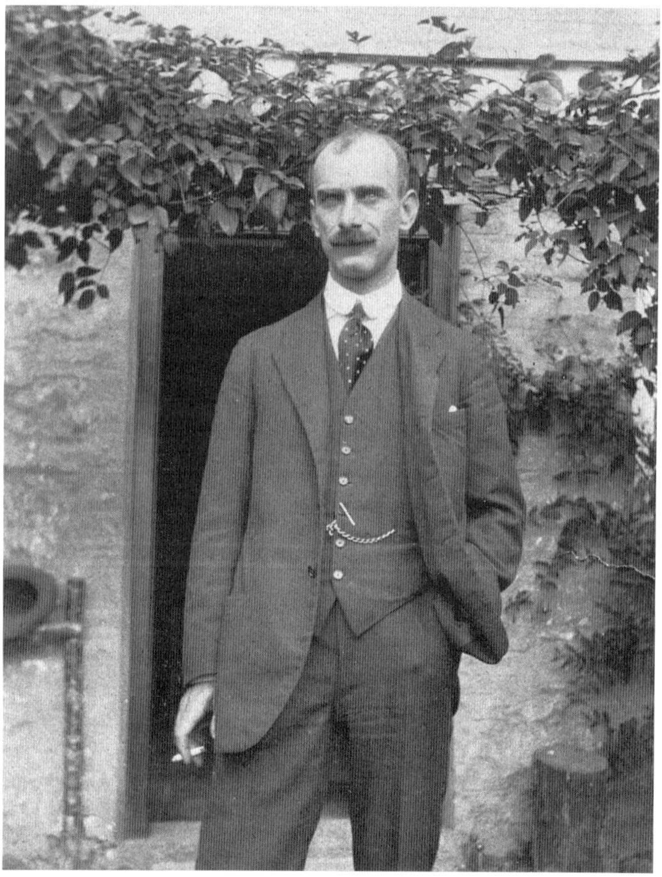

*Figure 5.2 Thomas Lewis in 1916 the year of his marriage, aged 34. Note the ever present cigarette.*

'broke the ice in this country being the first full time job in clinical medicine'.[223] In a letter to Fletcher he wrote:

> I am pleased not only because it gives me the freedom to devote my whole time to the only work I really care about but because I am confident that there is before us a great nay unique opportunity of striking a blow for purity of Medicine and the allied subjects ... it is a peculiar satisfaction to me to be associated with you.[491]

He was appointed at a salary of £1080 per annum rising to £1200, and was allowed to stay on the staff at UCH providing other duties did not exceed eight hours per week and with the surprising proviso that he must resign if the Committee said so. This was the end of his five years in private practice which he had never enjoyed, partly because he disliked taking money from sick people. In their second annual report for 1915–1916 the MRC described Lewis' work at the Military Heart Hospital in 1916 under the heading 'Department of Clinical Research' – the first time this title, later to be so well known, was used.

His personal life was also changing in an important way because in August 1915 he had become engaged to Alice Lorna Treharne James from Merthyr Tydfil. They were married in March 1916 and set up house in Hampstead. Up to then he had lived in rented rooms in Mornington Place, Camden Town which he had shared for several years with T.R. Elliott, and with the physiologist Dr Leonard Noon who died from pulmonary tuberculosis in 1913. Elliott and he were lucky not to have contracted the disease.

## Effort syndrome replaces other diagnostic terms

The dominant purpose of the Heart Hospital was to stem the very considerable loss of manpower from the Army which was due to soldiers being invalided with cardiac problems. Naturally some of these men did have organic heart disease especially in the 'V.D.H.' group where they comprised about one third, but these had been diagnosed and discharged at what Lewis called the 'First Sifting'.[282] The large remainder fell into the 'irritable heart' category. The terminology of this category was a matter of concern and was important in practice as well as academically. The terms 'disordered action of the heart', 'valvular disease of the heart', comprising many with innocent systolic murmurs, 'irritable heart', 'heart strain', and 'soldier's heart' all had, he said, 'the disadvantage that it presupposed the heart to be the primary seat of the mischief'. The term 'neurasthenia' was also used but it did not, in his opinion, help in management or give much insight into the cause. He proposed instead that the condition be called the Effort Syndrome, because the chief symptoms were 'unmasked or aggravated by exertion'.[146] This term had the great advantage that it did not label soldiers as having heart disease, and it was 'non-committal on the pathological side'.

The next step was to determine which soldiers with the effort syndrome could be returned to duty and which had to be invalided out. In other words, to determine their fitness or otherwise for service. Lewis and his colleagues found that the patient's history and physical examination were of no help. They soon came to rely on a man's capacity to undertake physical effort as the best way of judging fitness. Using standard army exercises of graded severity, the amount of work

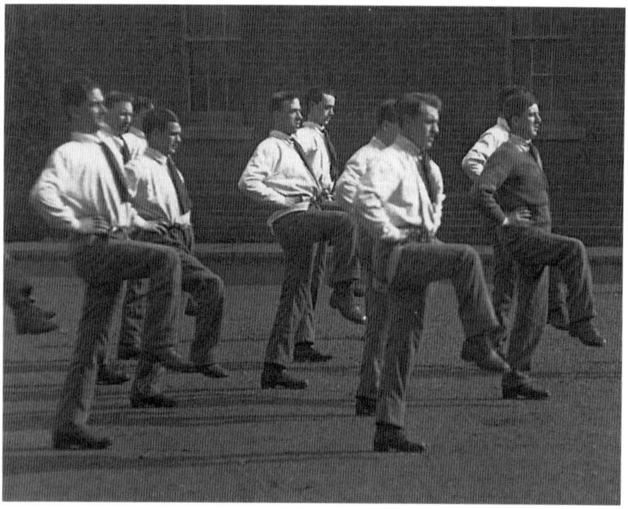

*Figure 5.3 Soldiers doing remedial exercises at the Military Heart Hospital.*

that a man could undertake without distress was gauged by observation, not by subjective symptoms. Over a period of several weeks those men who failed to progress beyond lower grade exercises were discharged as unfit, whilst the others were returned to full duty or light duty according to their exercise tolerance. Although this system was introduced to gauge fitness it turned out to be also a valuable therapeutic measure. In many patients there was a rapid improvement in symptoms as physical and mental fitness got better with progressive exercises. (Fig. 5.3)

On average the men had already been in hospital for 5.3 months before coming to Hampstead where their stay was only 2 months, with 64% being returned to service either at home or overseas.[149]

## Research into the effort syndrome • Respiratory alkalosis discovered

But observation and treatment, however important, were not enough for Lewis the clinical investigator. He initiated and directed no less than 20 detailed studies of various symptoms and signs in the effort syndrome and they were all completed in less than a year.[146] This was a remarkable experimental attack on the features of this poorly understood and under-investigated syndrome.[87] Breathlessness was studied by Drury who found a low normal figure for alveolar carbon dioxide. Chest pain occurred in three-quarters of patients and Meakins and Gunson found that half of them had chest wall hyperalgesia. Sweating was frequent and Cotton and Slade showed that it increased more in patients than in controls after injection of pilocarpine. Amyl nitrite was used to study flushing, which it enhanced. A slow decline of heart rate after effort was known to be a feature of the syndrome and a special study showed it to be a reliable criterion of fitness. Atropine injections indicated that vagal tone was unaltered, and Parkinson showed that full digitalization did not affect heart rate at rest or after exertion. Fraser used intravenous adrenaline and apo-codeine to investigate the stimulatory and inhibitory function of the sympathetic nervous system, both of which were increased. Other studies included fainting, giddiness, heart size, the electrocardiogram and blood pressure. But the most important finding which has influenced workers to the present day was in the field of blood chemistry. Lewis had already used this approach a few years earlier to investigate dyspnoea in cardiac and renal patients and again he had the invaluable help of Joseph Barcroft.[256] They showed that there was an 'absence of an adequate supply of buffer salts in the blood', in other words a respiratory alkalosis, and they considered that it went far to explain the otherwise inexplicable breathlessness in irritable heart.[259] Barcroft showed that when small quantities of carbon dioxide or lactic acid such as are produced by exercise were added to the blood of their patients it approached more towards an acid reaction than is normal and 'this approach is at once signalled by breathlessness, the respiratory centre being extraordinarily sensitive to the blood reaction'. Their finding also removed 'the temptation to cover our ignorance of the pathology of the malady' by ascribing it to instability of the central nervous system, and it was a warning against assuming that the symptoms were due to 'poorness of spirit and lack of zeal'. The concept that overbreathing was the cause of the symptoms was supported in World War Two by the psychiatrist William Sargant in a paper entitled 'The hyperventilation syndrome'.[312]

## Dermatographism, the white line on stroking the skin

Paradoxically, what turned out later to be an important study was a sign which had nothing directly to do with the syndrome. It had been said that the production of a white line or tâche on stroking the skin – dermatographism – was a feature of subjects with 'irritable heart'. It was in fact just a feature of young men, but having seen it Lewis was intrigued by its mechanism.[38] He showed that it still occurred when blood flow to an arm was arrested with a pneumatic cuff and reasoned that contraction only of capillaries, not arterioles, could blanch the skin in this situation. It had traditionally been the view among physiologists that capillaries were passive vessels and although there was some recent animal work to the contrary this was the first proof of capillary contraction in man. It was also important in two other ways. It heralded his later and extensive researches on the blood vessels of the skin and it was an early example of his gift for getting a significant result from a very simple experiment.

## Possible reasons for the effort syndrome

The difficult question as to the likely aetiology of the effort syndrome was being scrutinised too. Earlier studies by Allbutt and Mackenzie, and indeed by Da Costa himself, had shown clearly that the disability was often present even before the men enlisted in the Army. Parkinson found that this was so in half of their own

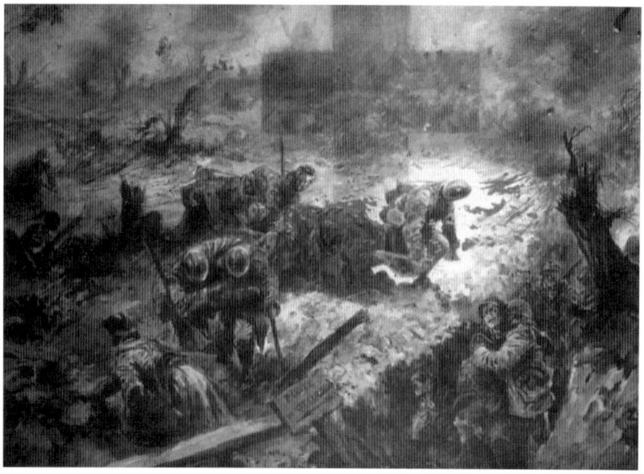

*Figure 5.4 A striking painting, by Lucien Jonas, of a French first aid post in a front line trench in 1917. 'The hard physical labour ... the constant wracking of nerves by violent noises ... bring continuous fatigue ... and ultimate breakdown ...' (Quotation from reference 216.)*

cases thus confirming that the syndrome was not peculiar to soldiers nor necessarily to conditions of war, and Hume, now a full Colonel, reported the same finding among 1000 cases at his centre in France.[89] Lewis was in no doubt that the syndrome was 'a very mixed group'. Among the chief classes one of the largest was that of 'constitutional weakness, nervous or physical or both'. Another large class comprised those who were 'played out by exposure, disturbed sleep and the constant strain ... which work in the front line brings'.[149] (Fig. 5.4) Other groups were those with unrecognised infections, or with delayed recovery from an acute illness. The influence of constitution was well shown in a detailed one year follow-up study of 525 subjects which showed the prognosis to be better in those in whom the syndrome had first appeared during active service. In these men 25% returned to full duty and 50% were discharged, whilst in those with an onset before enlistment the figures were 15% and 71% respectively. In June 1917 Professor F. Mariani from Genoa, Italy, visited the hospital and arranged for a paper by Lewis to be translated into Italian and published in the journal *Le mal del cuore*.[147] The paper contains the only photograph ever taken of Lewis working at his desk. (Fig. 5.5)

## Move to Colchester • A critical comment by Mackenzie

By 1917 the increasing demands of the war effort led to a shortage of medical officers and Drury, Gunson, Parkinson and Slade were posted to France whilst Meakins went to the Canadian hospital at Taplow. Temporary services were obtained from, among others, Lewis' former colleague, Captain A. Goodman Levy, whilst Professor Tileston from Yale became a voluntary worker. Centres in France were set up to deal with cases without having to send them back to England and just one centre saw 7000 patients in two years. Even so the Hampstead hospital was too small and in August 1917 it moved to the Sabraon Military Hospital at Colchester, Essex, where Lewis was appointed as consultant

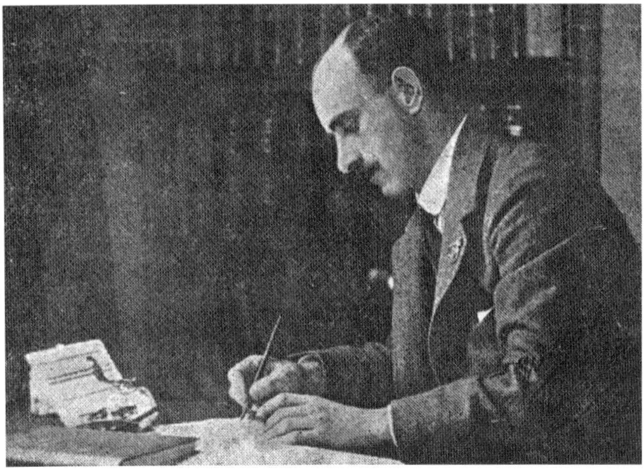

**Prof. TOMMASO LEWIS.**

*Figure 5.5 Lewis at his desk at the Military Heart Hospital, Hampstead. (From reference 147.)*

physician to the Eastern Command. He declined the rank of Colonel, preferring to remain a civilian so that he could 'tick off the Generals'.[377] Later on he described the origin of the military heart hospitals in a letter to Dr Maude Abbott[(8)] in Montreal.[388] In this he mentioned that he was never officially in control at Hampstead, but that being senior to the officers there and representing the MRC 'a certain measure of control naturally came to me'. He stated that the move to Colchester involving a change from 150 to 700 beds was made after pressure was brought to bear on the War Office by the MRC acting at his suggestion. He added that with the move, 'I stipulated for official control of the medical services and I obtained it'. She had asked about Osler and he replied that 'Sir William did not visit us more than a few times at the most at Hampstead' and came every six weeks at Colchester. He said that they saw very little of the consultants at Hampstead and this comment fits in with a statement made by Mackenzie in a letter written to Lewis in 1921:

> Over ten years ago I realised that little further progress could be made in our knowledge of prognosis and heart failure unless we got a better understanding of the laws producing symptoms. You may remember how I tried time and again to impress upon you and your colleagues at the starting of the Hospital for Soldiers Heart. None of you would listen to me and I saw you drifting away on a wrong path. I did my best to help you, but finding my suggestions unheeded, I ceased to visit the Hospitals and carried on the investigation among the patients who came to my consulting room. I then dimly realised where the defect lay and where lay the remedy.[447]

## Gives Croonian Lecture at the Royal Society and is elected a Fellow

This was the year when he delivered the prestigious Croonian Lecture of the Royal Society entitled 'Upon the motion of the mammalian heart'.[145] After regretting that the topic could not be linked to the war effort he summarized his work on the spread of the excitation wave and then proceeded to explain in a masterly fashion the structure and function of the cardiac chambers. He gave generous acknowledgement to the work of the late Walter H. Gaskell whom he had greatly admired.[139] Lewis was elected a Fellow of the Royal Society in 1918 and the pleasure was tempered by the regret that his father, who had eagerly anticipated the election, was no longer alive. His election had been delayed because Joseph Barcroft, who nominated him, had mistaken the wording on a notice sent to him by the Royal Society. The notice asked if he wished Lewis' candidature to be suspended and he replied no, not realising that this meant that the name of the candidate should be hung up on a wall in the Society's rooms for inspection. Barcroft wrote to congratulate him on the election and to apologise for the mistake and Lewis annotated his letter with the comment 'Unhappily it meant that Father never knew'.[343]

The Military Heart Hospital at Colchester fully justified its establishment by admitting up to 150 patients per week and altogether it dealt with 8000 soldiers. Lewis worked out that the reduction in hospital stay, now down to six weeks, which the exercise system had accomplished was saving £50 000 per annum at Colchester alone – equivalent to the entire budget of the MRC.

## American officers at Colchester

The United States entered the war in April 1917 and some months later American officers were sent to Colchester for training. Lewis was in regular touch with the Surgeon General's Office in Washington, at first with Theodore C. Janeway and then with Warfield T. Longcope, Lewis A Conner and William S. Thayer.[383] It was decided that there would be six officers under training at any one time, each one staying for two months. By now, at the end of 1917 and into 1918 there was such a shortage of medical officers in the British Army that none could be spared to work at Colchester and the American officers were indispensable to the work of the Heart Hospital. By the middle of 1918 the waiting list for admission was 379 and was increasing.[384] His former American pupils B.S. Oppenheimer and M.A. Rothschild were among the first to arrive and they then returned to the States to organise training at various places including the military hospital at Lakewood.[460] Other Americans who worked there and who later became distinguished in cardiology were Frank Wilson,[(9)] William St Lawrence and Samuel A. Levine[(10)] all of whom wrote papers on 'irritable heart', and also Harold E.B. Pardee and A.D. Edgar. Levine (Fig. 5.6) later wrote of his good fortune in being trained by Lewis and recorded his personal memories of a happy time at Colchester where Lewis took him and others on bird walks.[338] He sent Lewis a copy of his book *Clinical Heart Disease* with the inscription 'To Sir Thomas Lewis. With pleasant recollections of the Colchester days and the stimulus you gave us Americans'. Frank Wilson became very interested in ornithology and he often joined Lewis and his wife on their expeditions to watch and photograph birds. He became one of the world's leading electrocardiographers, working at Ann Arbor Michigan, and he and Lewis became life-long friends.[26] During this era Lewis continued to lecture at UCH and it is likely that Wilson worked there too, because he published a paper jointly with Ross A. Jamieson on musical aortic diastolic murmurs using the twin string phonocardiogram.[333]

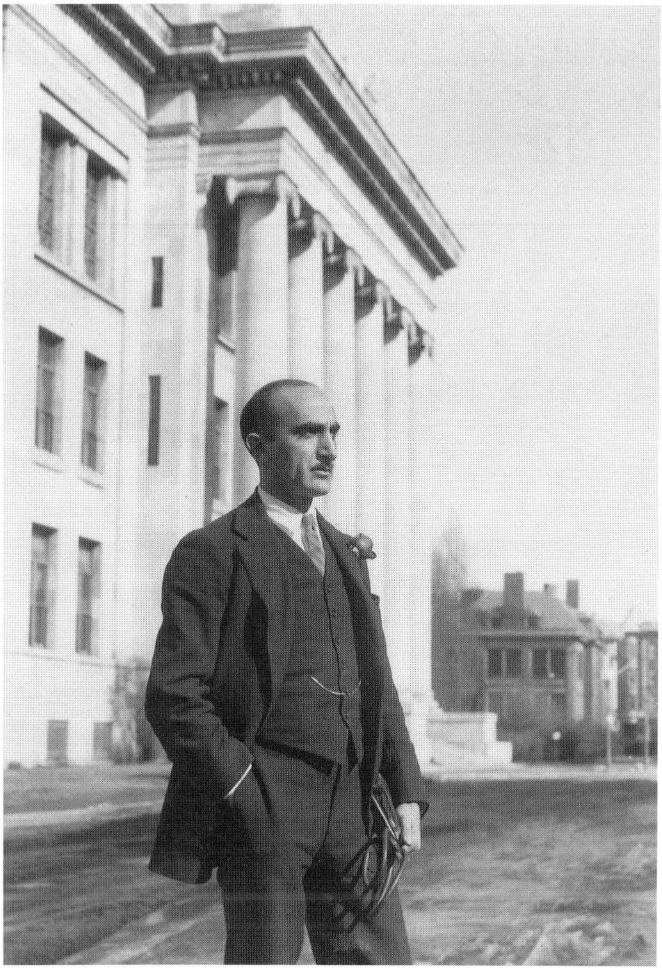

*Figure 5.6 Dr Samuel A Levine at the Peter Bent Brigham Hospital, Boston, in 1925.*

## Monograph on the Soldier's Heart and the Effort Syndrome

In 1918 Lewis wrote a 140-page book, *The Soldier's Heart and the Effort Syndrome* (Fig. 5.7, *overleaf*) for the instruction of medical officers who were either dealing with patients, or serving on recruiting and pensioning boards.[149] Although he called it just a collection of war-time notes it was in fact a really comprehensive and practical treatise on the subject. The symptoms and signs of the effort syndrome were described and contrasted with those of heart disease. There was a 30-page chapter on how to diagnose heart disease with a full discussion on the significance of apical systolic murmurs when for the first time we meet Lewis' lifelong prejudice against diagnosing mitral regurgitation or admitting that it can be

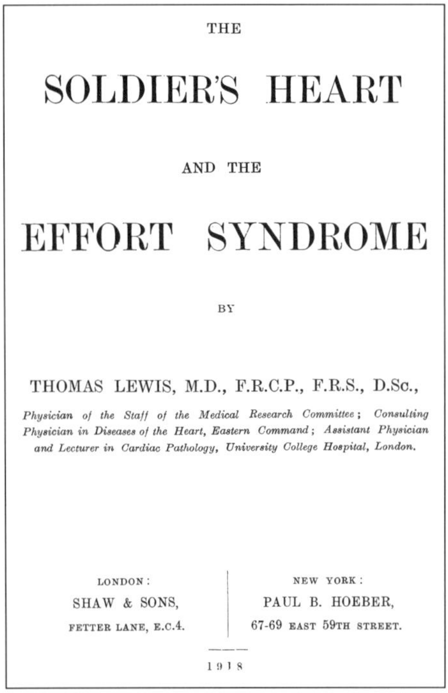

THE

SOLDIER'S HEART

AND THE

EFFORT SYNDROME

BY

THOMAS LEWIS, M.D., F.R.C.P., F.R.S., D.Sc.,

*Physician of the Staff of the Medical Research Committee; Consulting Physician in Diseases of the Heart, Eastern Command; Assistant Physician and Lecturer in Cardiac Pathology, University College Hospital, London.*

LONDON: SHAW & SONS, FETTER LANE, E.C.4.

NEW YORK: PAUL B. HOEBER, 67-69 EAST 59TH STREET.

1918

*Figure 5.7 Title page of the monograph in 1918 summarizing his work at the Military Heart Hospitals at Hampstead and Colchester. He had just been elected a Fellow of the Royal Society; note the letters F.R.S. used for the first time.*

important. But in the context of examining army recruits he was surely correct in advising that such murmurs should 'be neglected in arriving at a prognosis in young men'. The chapter on prognosis and treatment had an analysis of what happened to 860 cases of the syndrome, 34% being returned to full duty and only 9% discharged. A very helpful chapter dealt with medical reports on discharged soldiers indicating how to answer the questions properly on Army forms which if badly done 'entail endless trouble to the pension boards ... hardships to individual men ... and serious inroads upon the public purse'. The book had 21 tables of detailed analysis to support a clear and authoritative text and was enthusiastically reviewed in *The Times* of January 25 1919 when their medical correspondent referred to 'the great reputation of Dr Thomas Lewis (who) deals with that borderland of disease which has been the lure and stumbling block of so many previous workers'.

What indeed were the views of other workers about the condition, and especially about its causation? Prior to the war both Osler and Allbutt regarded it as a neurosis or cardiac neurasthenia. From his experience at Colchester, and in the American army, S.A. Levine rejected the term effort syndrome because the prominent symptom of chest pain did not occur on effort in normal people and together with others he proposed the term neurocirculatory asthenia.[337] Another American, A.E. Cohn, wrote 'In the expeditionary forces we were led, after reflection, to adopt the view that the irritable heart of soldiers was the expression of a neurosis'.[34] But there was good reason to consider separately the men whose illness started under long continued combat conditions. From his experience in France, Hume said that many sufferers were in no way neurasthenic, 'the majority of men who have served in the trenches have exhausted nervous systems'.[89] Lewis said that although the experience of war 'selects the weaklings and marks them down' even healthy men 'break when the trial is too long continued: there is a limit to the endurance of each and all'. Mackenzie chose to label the cause as 'general exhaustion', and as he pointed out it is a common disorder in civil life in which context it is related to the 'chronic fatigue syndrome' and 'myalgic encephalitis'. Recent studies by Peter F.G. Nixon have led him to identify Lewis and Barcroft's work on the blood reaction as the key to the pathogenesis of the effort syndrome, a term which he prefers to retain. Nixon states that chronic hyperventilation is the mechanism of the syndrome and that this leads to the body's alkaline buffering systems getting depleted by dyskinetic over breathing. He supports Hume's view that subjects with this syndrome are not neurotic, and he emphasises that it affects able people who get hyperventilation when they are subjected to inescapable stresses. This results in the control of breathing becoming uncoupled from the body's physical needs and attached instead to the mind's arousal system.[291] However other workers consider that hyperventilation is only part of the explanation and the debate about the pathogenesis continues. Dr Charles P. Wooley has done excellent research on the history of the syndrome from a cardiologist's point of view.[337]

The wards at Colchester continued to be fully occupied during 1918 and did not close until 1919 but Lewis left the hospital in June 1918 and returned to UCH. One of the patients at Colchester was an artist who later became very well known to the British public from his newspaper cartoons which he signed 'Strube'. He made a good cartoon of Lewis, (Fig. 5.8) with a pun on the famous Lewis machine

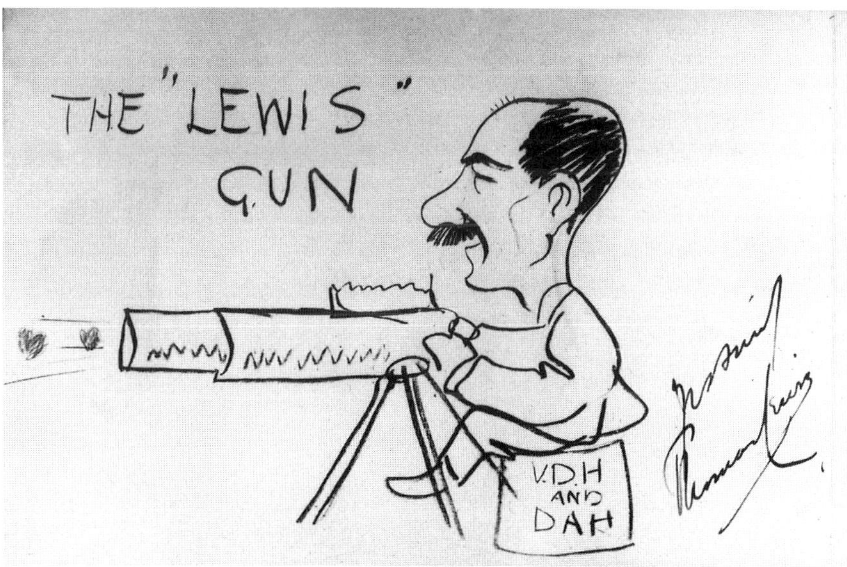


*Figure 5.8 A cartoon of Lewis drawn by the artist 'Strube'. It epitomizes Lewis' determined, even aggressive, approach to problems.*

gun of the time, showing Lewis attacking the terms D.A.H and V.D.H. Apparently Strube was not permitted to be discharged from the military hospital until he had made a cartoon of every member of the staff! Lewis had a letter at this time from his friend T.R. Elliott now in France as a Colonel in the RAMC who wrote:

> You are tired, my dear Lewis, and so am I – that's why we both want to get out in the quiet country. Even the victories of the last four weeks haven't altered my feelings. But you are not going to drop the ideals that you have followed through hardships in the last 15 years and you'll have to spend your working time in and near towns. Those who have not been killed in fighting must in simple duty spend the rest of their days doing what they can for England: and there is infinite work needed in medicine. American medicine is full of promise in her well trained younger men. She has dozens where we have one who is well equipped for work.[356]

His last research article on 'irritable heart' appeared in the *British Medical Journal* on March 30 1918, and it contained a striking photograph of a patient (Fig. 5.9) showing the typical tired, anxious, faces.[148] But Lewis ensured that work on the syndrome would continue into peacetime and his follow-up studies, started in 1915, went on until 1923 when 601 men living in London had each been observed for five years.[67] The results showed that 15% were quite fit, 18%

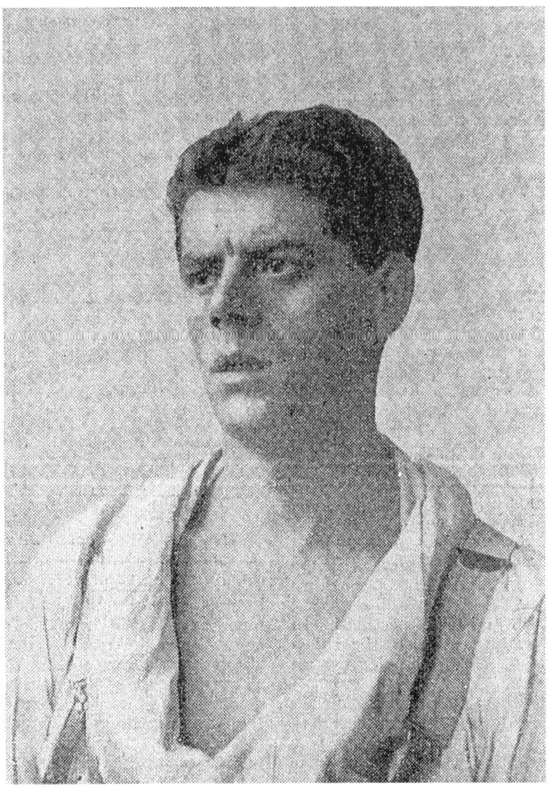

*Figure 5.9 Photograph of a patient aged 28 with long standing effort syndrome. 'The face expresses fatigue and the anxiety of early breathlessness'. (From reference 148.)*

improved, 56% unchanged, and 3% worse whilst 8% got a serious disease, most commonly tuberculosis. The worse the exercise tolerance, and the higher the patient's age, the less good was the prognosis.

## Assessment work for the Ministry of Pensions and the Cardiac Club founded

Having found from his experience that medical officers often dealt inadequately with cardiac patients Lewis conscientiously set about improving and re-organizing the assessment of men with cardiovascular disability. At Colchester he and his assistants gave 150 courses of instruction to doctors who sat on pension boards, and when he was back in London he lectured every week to the Resurvey Boards. Lewis' work during the war on the effort syndrome, and his continuing assistance to the Ministry of Pensions was of enormous value to the Government. It was recognised by his appointment in 1920 as a Commander of the British Empire (CBE)[(11)] and in 1921 by the conferment of a Knighthood.[(12)]

A cardiac diagnosis was common among the pensioners, and nationwide there were important problems of inaccurate diagnosis and lack of uniformity of assessment, due to inexperience and overwork in the pension service. Lewis tackled these problems by writing, in April 1920, to a cardiac consultant in every region of the country asking if they would be prepared to give advice to the Ministry of Pensions.[386] They all agreed and he then made the important recommendation to the Ministry that cardiac specialists were essential for instructional and assessment work at the Boards, and on his advice they appointed twelve honorary consultants in diseases of the heart to supervise the work in all regions of the country. By doing this Lewis gave the impetus for the organization of cardiology in Britain, which was initiated in 1921 when the Ministry held a conference of consultants in cardiovascular diseases. The main session was on administrative and technical matters, but it was followed by one on clinical problems which was a pioneer and important step towards the development of cardiology as a specialty.[40] The second one on February 3 1922 was attended by 14 consultants from nine regions, and there were discussions on endocarditis, arteriosclerosis and the use of quinidine.[458] These conferences were the first time in Britain that cardiologists had met as a group and they proved so useful that it was decided to continue the clinical sessions under a different arrangement. On February 21 William E Hume wrote to John Cowan with the suggestion that all consultant physicians with an interest in heart disease should get together at the next meeting of the Association of Physicians. They did this at Oxford on April 22 and 15 of them founded the Cardiac Club and elected Sir James Mackenzie as an honorary member.[40] It was appropriate that Lewis should be in the chair for the first General Meeting of the Club held at UCH on November 22 because it had arisen from his initiative in getting the Ministry to nominate cardiac consultants. Afterwards they always met on the day before the Association's meeting in the spring and this tradition was maintained until 1979. Lewis never gave a paper to the Club and he declined an invitation to do so in 1932 when the secretary, Evan Bedford, asked him to open a discussion on bundle branch block.[345] The Club became a vital force in British cardiology and by the time of its last General Meeting in 1936 it had elected a further 19 members. It then became, in 1937, the

Cardiac Society of Great Britain and Ireland, which in 1946 was re-named The British Cardiac Society.[30]

## Notes to Chapter 5

(1) Medical Research Committee: The National Health Insurance Act of 1911, which had been introduced to Parliament by Mr Lloyd George, had a clause whereby an annual sum calculated at the rate of one penny in respect of each insured person in the United Kingdom was to be contributed to a fund for research. The original idea was to give this money for work into tuberculosis, then a great scourge, but in 1912 the Departmental Committee on Tuberculosis recommended that the research carried out under the Act should not be restricted to tuberculosis. The Committee also said that the research should be the responsibility of a formally constituted Medical Research Committee. Unfortunately it is not known who initiated this important recommendation. At its onset the Medical Research Fund was given £55 000 per year.

(2) Walter Morley Fletcher, FRS, later Sir Walter, 1873–1933, had an outstanding career as a physiologist at Cambridge and his work on the biochemical basis of muscular contraction was recognised by his election to the Royal Society of London. He took a medical degree but did not practise. At the age of 41 he became the first secretary of the Medical Research Committee (later Council) and served in this post until his death from a cerebral abscess in 1933. The MRC thrived under his direction for he combined great organizing ability with scientific vision and a deep understanding of the needs of research workers. He could be combative in arguing for causes he supported and this led to the mistaken charge of arrogance. He had a generous nature with great personal charm and presence and he had a wide friendship.

(3) Thomas Clifford Allbutt, FRS, (later Sir Clifford), 1836–1935, was the Regius Professor Medicine in Cambridge. He was an authority on hypertension, and wrote a two volume work, *Diseases of the Arteries including Angina Pectoris* in 1915. Allbutt was an erudite physician and noted for his book, *Notes on the Composition of Scientific Papers.*

(4) John Parkinson, (later Sir John), 1885–1976, was one of the foremost British cardiologists of the 20th century. He trained under Sir James Mackenzie at the London Hospital and succeeded him as head of the cardiac department. Among other important contributions he championed the place of radiology in diagnosis of heart disease and is known for the Wolff–Parkinson–White syndrome.

(5) Thomas Forrest Cotton, 1884–1965, qualified in medicine at McGill University, Montreal and soon afterwards went to Europe to study under Professor K L Wenckebach. In 1913 he joined Lewis at UCH and continued to work with him in the Military Heart Hospitals at Hampstead and Colchester. He remained with Lewis until he was appointed to the staff of the National Heart Hospital London in 1924. He was a fine clinician, who was the first to recognise clubbing of the fingers as a sign of infective endocarditis.

(6) Francis Richard Fraser, (later Sir Francis), 1885–1964, qualified in Edinburgh in 1910 and then did postgraduate work in cardiology in New York with A E Cohn. After World War One he was on the staff of St Bartholomew's Hospital, and then became the first professor of medicine at the newly established British Postgraduate Medical School at Hammersmith Hospital, where he built up a world class department of medicine. The lecturers in his department included John McMichael, Paul Wood, Edward Sharpey-Schafer and Guy Scadding. His flair for leadership made him the obvious choice for the demanding post of director of the Emergency Medical Service in World War Two.

(7) Alan Nigel Drury, FRS, (later Sir Alan), 1889–1980, studied medicine at Cambridge and was sent by Sir Clifford Allbutt to the Military Heart Hospital at Hampstead where he worked with Thomas Lewis. After the first War he joined Lewis' department at UCH where he showed his skill as an electrophysiologist, becoming an indispensable member of Lewis' team. He was not a clinician and in 1927 he went to Cambridge where he studied the physiology of cardiac muscle, whilst continuing as a full-time worker under the Medical Research Council. In 1943 he became director of the Lister Institute in London and finally, from 1952–1960 he directed the Institute of Animal Physiology near Cambridge. Together with R T Grant he wrote a very fine obituary notice of Thomas Lewis for the Royal Society.

(8) Maude Elizabeth Seymour Abbott, 1869–1940, was a Canadian physician who became a pathologist at McGill University. She was encouraged by Sir William Osler to undertake a study of congenital heart disease and her 1936 *Atlas of congenital cardiac disease* was widely acclaimed. The International Association of Medical Museums was largely her creation.

(9) Frank Norman Wilson, 1890–1952, was an American physician who became a world leader in electrocardiography working at Ann Arbor, Michigan. Much of his research was devoted to the study of the ventricular complex in the electrocardiogram, and his grasp of mathematics enabled him to formulate important basic concepts of bioelectric phenomena. He devised the V lead central terminal which founded unipolar electrocardiography. From 1918 onwards he and Thomas Lewis were close friends who shared a common passion for ornithology.

(10) Samuel Albert Levine, 1891–1966, was a notable American cardiologist who wrote a standard work, *Clinical Heart Disease* in 1936. In particular he made important contributions to the study and treatment of coronary heart disease. 'Sam' was a true anglophile and he gave the St Cyres Lecture at the National Heart Hospital, London, in 1948 on *Auscultation of the Heart*. He greatly admired Thomas Lewis, with whom he worked at Colchester during World War One and he founded the Thomas Lewis Lecture of the British Cardiac Society.

(11) The Order of the British Empire is a British order of chivalry which was founded in 1917. The order of rank is: Member (MBE), Officer (OBE), Commander (CBE), Knight Commander (KBE), Knight Grand Cross (GBE).

(12) A Knighthood is an ancient honour conferred by the British monarch. Lewis was a Knight Bachelor which is a non-hereditary title.

# Chapter 6

## Department of clinical research established • Atrial fibrillation and the circus movement • *Mechanism and Graphic Registration of the Heart Beat* • Experimental and clinical studies with quinidine

When the war was over, Walter Fletcher wrote to the Dean at UCH Medical School in December 1918 saying that the Medical Research Committee would like to re-establish a department in the school 'having as its primary object the advancement of knowledge of the cardiovascular system'.[486] This was agreed to and in January 1919 Lewis was appointed a full Physician to the hospital and also Physician-in-Charge of the Cardiographic Department. This was a hospital service department, like the X-ray department, but his research work had the separate MRC title, 'Department of Clinical Research'.

There now arose a problem regarding his books. In 1915 he had written to Fletcher saying he had some spare time and had started on new editions of his three books, in particular 'a pretty big task' on *The Mechanism of the Heart Beat.* 'I should be glad to feel that the work entailed is recognized by your Committee as it will mean a good deal of my time. I have always regarded these books as part and parcel of my scheme of work'.[489] In his reply Fletcher had said, 'the Committee would recognize that the preparation of your book falls properly within the scope of your relations with them'.[185] But Fletcher now complained to Lewis that the monograph on *The Soldier's Heart* contained no reference to the MRC except on the title page, even though the work had been done under the auspices of the Committee. In a two page handwritten disclaimer Lewis, in referring to the complaint, said, 'In our conversation you expressed this somewhat strongly', adding 'my reply was primarily intended to contravert your statement…' There is a pencilled note in the margin by Fletcher, 'not made', but there is no reply from him.[492] As we shall see there were to be further complaints by Fletcher on similar lines in the years ahead. Lewis was, however, meticulous in other directions, such as requesting leave; asking what to do with £71 of teaching fees in one year (reply – 'keep them'); seeking permission to give a lecture in Sheffield, and asking if he might purchase various items of equipment.

### Personal finance and salary

At this time his personal finances were becoming a problem. He now had a house of his own, with a wife and family to support – their first child Patricia was born in December 1918. In a letter to Fletcher he says that he could not live on his salary alone and had never expected to do so and save money. He had 'relied on private sources of income to see me through ... but the war has hit us as a family pretty heavily ... living as I do in constant association with practising physicians many expenses are unavoidable'.[493] Fletcher replied that when the MRC became a Council, not a Committee, under the Privy Council on April 1st 1920 all salaries would be reviewed and later that year all salaries over £1000 p.a. (his was £1040) got a bonus of £658.This was a good salary for those days, but certainly less than a physician would earn in private practice.

## The importance of diagnosing heart failure, not valve lesions

His work at the military hospitals and for the Ministry of Pensions had an unexpected bonus which he referred to in a British Medical Association lecture at Sheffield in 1919 entitled 'On cardinal principles in cardiological practice'.[151] This experience had given him the opportunity to see the routine work of many doctors when dealing with cardiac patients. In his previous hospital work he had met only hospital consultants and indeed, as Paul White had noticed, his main interest seemed to be in the laboratory. He now realized that a majority of practitioners were preoccupied with finding cardiac murmurs and diagnosing valvular disease of the heart, even from just an isolated systolic murmur. He told his audience in this lecture that the most important cardinal point concerned not murmurs but the symptoms and signs of cardiac failure with especial attention being paid to exercise tolerance. Knowing the amount of work which would bring forth distress was, he said, half the battle in getting early evidence of an impaired circulation. But by contrast with the symptoms, the *signs* of congestive failure in the neck veins and liver occurred late and not until the disease was in an advanced state.

## Emphasis on finding suitable jobs for cardiac patients, and rehabilitation

A problem which clearly made a deep impression on him was that of finding appropriate employment for disabled men, and his involvement with this question shows well the warm and compassionate side of his nature. He knew how difficult it was for a working class man to change his job and having noted that 'cardiac cases are for the most part conspicuously willing workers' he said, 'It is a shameful thing that these unfortunates are put by hard necessity to tasks far beyond their endurance'. And he was certainly a pioneer in rehabilitation with his remark, 'We greatly need in this country a system by which disabled workers are placed and cared for in suitable employment'.[151] He wrote to the Ministry of Health saying, 'the need of suitably placing disabled men is a very wide and very urgent one. It is one I have repeatedly referred to publicly and in memos to the Ministry of Pensions and the MRC'.[494]

There was now a great deal of work to be done and several important tasks demanded simultaneous attention. He had to re-establish his department and its research work, revitalize the journal *Heart*, continue the Ministry of Pensions work and produce a new edition of his main book.

## Writes the second edition of his monograph, *The Mechanism of the Heart Beat*

He seems to have been surprised by the demand for the first edition of *The Mechanism of the Heart Beat* which he regarded more as a monograph than a textbook and it showed him the need for a comprehensive work on electrocardiography. When he had first planned a new edition in 1915 he anticipated that this would take him three months to do. It is a measure of his capacity for intense concentration and sustained hard work that he felt three months would suffice for a task which could easily have occupied a year or more for another author. The task was now even bigger, but in under six months the second edition was published in 1920 (Fig. 6.1) with the new title *The Mechanism and Graphic Registration of the Heart Beat.*[154] The text was rewritten and many of the 349 figures were new. Nearly half of the 801 references were to papers published after the 1911 edition, and the bibliography was unique in giving the page

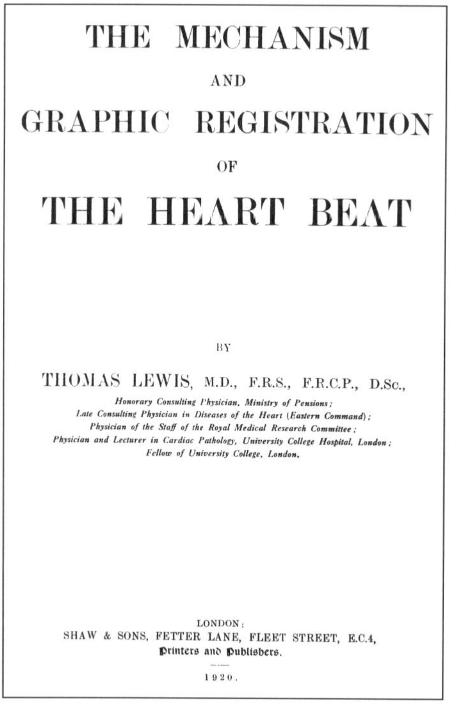

THE MECHANISM

AND

GRAPHIC REGISTRATION

OF

THE HEART BEAT

BY

THOMAS LEWIS, M.D., F.R.S., F.R.C.P., D.Sc.,

*Honorary Consulting Physician, Ministry of Pensions;*
*Late Consulting Physician in Diseases of the Heart (Eastern Command);*
*Physician of the Staff of the Royal Medical Research Committee;*
*Physician and Lecturer in Cardiac Pathology, University College Hospital, London;*
*Fellow of University College, London.*

LONDON:
SHAW & SONS, FETTER LANE, FLEET STREET, E.C.4,
Printers and Publishers.

1920.

*Figure 6.1 Title page of the second edition in 1920 of* The Mechanism of the Heart Beat, *now renamed and largely rewritten.*

numbers where the papers were referred to in the text. It must have been a huge task for one man just to read and compile the references, not to mention selecting the figures, writing the text and getting it all ready for the publisher. The preface gave him the opportunity to point out that diagnostic methods, and in particular bedside tests, had little value until their reliability had been tested objectively. 'A physical sign or method serves no purpose in the pursuit of science until the measure of its fallibility is taken'. He was also able to present his belief that a main defect in scientific medicine at that time, 'clinical pathology' as he then called it, was a reliance on hypothesis rather than factual observation:

> Inexact method of observation, as I believe, is one flaw in clinical pathology today. Prematurity of conclusion is another, and in part follows from the first; but in chief part an unusual craving and veneration for hypothesis, which besets the minds of most medical men, is responsible. Except in those sciences which deal with the intangible or with events of long past ages, no treatises are to be found in which hypothesis figures as it does in medical writings. The purity of a science is to be judged by the paucity of its recorded hypothesis. Hypothesis has its right place, it forms a working basis; but it is an acknowledged makeshift, and, as a final expression of opinion, an open confession of failure, or, at the best, of purpose unaccomplished. Hypothesis is the heart which no man with right purpose wears willingly upon his sleeve. He who vaunts his lady love, ere yet she is won, is apt to display himself as frivolous or his lady a wanton. For this reason oftentimes I was particular to set forth evidence upon evidence for a given conclusion in the book, feeling that no doctrine is sufficiently supported if yet another serious argument may be urged in its favour. For the same reason the leading theses chosen were those founded upon abundant evidence.[155]

The book had an enthusiastic one page review in *The Lancet* which properly pointed out however that 'graphic records help us but little in that great group of sufferers whose cardiac mechanism is apparently normal but inefficient'. The reviewer took the opportunity too of writing a short but stimulating account of the state of cardiology at that time pointing, among other topics, to the need for preventing heart disease and the necessity of discarding some unproven physical signs. This review is a useful source for historians of cardiology.[3] Sir James Mackenzie, too, was impressed with the book and he wrote to Lewis on June 3 1920 to say;

> I have just received a copy of your second edition of the *Mechanism* and congratulate you on a very fine piece of work. The book is a model of how medical books should be written and it is a pity that the same care and study is not given to other organs of the body, for even the nervous system is not studied with the skill you have displayed.[446]

## Research work on arrhythmias resumed, with Alan N. Drury as a full time research worker

The department's research work was concerned once again with cardiac irregularities. Lewis had decided in 1914 to investigate further the nature of atrial fibrillation and was able to start work on this at once in the autumn of 1918 with the help of his one remaining assistant Tom Cotton. (Fig. 6.2, *overleaf*) Cotton, now aged 31, was a Canadian physician who had worked in Lewis' laboratory in 1913

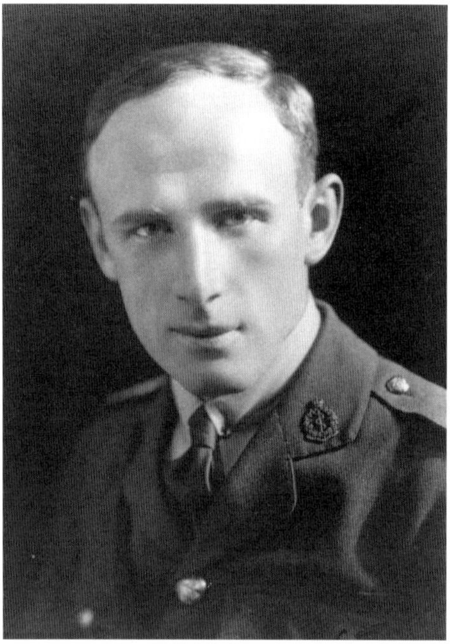

*Figure 6.2 Thomas Forrest Cotton, a Canadian physician who was one of Lewis' early research assistants*

and remained with him throughout the war. Early in 1920 Dr Alan Nigel Drury was appointed as the department's first full time research worker and he was an invaluable member of it until he left six years later to embark on his own distinguished academic career.[91] Although Drury had briefly worked under Lewis at Hampstead as a newly qualified doctor his recruitment was not deliberate. It came about after he had called on Lewis to ask for some advice. In the autumn of 1920 Drury went to work with Einthoven in Leiden for four months, and the length of his stay indicates clearly that Lewis wanted him to get a mastery of all aspects of the string galvanometer. Lewis was conscious of his own lack of understanding of electricity and physics – a consequence of having been educated at home. Drury said that the latest galvanometer that Einthoven had made was the best that had ever been developed, but it was very difficult to construct. 'There was, as Einthoven had warned me before I decided to go, a certain secrecy about certain aspects of the technique which was a definite bar to learning all I wanted to know'.[91] In particular Drury was excluded from the laboratory on Fridays, and years later he found that this was the day on which Einthoven made radiotelegraph transmissions with a special galvanometer to his son in the Dutch East Indies, which he hoped would become a commercial possibility. A second full-time appointment to the department was also made in 1920 when Dr Ronald T. Grant[(1)] came from Glasgow, where his interest in cardiology had been aroused when he learnt to use the Mackenzie polygraph during a house job after leaving the Army.[84] He was introduced to Lewis by Dr John McNee[(2)] then working in Elliott's department.

# Circus movement proposed as the mechanism of atrial flutter and fibrillation

Lewis now embarked on an intensive study of clinical and experimental atrial arrhythmias which occupied him for two years. Having described atrial fibrillation some years ago he was now keen to identify the electrophysiological mechanism underlying it. In addition he had become intrigued by atrial flutter with its regular unvarying atrial rate of about 300 per minute (Fig. 6.3) which could persist for years, in contrast to the other regular arrhythmia, paroxysmal tachycardia which usually lasted only for hours or a few days.

Having identified atrial fibrillation with the electrocardiogram – or 'the galvanometer' as he usually called it – it was natural for Lewis to enquire after its underlying mechanism. C.J. Rothberger and H. Winterberg in Vienna, whose opinion was much respected by Lewis, had shown experimentally that there was a close inter-relation between atrial flutter and fibrillation and Lewis knew that clinically there was a close affinity between the two because digitalis converted flutter to fibrillation. Nevertheless he thought that the nature of flutter was 'altogether mysterious'. A suggestion as to the cause of atrial fibrillation had already been made in 1914 by George R. Mines, whose experiments were based on earlier work by Alfred G. Mayer. The latter had shown that a continuous circulating wave going on for days could be produced by stimulating the bell of the Medusa jellyfish.[158] The original discovery that the bell of Medusa was excitable had been made 30 years before by George J. Romanes.[59] Lewis had been acquainted with

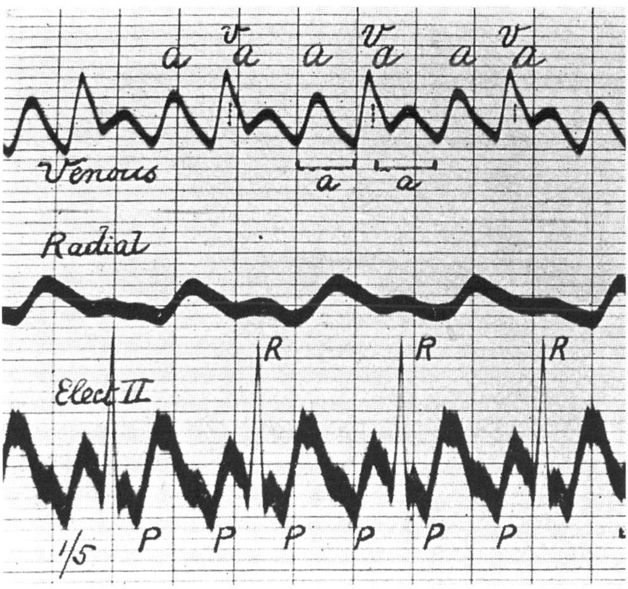


*Figure 6.3 A fine recording of the jugular venous pulse, arterial pulse and electrocardiogram in a patient with atrial flutter. (From reference 168.)*

Romanes' work for nearly 20 years, having obtained the 1898 seventh edition of his book *Animal Intelligence* whilst an undergraduate. In 1910 he must have been attracted to the idea of a circulating impulse because he purchased the 1885 second edition of Romanes' book *Jelly-Fish, Star-Fish and Sea Urchins being a research on primitive nervous systems.* His copy of the book is well annotated in pencil with one note reading, 'contraction wave originating an impulse' and another, 'contraction discharging impulse formation'. G.R. Mines used rings of atrial muscle from dogfish and rays and was able to induce circulating rhythms or circus movements and he postulated, as did Walter E. Garrey who called them 'circus contractions', that these rhythms were the cause of fibrillation. Lewis reviewed these studies in 1913 and disagreed with their conclusion.[138] Later he put forward the idea that 'irritable foci in the muscle underlie fibrillation'.[158] But when he and Cotton examined fibrillation in the dog from this viewpoint they found their observations to be 'for the moment unintelligible'.[158] So therefore the simpler arrhythmia of atrial flutter was, with a good deal of difficulty, induced by induction shocks and it was closely observed by placing several electrodes on the atria. Instead of finding the usual radial spread of the wave, 'a very different state was discovered'. A wave emerged from below the inferior vena cava, and having passed upwards it turned backwards round the superior vena cava. Then a wave appeared again at the inferior vena cava. Was it a new one coming from an irritable focus or a continuation of its predecessor? Calculation of its velocity and path of travel showed it to be a continuation, or re-entrant wave.[157] So Mayer's original and brilliant concept of circus movement with its extension by Mines and Garrey was undoubtedly the mechanism of atrial flutter. Lewis wrote a very interesting account of how the concept of the circus movement had developed, including a long statement as to the way in which his own ideas had changed. Among other comments he wrote, 'We are not indebted to Mines for proof of the circus movement, but to Mayer: we are not indebted to him for the first suggestion that fibrillation has circus movement underlying it, but to MacWilliam.'[158] But it was now necessary to show that the human arrhythmia had the same basis. This was done by making simultaneous recordings from three electrodes placed on the chest wall in such a way as to form a triangle. This enabled the electrical axis of the flutter wave to be calculated at 1/50 second intervals and it proved to rotate through 360 degrees in each cycle just as one would expect with a circus movement. (Fig. 6.4) The idea was then extended to atrial fibrillation. Rothberger accepted the concept of circus movement in flutter and fibrillation but denied that one could measure the axis of fibrillating atria. Lewis pointed out that chest leads, not limb leads, must be used to do it.[169] He had been the first, in 1910, to show the value of placing an electrode over the region of the right atrium to emphasize atrial activity and this was another occasion when his pioneer use of chest leads was employed, albeit only for atrial, not ventricular, activity. (Fig. 6.5) The leads at that time had to be bipolar, not unipolar which came much later. The two electrodes were placed a few inches apart with the positive electrode over the site selected for the recording. He also used leads over the left chest, but not for analysis of the ventricular complex. Lewis was justifiably pleased with confirming this mechanism not just for its own sake but because it supported his concept of combining experimental and clinical studies in the discipline of clinical science. Flutter was discovered and defined clinically, and once its mechanism had been worked out in the dog it enabled final confirmation to be obtained in man. It is worth noting that he had started out with the idea that fibrillation

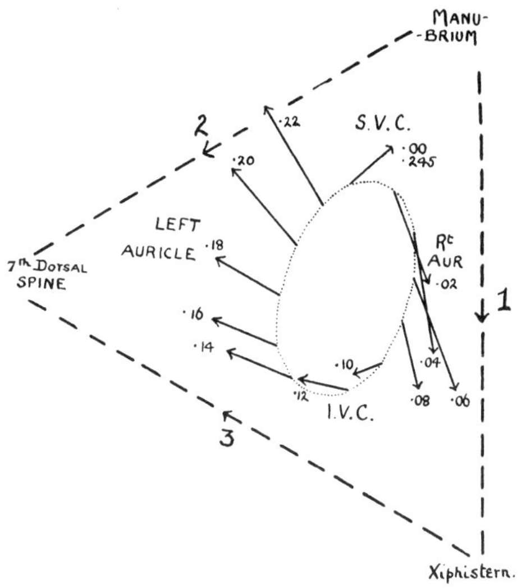


*Figure 6.4 The electrical axes of a flutter wave are plotted sequentially by using three electrocardiographic leads in the sagittal plane. The diagram shows that there is a circus movement around the mouths of the superior and inferior venae cavae, (SVC and IVC). (From* Heart *1921;8:351.)*

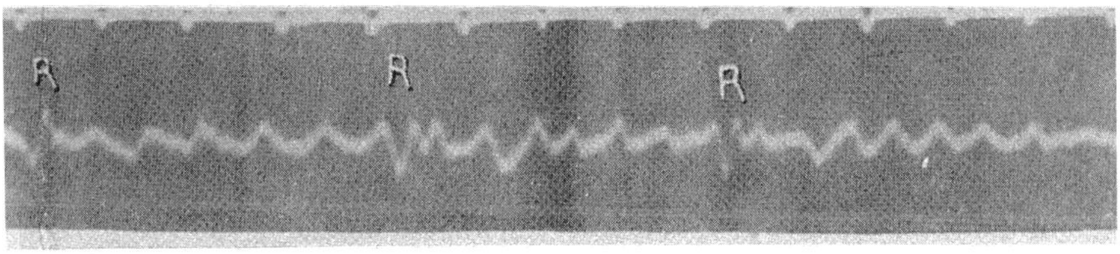


*Figure 6.5 A pioneer use of a precordial lead in 1910, taken from a pair of contacts to the right of the sternum. In this instance it was used to show that the 'f' waves of atrial fibrillation were maximal over the right atrium. From reference 121.*

was due to the formation of stimuli at multiple foci in the atria. But this concept had to be abandoned in favour of circus movement, and it forced him to have a correction slip placed into the second edition of the *Mechanism and Graphic Registration of the Heart Beat,* at page 341, saying that 'auricular fibrillation is not due to the activity of many centres ... the excitation wave is broken up and travels along sinuous and varying paths re-entering fibres through which it has already travelled...the hypothesis which Mines and Garrey have advocated now definitely holds the field'. His main co-worker in these studies was Drury, and they were joined by Harold A. Bulger from Boston, Harold S. Feil from Cleveland, William D. Stroud from Philadelphia, and Constantin C. Ilieuscu from Bucharest. The work was published in a series of papers entitled 'Observations upon flutter and fibrillation' which came out in nine parts in *Heart* in 1920 and 1921, together with six other papers on the subject. One can understand why Drury said, 'Lewis drove himself relentlessly. The pace was terrific and he left his co-workers panting.'[49,50] The work was summarized by Lewis in his Oliver-Sharpey lectures to the Royal College of Physicians in April 1921, entitled 'The nature of flutter and fibrillation of the auricle'.[157]

## Experimental and clinical studies of quinidine

This academic work on the mechanism of atrial fibrillation happened to coincide with an important therapeutic advance, namely the discovery that quinidine could halt fibrillation and restore normal rhythm. This was the first time that any drug had been shown to actually terminate an arrhythmia and it came about, as often happens with new medicines, by a chance observation. A few years earlier a patient of Professor K.L. Wenckebach convinced him from a personal observation that quinine could terminate paroxysms of atrial fibrillation.[85] This led W. von Frey in Berlin to investigate in 1918 all four alkaloids present in the bark of the cinchona tree and to show that quinidine was the most effective. The war delayed Frey's paper getting to Britain but as soon as he read it Lewis seized the opportunity offered by this new drug. By using his technique of recording atrial activity very precisely with chest leads placed near the sternum, 'a special clinical method of recording', Lewis was readily able to measure changes in atrial rate in man whereas Frey had had to rely on whether or not the arrhythmia stopped. (Fig. 6.6) The superiority of quinidine was confirmed by showing that it slowed atrial conduction much better than the other three cinchona alkaloids. That study was done by Grant and Iliescu who also showed that the reputed effect of quinine was due to the presence of quinidine in the commercial preparations.[69] So if Wenckebach's patient had taken pure quinine this great discovery might never have been made. Quinidine came along at just the right time to give useful support to the hypothesis of circus movement. Lewis pointed out that for circus movement to be maintained there had to be a gap between the head and the tail of the circulating wave. (Fig. 6.7) If the gap closed the movement would cease. Quinidine was shown in his dog work to prolong the refractory period and if this effect were to outweigh its opposite action on slowing conduction then the gap

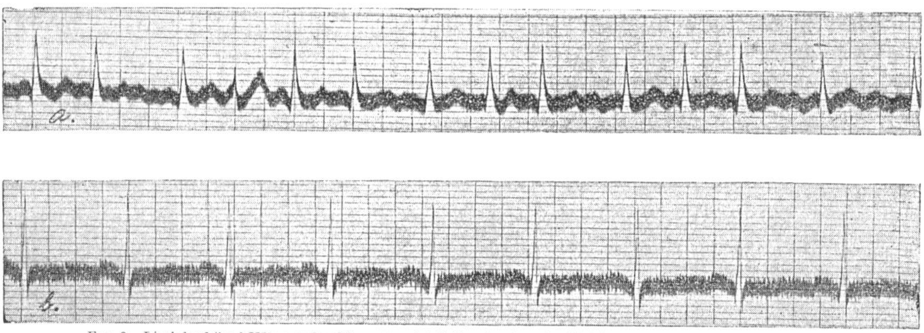


FIG. 2.—Limb lead (lead III) records of Case XII. (a) Before treatment. (b) After appearance of normal rhythm.

*Figure 6.6 The use of quinidine was intensively studied in Lewis' laboratory, and these electrocardiograms show reversion from atrial fibrillation (a) to sinus rhythm (b). (From* BMJ *1921:II;512.)*

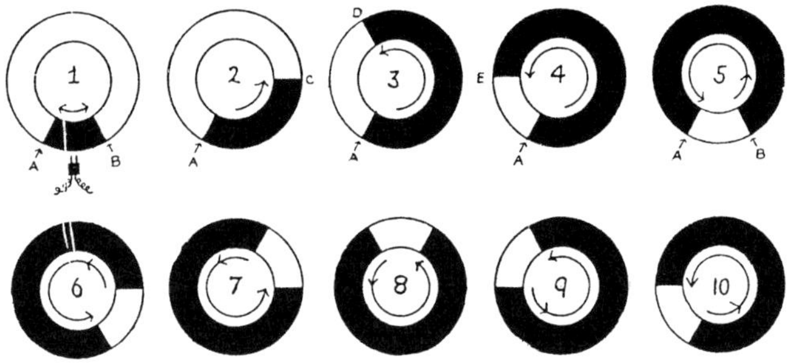


*Figure 6.7 A diagram to show the establishment of a circus movement in a ring of muscle. A gap is maintained between the head and the tail of the wave of excitation. (From reference 157.)*

would close and normal rhythm be resumed. It was a convincing argument and 'the whole of the work went forward without suggestion or other aid from pharmacology'.[202] In other words the clinical research worker was just as competent to do pharmacological work as was the animal pharmacologist in the basic science laboratory. Lewis acknowledged that the proof of a circus movement came from the work of Mayer, but he himself rightly got the credit for establishing it as the mechanism of atrial fibrillation and flutter because of his fine experimental work. (Fig. 6.8) It needs to be asked whether his hypothesis has stood the test of time. It is now accepted that flutter certainly is a circus movement with re-entry around the mouths of the great veins. Fibrillation however consists of multiple wavelets moving around electrically charged areas, and may be described as a form of circus movement but not one which uses fixed anatomical pathways.

The work on quinidine included a thorough study of the clinical aspects of the drug.(160–162) The effects of varying doses, either single or repeated was noted as was the solubility of different preparations. It was shown that the unwelcome rise in ventricular rate with quinidine could be beneficially prevented by giving digitalis simultaneously, thus settling a previous dispute as to whether the two

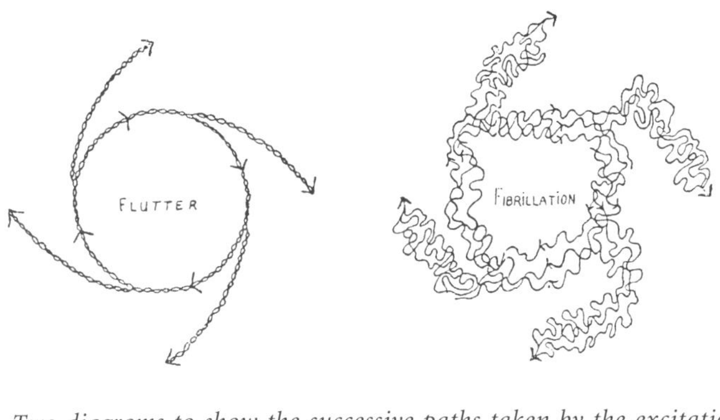


*Figure 6.8 Two diagrams to show the successive paths taken by the excitation wave in atrial flutter on the left and in fibrillation on the right. With flutter the path is accurately repeated from cycle to cycle, but with fibrillation the path is ever varying though it progresses in a clockwise fashion around a central area. (From reference 157.)*

drugs should be given together. Lewis and his colleagues pointed out that ventricular extrasystoles commonly occur during treatment and they emphasized the danger of ventricular tachycardia – of which he had elsewhere published impressive recordings. In particular Lewis drew attention to the fact that reversion to sinus rhythm with quinidine showed that hearts with even chronic atrial fibrillation do have the capacity to beat normally. But in only a small percentage of patients was it possible to restore sinus rhythm permanently, and he indicated the danger of embolism with resumption of normal rhythm.

## Notes to Chapter 6

(1) Ronald Thomson Grant, FRS, 1892–1989, was 27 when he started with Lewis, having served in the Army during the War. He worked first on the effect of quinidine in atrial fibrillation. He then became a good cardiac pathologist, cutting and staining all the microscopical sections himself, and studying the bicuspid aortic valve. His main work lay in the follow-up study of soldiers with heart disease. He stayed with Lewis for 14 years and then became the director of the new department of clinical research, funded by the Medical Research Council, at Guy's Hospital in London, where he did important work during the second world war on the problem of shock. This work took him at the age of 52 to the front line in Italy, when he formed the Royal Army Medical Corps Traumatic Shock Research Unit.

(2) John William McNee, (later Sir John), 1887–1984, worked in the Medical Unit at UCH Medical School where he undertook important work on the liver and spleen. He was then appointed as Regius Professor of Medicine in Glasgow.

# Chapter 7

## Visits Einthoven in Leiden • Endocarditis research • Congenital heart disease • Visit to the United States of America

NOW THAT he was back at work with the electrocardiogram, Lewis was anxious to know what Einthoven thought of his long paper on the spread of the excitatory process in the vertebrate heart given at the Royal Society in 1916.[144] This led in September 1918 to a renewal of the correspondence after a gap of three years. This long interval might be explained by the belief that when Lewis worked on one subject his mind was closed to others, or possibly he had been unable to write even though Holland was neutral. Certainly he was glad once again to have Einthoven's uniquely valuable help and wrote:

> I not only appreciate the kindly way in which you speak of the paper, but appreciate and value equally your criticisms. Criticism of such a kind is most helpful always ... and I only wish that in these later days of Physiological Science it were more frequent.[317]

But although the letters are full of technical detail they also show very clearly the warmth of friendship between the two men. Einthoven, now aged 58, says he has frequent headaches and fears he is growing old and also says that he is astonished at the amount of scientific work that Lewis can do whilst seeing patients every day. Lewis replies that whilst he is grieved to learn of the headaches he cannot believe Einthoven is older in his mind because he writes so clearly, adding, 'And now my dear Professor you must not think that I work so very hard. I have never seen many private patients and in the future I will not see any.'

A year later Lewis received an invitation to give a lecture in Leiden and he wrote to say how stimulating it would be to come again to 'the Mecca of electrocardiography.' The lecture, on his circus movement work, was given on March 17 1921 and was followed by one in Amsterdam. He stayed with Einthoven (Fig. 7.1) (*overleaf*) and clearly enjoyed the hospitality of the Einthoven household with 'your many kindnesses to me' and he admired the excellence and activity of Einthoven's laboratory. (Fig. 7.2) (*overleaf*) However, he declined to have his lecture published and this was for two reasons: firstly, the work was already in print and 'I never publish the same matter twice' and secondly – and an interesting confession after his previous disclaimer – 'I have been writing original articles for several months now and am already tired ... I am feeling the strain of this year's work'.[318] Soon afterwards Einthoven came to London to lecture at the Royal Society of Medicine and greatly enjoyed meeting Mrs Lewis and 'my stay in your hospitable house'. Lewis and his wife gave a supper party so that Einthoven

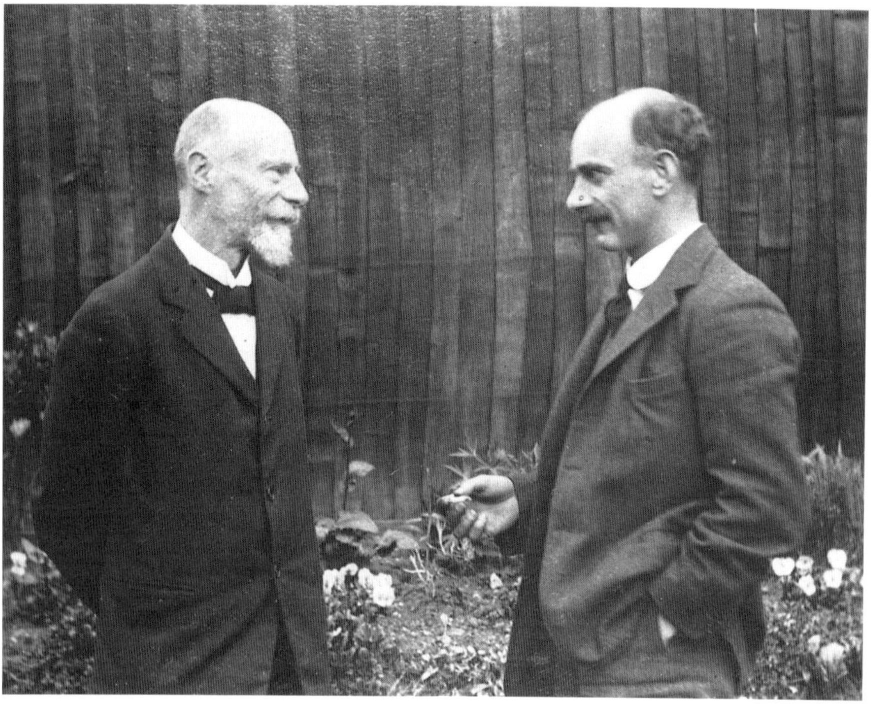

*Figure 7.1* Willem Einthoven with Thomas Lewis in Leiden April 1921.

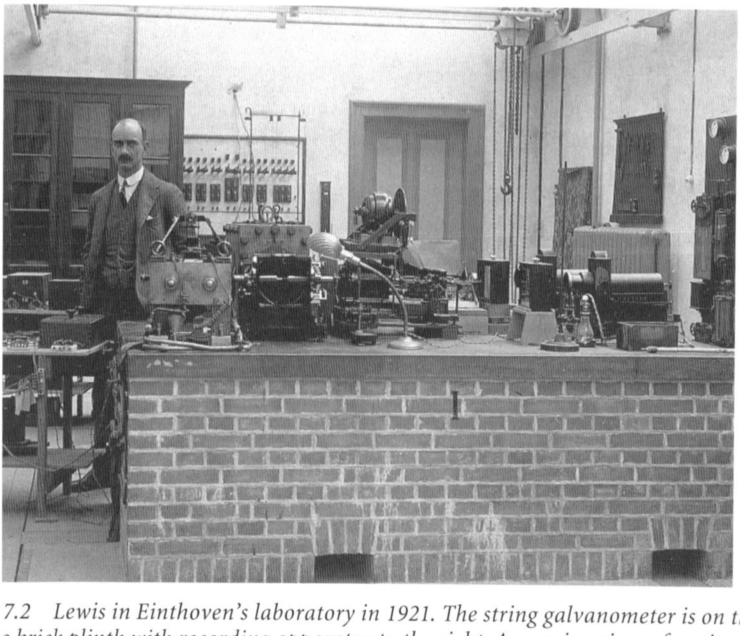

*Figure 7.2* Lewis in Einthoven's laboratory in 1921. The string galvanometer is on the left of the brick plinth with recording apparatus to the right. A massive piece of equipment.

could meet physiologists. They gave another for younger doctors which was attended by Drury who had just returned from four months in Einthoven's laboratory. Lewis was conscious of his lack of understanding of electricity and physics, and Drury was being trained to fill these gaps. This arrangement shows that Lewis intended to continue his work in electrocardiography but as it turned out this was almost the end of that era. After 1921 his own new work in this field was limited to a study on the effect of vagal stimulation in the dog on intra – auricular block and a final paper in 1925 with Arthur M. Master on AV conduction in the mammalian heart. Drury did continue with experimental work mostly on conduction in atrial muscle. However there were still important conclusions to be drawn from all his previous work and Lewis presented them in two nominated lectures.

## The Linacre Lecture and the Mellon Lecture

The Linacre Lecture at Cambridge in May 1921 was entitled 'The law of cardiac muscle with special reference to conduction in the mammalian heart' in which he compared the size, glycogen content, conduction rate and rhythmicity of the four types of cardiac fibre: Purkinje, auricular, ventricular and nodal.[156] By knowing one of these features it was possible to predict what one of the others might be. The rhythmicity of Purkinje fibres, for example, was unknown but one could predict it to be low and therefore get an explanation of the puzzling phenomenon of 2:1 block with tachycardia. The Mellon Lecture at Pittsburgh in 1922 was on 'Interpretations of the initial phases of the electrocardiogram with special reference to the theory of "limited potential differences".'[159] In this paper he put forward the concept that the ventricular muscle comprises a large number of small units, such as the muscle fibres themselves, and that the electrical curve inscribed by the muscle as a whole is a composite picture of the currents developed by these individual units. This new hypothesis opposed the older one of 'distributed potential differences' which maintained that the ventricular muscle constituted only one electrical unit. This was a very important paper and it has often been referred to since then.

The year 1922 was significant in the history of electrocardiography because it saw the death on March 11 of Professor Augustus Désiré Waller, the first person to record the electrical activity of the human heart. There has been some doubt as to who invented the word electrocardiogram but Einthoven definitely gave the credit to Waller.[27] At his demonstrations to scientific audiences Waller often used his pet bulldog as the subject, (Fig. 7.3, *overleaf*) standing him in jars of saline in order to record his electrocardiogram. Jimmie became well known when a member of Parliament alleged in the House of Commons that a cruel experiment had been performed on the dog without a licence![18] Lewis wrote that Waller's discovery 'will remain a milestone in the history of this branch of knowledge' and he praised his 'brilliant powers of exposition' and 'his unusually keen intellect'. However he added that 'those who explored the same field could not always see eye-to-eye with Waller in his later views'.[163] This probably refers to Waller's comment 'I do not however imagine that the string galvanometer ... is likely to find any very extensive use in the hospital...'.[27] Nevertheless it is possible that Waller would have shared the Nobel Prize with Einthoven, had he lived until 1924.

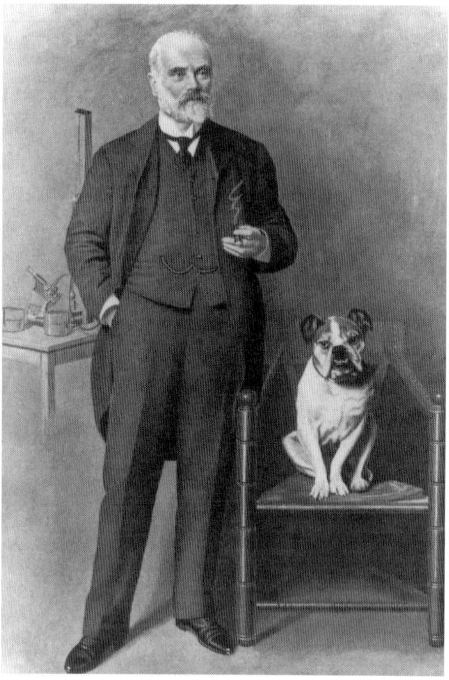

*Figure 7.3 Professor A.D. Waller with his famous bulldog, Jimmie, who was used to demonstrate the electrocardiogram to audiences. (From the magazine* Mayfair *in 1915.)*

## Editing *Heart*

The surge of work in the immediate post war years that left Lewis tired and feeling the strain included the editorship of *Heart*. The journal had not appeared in 1916 and volume 6 was completed in 1917 with several papers on 'Irritable Heart'. Volume 7 got off to a slow start with only two small issues, respectively of 35 and 70 pages,in each of 1918 and 1919. But the next two issues of Volume 7, that came out in 1920, had 248 pages with six papers by Lewis and his assistants. In 1921 there was enough material to fill five issues totalling 480 pages and this was a major editorial task. Furthermore, of the 22 articles in these issues, 14 came from Lewis' laboratory and those with his own name on them were usually long, ranging in these instances from 20 to 58 pages. Other papers came from five different centres in the States, with Frank Wilson writing from Ann Arbor on experimental bundle branch block, whilst one on ventricular tachycardia in relation to coronary occlusion by G Canby Robinson and George Herrmann came from Washington University medical school.

## Rejects a paper for *Heart* by Mackenzie

There was one paper that did not get published, and surprisingly it was by Mackenzie. He was now working at the Institute for Clinical Research[1] which he had founded at St Andrews in Scotland in 1918. Although the manuscript of the paper has not been kept, we know from the correspondence what the main points were. Mackenzie had sought to show by giving atropine to digitalised patients with atrial fibrillation that digitalis slows the heart by its action on the vagus. Lewis did not accept the evidence and said that the results could as well be interpreted as a mainly direct action on the cardiac muscle, and returned the paper.[387] Mackenzie was naturally upset and wrote two letters of about 1100 words each to explain his position. The chief reason for his disappointment was not so much a technical one about the effect of atropine, but because he regarded this paper as an important statement concerning his theory about the laws governing the production of symptoms. In his first letter he wrote:

> My dear Lewis, You have failed to comprehend the purport of the paper I sent to you... In the paper I dealt briefly with prognosis and heart failure. Neither of these subjects are really understood...Over ten years ago I realised that little further progress could be made in our knowledge of prognosis and heart failure unless we got a better understanding of the laws producing symptoms...Have you ever realised why I gave up a lucrative practice to live in–well, not poverty, but in much reduced circumstances? It was to carry this investigation further. My whole time has been devoted to this object and we have succeeded in discovering what I have been groping after for years...Already we have carried the subject so far that we see the beginning, not only of a new symptomatology, but a new pharmacology, and a new neurology.[447]

Lewis seems to have understood this and to have sympathy with it because he wrote, 'What I want you to consider is whether the present illustration will not in the long run damage rather than help your general hypothesis'.[387] But, as one might expect, Mackenzie remained unconvinced and in a second letter he wrote:

> My dear Lewis, I had thought of dropping this correspondence ...but I came across an old letter which brought back memories to me of our relations in the early days in Bentinck Street, and reminded me of how much I owed you in establishing my views upon a sound basis, and I thought it was a pity that those days, which are to me so pleasant to look back upon, should be marred by any disagreement.

Mackenzie then said that he looked on this paper as being the most original he had ever written and that although many journals would have been glad to have it, he was offering it to *Heart*, 'although not a very popular centre for propaganda' because Lewis had stood by him in the past. He continued:

> So you can imagine what my surprise was when this, which I thought was conferring a great favour on you was refused. Although I do not expect that at present you will accept our theory, I would like you just in the course of time to be turning over its possibilities... I know you so well that I do not doubt for one moment that you had a very high motive in returning my paper, but it seems to be that your principle is a very wrong one. We are all very much at sea about heart matters, and our views today may be quite altered in a very short time. If for instance when you described the inverted T wave and the widened PR interval as signs of grave significance, someone with ten times more experience than you had stated that these signs were not of grave significance, would you have been justified in rejecting the paper? If so, you might as well put upon the forefront of your journal 'No articles will be accepted which are not in accordance with the (temporary) beliefs of the Editor'. I merely present that view for your consideration. As this, I suppose, is to be the end of our collaboration, I can assure you that I will follow with interest your future progress, and no-one will rejoice more than I at your successes.[448]

If there was a reply from Lewis it has not been kept, but Mackenzie showed clearly that their friendship had not come to an end when he wrote only a few months later to say he had enjoyed reading the Linacre Lecture. 'I don't know when I read an article with so much pleasure as your Law of Cardiac Muscle. It is a type of paper which is unfortunately rare in medicine'.[449] Happily their good relationship continued and when the Mackenzies moved back to London, after six years in Scotland, Lewis and his wife used to visit them at their home. Mackenzie's monograph *Angina Pectoris* was published in 1923 and he wrote to Lewis on August 17:

> It was you who started me on this work about ten years ago. I have analysed the records of over 2 000 cases and written to hundreds of doctors and patients to see what happened. I am not satisfied with the work but it is the best I could do.
>
> Rotherberger has translated my book on Diseases of the Heart into German... He says he doesn't accept my views on angina, but it is evident he hasn't the ghost of an idea what these are. He is much exercised to show the world he said auricular fibrillation before Lewis! I trust Mrs Lewis and the family are doing well.[450]

In 1924 Lewis wrote a review of the monograph and Mackenzie wrote to say, 'It is an excellent review. Case 28 is myself and Case 58 my brother'. In the same letter he went on to compare the value of clinical judgement in the management of patients as against what he called 'machinery'. He had never quite come to terms with the use of the electrocardiogram, nor of X-rays either for that matter, and he said, 'Medicine today is like a child delighted with its toy but not old enough to reason'.[451] In a previous letter, in 1918, Mackenzie had written, 'Did you see the report of the Heart Hospital taking 10 000 electrocardiograms? And did you ever come across a better instance of blundering mis-spent energy?'.[445]

## Lewis' method of work

Drury (Fig 7.4) wrote an invaluable account of what it was like to work for Lewis at that time, in the early 1920s:

> I spent six breathless years with him. I purposely use the adjective breathless. Each year the research objective was known. When work went well, it was 'faster faster' and when difficulties cropped up there was a tense atmosphere of impatience and anxious probing till they were overcome and the smooth fast pace realised again. He considered that the week consisted of five-and-a-half days for laboratory work and the evenings and week-ends for work at home, and what could be done at home should not take up laboratory time. With one technician, whose capacity was limited, all the details of the experiments, the working out of the results, all the photographs and diagrams published were done either by himself or ourselves. The typing of the manuscripts was the only part delegated. About a month before his annual leave, all laboratory work was stopped and a period of 'writing up' followed in order to see what was ripe for publication, and what further experiments would be required. Lewis wrote quickly and what he wrote required little revision. Others of us were not so endowed so that while this period may have been one of relaxation to him, to us it was very exacting. He insisted that the writing up should be 'just right' and it seemed to take a lot of effort from us, and a lot of blue pencil from him to get it so. Then he went for his annual holiday. It was then that the tense

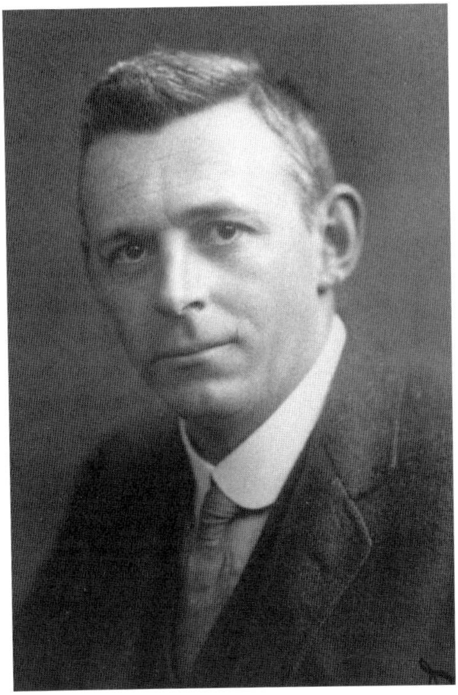

*Figure 7.4 Alan N. Drury was Lewis' most important associate in his electrocardiographic research in 1920–1922.*

atmosphere in the laboratory relaxed and we tried to get our breath to cope with all the problems that we knew he would think out during his holiday, and the mice in the laboratory literally came out to play.

A succession of young scientists from England, America, and the continent came and were thrown abruptly into this fast moving stream; clutching to straws like myself and the technician they quickly learnt to swim or were disregarded. In point of fact pretty well all learnt to swim and to become very capable assistants, with great advantage to themselves in their subsequent careers.

Lewis drove himself relentlessly and one had to be as relentless as one could in driving oneself. I do not think that research results came from any laboratory in such a steady and constant stream or that anyone changed the outlook in a subject so rapidly as Lewis did in cardiology. We learnt or could learn how to think clearly, to plan experiments, and to believe that research was only worth doing if one gave one's whole life to it. That we should never take up a problem unless we were prepared to carry it through, otherwise we should only 'foul the nest'. That if we had the capacity we should try and skim the cream off the milk and leave the skim to others. It was an invaluable and breathless experience.

Does this reminiscence portray the character of Lewis – of course it does not, it is simply what I remember of the way the work went on in the section of the laboratory I worked in during the years 1920–1926. As I know full well from my friendship with Lewis, when he entered the laboratory he took off his ordinary coat and put on his laboratory coat which was cut in a style he thought a

> laboratory coat should be cut. It was austere and tight fitting; it commanded respect and attention.[49]

After Drury left in 1926 he remained on the staff of the Medical Research Council and had a distinguished subsequent career.[91]

## A pioneer study of prognosis in heart disease

Soldiers who were discharged from the Army on medical grounds had to attend the pension boards at intervals and Lewis had realized, even during the war, that this would offer a unique opportunity to study prognosis, a neglected branch of medicine. It had been neglected, he pointed out, because it was impossible in hospital practice to follow up more than a third or so of patients, too small a percentage to be of value, but now most of them could readily be traced. This offered 'an unprecedented opportunity to our profession ... thousands of patients will remain under observation for many years or the rest of their lives ... a mass of information of a valuable kind can be collected'.[149] A special outpatient clinic was set up at UCH for this purpose and it was organized by Miss Elizabeth Bain who had joined Lewis' unit at Hampstead in 1916 and served for several years as a voluntary worker. She was then paid by the MRC to do the military follow up and became the secretary to Lewis' department at UCH. There is no doubt, as Lewis acknowledged in one of his annual reports, that this project owed much of its success to her skill and energy. She left in 1925 when she married an American research worker, Dr Alfred M. Wedd. The project was directed by Cotton, who had been at both Hampstead and Colchester, until Grant took over from him in 1921.

## Infective endocarditis

Cotton became impressed by the frequency of clubbing of the fingers in the patients with valvular disease, and he was one of the first to show that this was a sign of infective endocarditis.[36] He also drew attention to the high incidence of infective endocarditis in valvular disease which he estimated at 8%.[35] His observations were probably the stimulus for Lewis to begin a study of this disease in which, he said, he had long been interested and 'especially in the very slow but seemingly inexorable march upon which it conducts the sufferer to his death'.[190] This study which started in 1922 seems to mark an important turning point away from his intensive electrocardiographic studies of myocardial physiology and arrhythmias, and towards problems that could be investigated by simpler means. Grant was his collaborator and first of all they tried to discover what had happened to the fresh bacterial vegetations which they knew from the clinical histories must have been present six months or more previously. They found fibrous scar tissue at the base of the vegetations and then asked was this healed infection or an old disease of the valve. This question was directed especially at some instances of aortic valve disease where two cusps were welded together. Was this a congenitally bicuspid valve or one deformed by fibrosis of healed vegetations?

# The bicuspid aortic valve

The enquiry led to a thorough study of the bicuspid valve and its relation to bacterial endocarditis. By looking at serial sections of normal valves and uninfected congenital bicuspid valves they were able to show that the position of the annulus in relation to the media was quite different in the two, and this enabled even a grossly distorted valve to be identified as congenital or acquired. (Fig. 7.5) They concluded that at least 23% of adult subjects with congenital bicuspid valves acquired bacterial endocarditis.[242] The congenital deformity favoured platelet thrombi in which the bacteria were able to get a foothold. (Fig. 7.6, *overleaf*) Although earlier writers had noted the association between bicuspid valves and infection this was the first study to identify the especial pathology and to quantify the risk of endocarditis. Their series of 31 autopsy cases was also notable in being not only consecutive cases but also ones who had been studied during life. At this time Maude E Abbott in Montreal was doing an important and pioneer enquiry into congenital heart disease, a study which Osler had recommended to her, and she had a correspondence with Lewis over several years. In 1922 he asked about the frequency of bicuspid valves and at her request sent material for the Canadian Army Medical Museum Catalogue. In 1924 Abbott sent a four page letter in which she says that Lewis' article 'entirely ignores my own practically identical contribution from the statistical side...it is not even among the general references'. This was in reply to a letter from Lewis saying he had heard that she had a grievance towards him for not acknowledging her material. Who told him: Cotton perhaps? But a month later Abbott wrote to say she was glad to learn from Lewis that he had accidentally omitted to refer to her article which was in Osler's *System of Medicine*.[340]

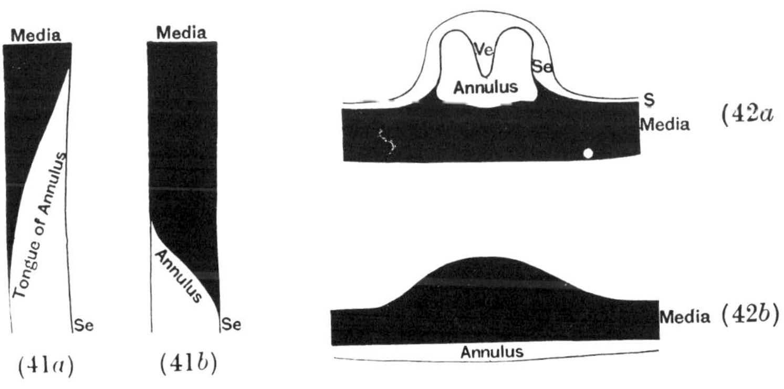


*Figure 7.5 Diagrams of sections through the aortic commissures to show how the relationship of the annulus to the media distinguishes a congenitally bicuspid valve (b) from a normally formed one (a). (From reference 190.)*

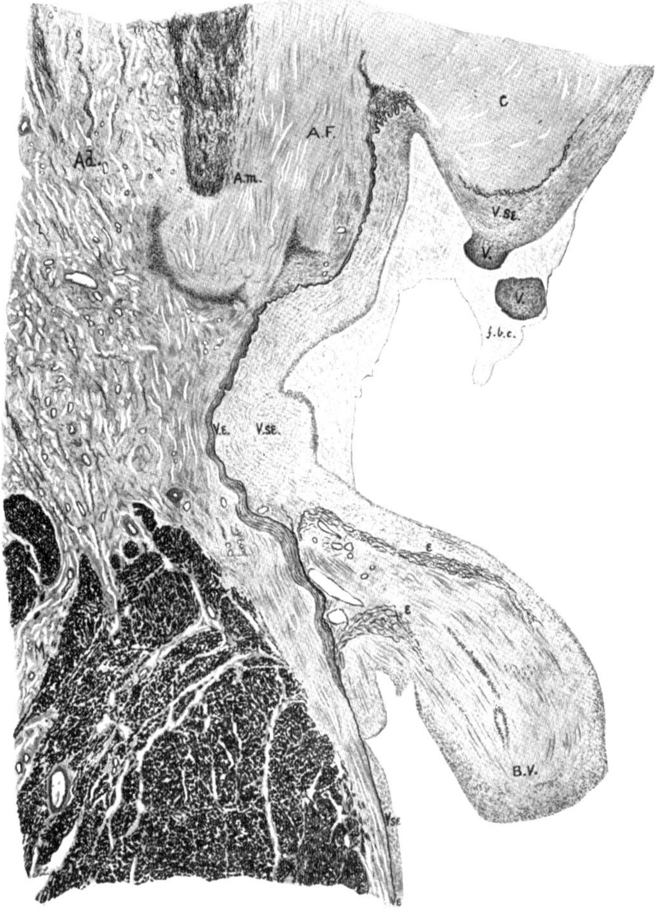


*Figure 7.6 Vertical section ×17 through the centre of an aortic commissure in a case of endocarditis. B.V. is tissue forming the base of the vegetations. This drawing was made by Lewis who often illustrated his papers with his own excellent drawings and photographs. From reference 242.*

## Congenital heart disease

Congenital heart disease interested Lewis for the whole of his life, and having discussed his bicuspid valve study it is appropriate to mention his other work and involvement with this subject. Some years previously he had prepared specimens of hearts from various species such as fish and amphibians, using the wax impregnation technique, to show the evolution of the cardiac chambers and great vessels. His association with the London Zoo may have been the stimulus to do this and certainly it would have been the source of his material. He placed these specimens in the medical school museum together with a dozen or so hearts from patients with congenital heart disease. His good annotations gave careful explanations for anomalies such as persistent ductus arteriosus and pulmonary stenosis and there was an especially fine example of cor triatrium with reasons given for the extra septum.

The chapter on congenital malformations in his *Diseases of the Heart* occupies only seven pages but it shows him to have a good understanding of the subject, perhaps surprising in view of his lack of interest in purely descriptive observations.[188] Here are some examples:

Single ventricle is usually associated with malposition of the great arteries and pulmonary stenosis. Abnormal blood pigments mimic central cyanosis. Atrial fibrillation occurs in older patients with atrial septal defect whilst the ostium primum type is associated with 'defect of the mitral valve and mongolian idiocy'. 'Attacks of an epileptic nature or of coma' occur with severe cyanosis. This last comment refers to the cyanotic attacks in tetralogy of Fallot – though he disliked eponymous titles, and did not use this one.

In the fourth edition of the book, written in 1945,[237] he states that 'ligation of the uninfected ductus ... is justifiable in the hands of the experienced' and it is known that he referred one of his own patients for operation to Mr Oswald S Tubbs at St Bartholomew's Hospital. Coarctation of the aorta held an especial interest for him and in 1933 he wrote a comprehensive account of it based on nine personal cases.[184] He emphasized that the condition is often missed and tells how five cases were found 'to our considerable astonishment' when the femoral pulses of his own patients with hypertension were systematically examined. He mentions that one of these patients had been at the Hampstead Military Hospital and had eluded the diagnostic skills of Sir William Osler, Sir James Mackenzie and Dr Francis R. Fraser.

He was the first person to emphasize the important diagnostic feature that on X-ray examination the aortic arch cannot be traced beyond its ascending portion. Noting that patients live normal lives for many years in spite of their high blood pressure he states that, 'It is a convincing illustration of the fact that heart failure does not follow from simple and prolonged overwork'. This comment was made in support of his entrenched view that it was mainly disease of the myocardium, and not mechanical lesions, that lead to failure. Of his three autopsy cases, one had endocarditis and two had severe coronary disease. He maintained an interest in the clinical diagnosis of congenital heart disease, and during his last years at work in 1943–1944 he regularly examined patients from the Hospital for Sick Children, Great Ormond Street, London. His final paper published four months before his death related the autopsy findings in a baby with congenital tricuspid stenosis in which he showed, by histology, that the former concept of fetal endocarditis as a cause of valve lesions was fallacious.[234]

## A second visit to the United States of America

In the spring of 1922, Lewis set off on his second visit to the United States accompanied this time by his wife. He had a great reputation there from his books and articles and in addition he was well known to many individuals. On the title page of *Heart* there were the names of 21 American physicians from 15 cities who helped in the selection of papers and by now he had had 12 research workers from the States. Although the visit was primarily a lecture tour it was obviously on his conscience that this might not be a proper use of the MRC's time and money because he told Fletcher that it was going to be taken as his annual holiday. But actually the prestige of his visit would have reflected very favourably on the MRC whose name appeared on the published lectures. He was away for two months, going first to Philadelphia on May 5 to give the Nathan Lewis Hatfield Lecture, next to Pittsburgh on May 8 for the Mellon Lecture and then to Portland Oregon from May 15–21 for two Noble Wiley Jones lectures. The Mellon Lecture which has already been mentioned was on academic electrophysiology and has often been quoted in the later literature on that subject. The other three lectures, which were concerned with the actions of atropine, digitalis and quinidine in atrial fibrillation were published in the *American Journal of Medical Sciences*, then remarkably in its 102nd year.[160–162] He was able in particular to summarize the work in his department on the clinical aspects of quinidine therapy in which Dr Alfred M. Wedd of Pittsburgh had been one of his co-workers. When Lewis got off the train in Pittsburgh he was asked by Wedd to go immediately to see a wealthy patient who was not responding well to quinidine treatment. The problem was solved when Lewis increased the dose.[377] The next destination was Ann Arbor where the University of Michigan awarded him an honorary degree of Doctor of Science. They stayed with Frank and Juel Wilson, and their mutual devotion to ornithology and friendship were more important reasons for this visit than was electrocardiography. (Fig. 7.7) Together they

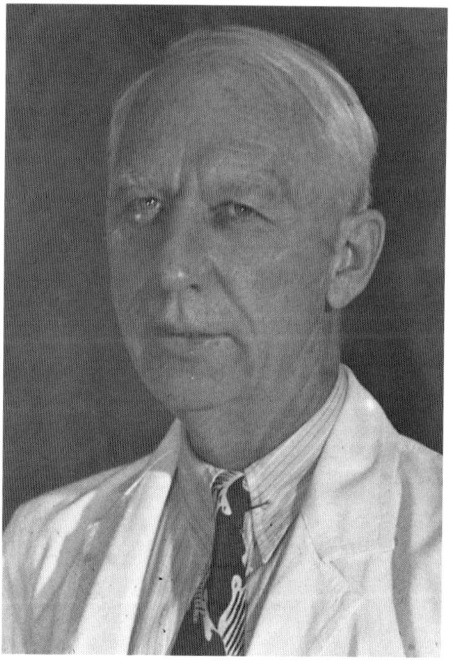

*Figure 7.7 Frank N. Wilson, the renowned American electrocardiographer was a close friend of Lewis and they shared a passion for bird watching.*

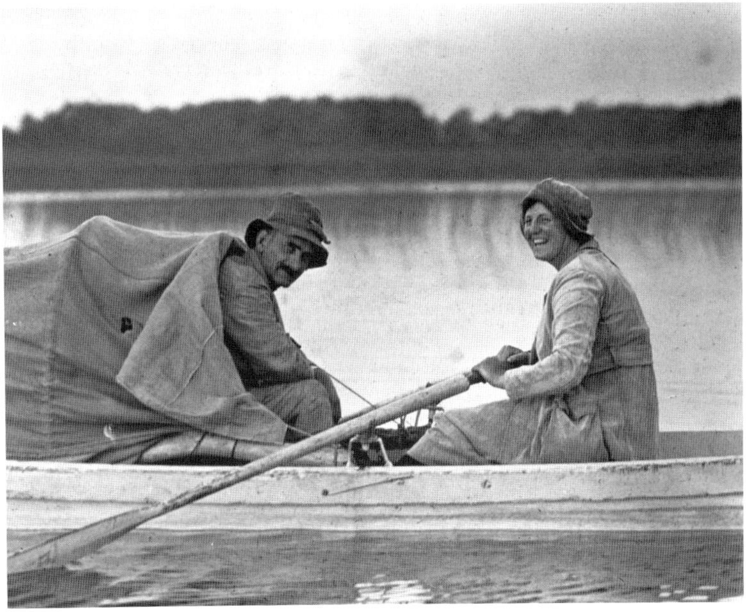

*Figure 7.8 The Lewises on a lake near Ann Arbor. The boat has a hood for bird watching. Photograph probably taken by Dr. Frank Wilson.*

pursued their hobby in a rowing boat on a nearby lake, hoping especially to see the black tern which had become rare in Britain. (Fig. 7.8) Wilson later wrote a good account of his time in England with Lewis:

> He is a small, shy Welshman with watery blue eyes and a rather brusque manner, who is capable of the most intense concentration. I have often seen him sit down to write a scientific paper in a small room in which half a dozen officers were carrying on a noisy conversation. He was often very affable and agreeable, but when he did not wish to be interrupted at his work he was extremely curt to casual visitors, regardless of their eminence. During the first decade of his career he had buried himself in his laboratory working at a high speed until late at night without interruption except for the inevitable afternoon cup of tea and a sandwich with a glass of milk brought in by the laboratory diener at dinner time.
>
> The amount and excellence of Dr. Lewis' work brought him fame at an early age, and a great many students from all parts of the world, but particularly from America, came to work with him. Many of these were capable and earnest, but others came out of curiosity or in order that on returning home they might gain prestige by claiming that they had worked in his laboratory. Experience with men of this kind was, I am sure, responsible for his lack of cordiality to chance visitors. I am deeply indebted to him for help and advice. On numerous occasions I have learned that long before and without my knowledge he had gone far out of his way to speak a good word for me or to advance my interests in other ways. I know that he has done the same for many others. I am indebted to him also for an avocation that has given me much pleasure. He once told me that when he married he felt that he could not stick to his laboratory quite as closely as before and so he looked about for some recreational activity in which both he and his wife could take part. Having long been interested in birds, and having had some experience with photographic processes in

> his work, he decided that they might take up bird photography. For many years he devoted his week-end holidays to this pursuit. He worked at it with the same perseverance and intensity that characterized his ordinary activities and, as in his laboratory work, produced results of unsurpassable excellence.
>
> In the spring of 1918 I had the pleasure of assisting him in his photographic activities. During April, May, and June of that year the great battles in France crowded the British transports with wounded, and there was no room for cases of the kind treated at Colchester. We spent almost every afternoon during that period searching the beautiful English fields, woods, and hedgerows for birds that could be induced to pose for the camera. The evenings were spent in the dark-room developing the plates and criticizing the results. In this way I came to know Thomas Lewis intimately and to admire more and more his boyish enthusiasm, his tireless energy, and his brilliant mind. On these excursions I learned the technique of photographing birds, and this pursuit has given me great satisfaction and an abiding interest in natural history and conservation.[334]

During and after this round of professional engagements, Lewis and his wife found time to go sightseeing in the States. They visited Yosemite National Park, where his parents and Clifford had been ten years beforehand, Grand Canyon in Arizona, and Niagara Falls. They travelled home from New York where no doubt they met the many friends that Lewis had there. Indeed Lady Lewis would have met some of them such as Bernard Oppenheimer and Marcus Rothschild during her visits to Colchester.

## Note to Chapter 7

(1) The Institute for Clinical Research at St Andrews Scotland was established by Sir James Mackenzie in 1918 at the age of 65 and he remained its director until 1924. It had been his lifelong belief that a study of the early stages of disease, characterized only by symptoms, had been neglected in favour of the later stages when physical signs were present. He founded the Institute in order to give detailed study to the significance of symptoms by long term follow-up of patients. He selected St Andrews because it was a small town with a relatively stable population. It was also in his own country of Scotland and it had a university. He soon had the enthusiastic co-operation of the general practitioners in the town, but increasingly severe angina forced him to return to the warmer climate of London in 1924. Mackenzie's imaginative concept is mirrored in the Framingham Project in the United States, where the small town of Framingham in New England was chosen in order to make a very long term follow up of originally healthy people, in order to determine factors which predispose to the development of heart disease. It is interesting that Dr Paul D White who was one of the early supporters of the Framingham Project had visited St Andrews in 1922 to study Mackenzie's work and ideas.

# Chapter 8

## War injuries used as research models • The triple response of the skin to injury, the H substance • Monograph on blood vessels of the human skin • Physiology and medicine • Third edition of *The Mechanism* • Nobel Prize for Einthoven • Death of Mackenzie • Controversy over dog experiments

THE MEDICAL Research Council's annual reports followed the calendar of the university year by running from October, and the work in Lewis' own department had the same pattern. From 1922 to 1923 the main topic he chose for his research emphasizes the break with electrocardiography. Together with Drury he made an intensive study of the local and general circulatory changes which occur with an arteriovenous anastomosis. The stimulus for this work came about from seeing a man who had developed such a lesion after being hit in the groin by a bullet. Whilst demonstrating to the students that pulsation in the arteriovenous aneurysm could be stopped by occluding the femoral artery he noticed that the pulse rate fell promptly and the blood pressure rose. His 'curiosity was deeply aroused' and this single patient led to a long series of observations both in man and dogs.[197] They included the finding that atropine prevented the slowing of rate when the anastomosis was closed – an excellent demonstration in man that there is a reflex response of heart rate through the vagus nerve to a rise of blood pressure, shown a few years later by Hering to be largely mediated from the carotid sinus. His patient had intense capillary pulsation and this phenomenon was also studied in cases of aortic regurgitation, a similar haemodynamic situation, when he had 'the valuable assistance of Miss E.P. Wolf of Chicago'.[165] Dr Elizabeth Pauline Wolf, later Dr E.P.W. Blitzen, was the fourth woman to be one of his research workers. Unlike others at that time Lewis clearly did not discriminate against female doctors. Another patient with a war wound provided the opportunity to compare the electrical and anatomical positions of the heart. A soldier had survived with a bullet embedded in the muscle of his heart and its change of position with respiration could be accurately measured by X-ray. (Fig. 8.1, *overleaf*) As it turned out this positional change could not be correlated with the change in axis on the electrocardiogram, but it again provided an example of how Lewis could exploit a clinical situation to provide basic information.[164]

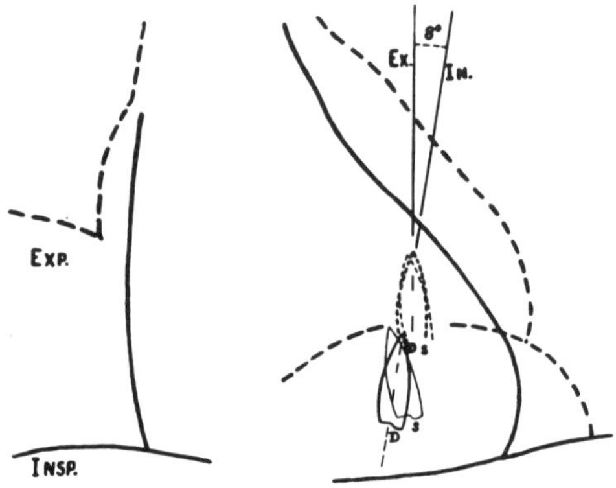


*Figure 8.1 Radiograph of the heart in an ex-soldier showing a bullet embedded in the ventricular septum. Its movement is traced in systole and diastole, and with expiration and inspiration. (From reference 164.)*

## Vascular reactions of the skin to injury

The work on capillary pulsation was followed by a long and very important series of studies on the vascular reactions of the skin to injury which were published in ten parts from 1924 to 1927. This research had really started in 1915 (though published in 1917) when, with Cotton and Slade, Lewis had been the first to demonstrate conclusively that human capillaries were capable of active contraction.[38] Physiological teaching at that time held them to be passive tubes, though Lewis found afterwards that Salomon Stricker had observed capillary contraction in tadpoles' tails in 1865. One might ask why he took up the subject again at this time. Certainly he had been impressed by the paper of Henry H. Dale and A.N. Richards in 1919 on the vasodilator action of histamine and their conclusion that the walls of capillaries as well as arterioles possessed tone. Dale had isolated the 'new' substance histamine from ergot ten years beforehand and had shown its biological importance, for example in producing anaphylactic shock.[55] Another factor may have been the publication in 1922 by Professor August Krogh[(1)] from Copenhagen of his monograph on *The Anatomy and Physiology of Capillaries.*[103] Lewis' own copy of this book is liberally annotated with comments, mostly of a critical nature, 'indeed!', 'no clear reason given', 'Dale and Richards state the opposite', 'not at all a fair statement'. But the most significant notes occur where Krogh summarizes the modern study of capillary contractility and appears to give priority to Ulrich Ebbecke in 1917. At this point Lewis has inserted 'January' for his own paper and 'October' for that of Ebbecke. These notes and also comments in his papers elsewhere indicate that Lewis did not have a high opinion of Krogh's work and he may well have been stung into action by the book.

Whatever the reason, he started off by looking again at the white line which follows a gentle stroke on the skin. He showed that the capillary contraction which caused it could take place against a pressure as high as 60 mmHg, created in the arm veins by a pneumatic cuff, and could also resist nearby arteriolar dilatation produced by histamine injection. The enquiry was then extended to a feature which he had seen in his earlier study, namely that if the skin was stroked heavily, to the point of pain, there developed a red line surrounded by a red 'flare' The red line, like the white line, had crisp margins indicating its origin in the capillaries but this time due to dilatation not contraction, because the heavy stroke had produced a 'paralytic condition' of their walls. In contrast to the red line which became slightly cyanotic after a while the flare remained bright red all the time and this, together with its ill defined margins, suggested its origin in dilatation of the arterioles. When the circulation to the limb was arrested with a cuff – 'the occlusion test' – the flare did not appear because the arterioles could not convey blood to the capillaries but the capillaries themselves could still dilate and give the red line. Another piece of evidence well worth mentioning for its elegance, simplicity and conviction – one might almost say they were Lewis' hallmarks – consisted of creating the red line and flare and then placing the white line at right angles across it. The white line abolished the flare where it crossed it because it contracted the passively dilated capillaries but it could not influence the active 'paralytic' dilatation which caused the red line. A previous nerve injury prevented the flare from appearing showing that it was dependent on the terminal parts of the peripheral nerves. Then attention was paid to the third reaction which follows a heavy stroke, namely the wheal. (Fig. 8.2, *overleaf*) This swollen ridge of skin develops later than the red line and was shown by simple tests to be due directly to increased permeability of the minute vessels and not as a secondary result of fluid leaking out when they became distended. For example, negative pressure applied to the skin does not produce a wheal, and indeed it prevents one from forming. One such test consisted of putting a pressure of 50 mmHg onto the skin. This prevented the vessels from dilating but the wheal still developed.

## The triple response of injured skin and the H substance

It was now established that the full response to a stroke consisted of three associated but independent reactions namely, a local dilatation of the minute vessels, an increase in permeability of their walls and a widespread arteriolar dilatation. To this complex three-fold reaction he gave the name 'triple response'. When this response was explored further he realized that it was not peculiar just to the stimulus of a stroke but that essentially similar reactions could be obtained by many different forms of physical injury such as cutting, burning and freezing. The triple response was in fact a fundamental response of the skin to injury. The question then arose as to whether a common factor could act on the vessel wall in two different ways, and also on the nerve endings in the skin to create the flare. An obvious possibility was the liberation of a substance from the tissues by injury. The idea was tested by pricking histamine into the skin of the arm. It produced the typical triple response and by comparing the natural response with the histamine reaction, especially during circulatory arrest, it could be shown that each part of the triple response was due to an interposed chemical factor. And so from a simple beginning there arose his famous conclusion that injury releases from the tissue cells a factor which he termed 'H substance'. It was so labelled because it was impossible to prove whether or not it actually was histamine. A full account of this work, with a complete list of references, is to be found in Lewis' monograph, *The Blood Vessels of the Human Skin and their Responses.*[172] A later and

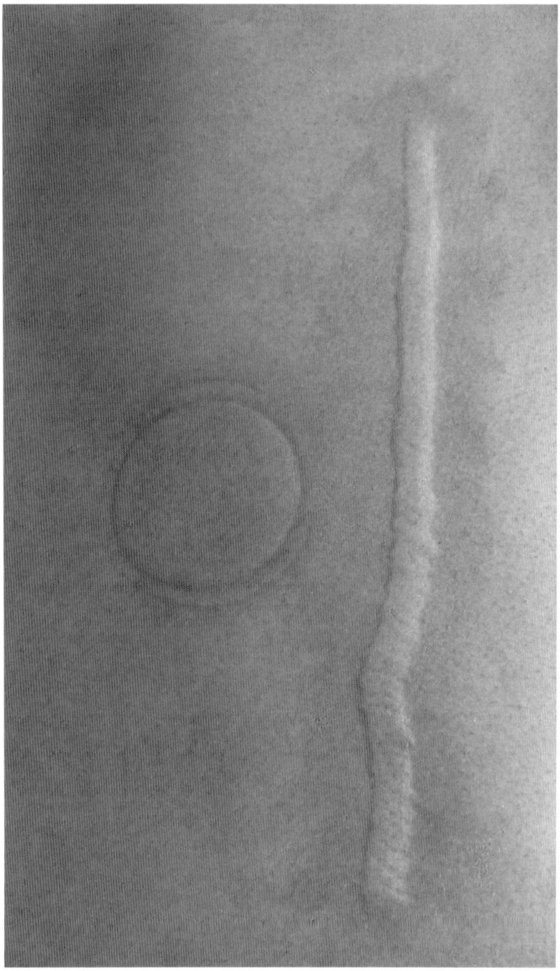

*Figure 8.2 In an urticarial subject a firm stroke has produced a large wheal, but a negative pressure with a suction cup of minus 90 mmHg to its left has not given rise to a wheal. (From reference 172.)*

unanticipated clinical application of the triple response is that it tells whether a neurological lesion is in the spinal cord or posterior root ganglion, or whether it is distal to them.

As a final comment on this work one may ask: Why did he decide to experiment with histamine – a substance that led at once to the right conclusion? The reply to this question is fortunately given by Lewis himself. He wrote that there was a choice of several agents known to produce whealing, including atropine and morphine among others, but he and Grant inclined towards histamine which was known to act in a very high dilution and had been isolated from mammalian tissue. They consulted their MRC colleague Dr Henry Dale, who had done the isolation and he made the same choice. Lewis thought that although the choice of histamine might have been a happy accident, it was not wholly accidental and said that:

> In scientific work the atmosphere often becomes gradually prepared for a given speculation or conclusion; a stage is reached when a conclusion is approaching inevitability, although this cannot always be seen till afterwards; it is only a matter of time and the conclusion will be formed. The truth of this statement is often illustrated by the almost simultaneous statement of the same conclusion by men working independently and providing distinct lines of argument. This was so in the case of histamine; histamine was so to speak in the atmosphere when questions relating to injury were discussed. The work of Dale ... and of Cannon and Bayliss ... was bringing histamine into the foreground of discussion on shock, resulting either from anaphylaxis or wounds.[198]

Henry H. Dale worked at the National Institute for Medical Research – an institute of the Medical Research Council – initially as head of the department of biochemistry and later as director of the institute. (Fig. 8.3) He and his wife Ellen were good friends of the Lewises; they lived near them in Hampstead, and the two wives often met. When Dale received a knighthood in 1932 he replied on behalf of his wife and himself to Lewis' message of congratulation by saying:

> I don't think she will like to be called Lady Dale by friends as dear as you both have become to us. 'H.H.' has been good enough for my intimates since my school days. So I make bold to send love to you and Lorna.
>
> Yours,
> H.H. Dale[354]

Another eight papers on the vascular reactions of the skin to injury followed the two which had delineated the triple response and H substance. They included

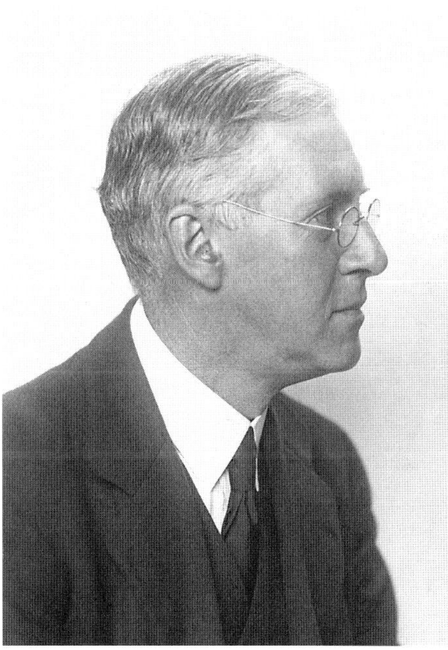

*Figure 8.3 Sir Henry Dale, a valued friend of Lewis who admired his scientific achievements.*

work on the pathology of telangiectases, on annular oedema of the skin, the effects of ultraviolet light, and on an anaphylactic skin reaction. One of his collaborators in 1926 was Dr Yngve Zotterman, a physiologist from Stockholm whose autobiography *Touch, Tickle and Pain*[339] contains only a brief reference to his stay at UCH but who gave me a personal account of it. He said that he enjoyed working with Lewis and that he was not intimidated by him as others were. In addition he found it very pleasant to meet Lady Lewis whom he described as a beautiful woman. Zotterman recollected that Lewis used to arrive each morning with a box of 'Craven A' cigarettes. By tea time they were gone and his assistants would offer him one of theirs. Zotterman smoked Turkish cigarettes but he was soon given to understand that the chief did not like them and that 'Craven A' would be preferred.

## Further work on the H substance and a monograph

Having shown that the triple response was due to the release of a histamine-like substance, Lewis was keen to extend the finding into the formulation of a general law, namely, that every form of injury to the healthy skin calls forth a series of responses dependent upon the same fundamental and natural chemical stimulus. But he felt unable to promote this generalization until he had explained how it was that the skin developed vesicles with herpes zoster when there was no primary injury to the skin. He especially had in mind these instances where herpes occurs with an injury or malignant disease of the spine when he supposed that there was no virus to travel along the nerves and attack the skin directly. We now know that his supposition was wrong – virus is in fact present in the vesicles of such cases. But this led him to show in cat experiments that the well known vasodilatation following antidromic nerve stimulation was due to the release peripherally of a histamine-like substance and therefore to claim that herpes zoster was due to antidromic impulses passing down the sensory nerves.[246] This was an error, arising from a false premise, but it illustrates his determination to try to explain important clinical phenomena and also his willingness to confront problems which would not easily fit into a hypothesis. Grant made a comment on this work:

> I felt his arguments were a bit specious and told him so adding that if I had committed a crime I would like to have you, Sir Thomas, as my advocate. He didn't like it. He disliked the suspicion that he was pushing his argument more than he should be. But he did that on purpose because his policy was that usually you had one hypothesis that works and you should keep it and follow it as long as possible. But in this instance it had begun to fail.[366]

The whole period after the war, of research into the skin, which yielded so much new information occupied only four years and in June 1926 Lewis summarized the experimental side of the work in his Croonian Lectures to the Royal College of Physicians. These were not written up because their content was available in several papers and as we have already noted he never published the same matter twice. By the end of 1926 Lewis had completed his 322-page monograph *The Blood Vessels of the Human Skin and their Responses* (Fig. 8.4) which was published in 1927.[172] It was reviewed in a 1600 word editorial in the *British Medical Journal* signed by Dale. This was unusual as most editorials were anony-

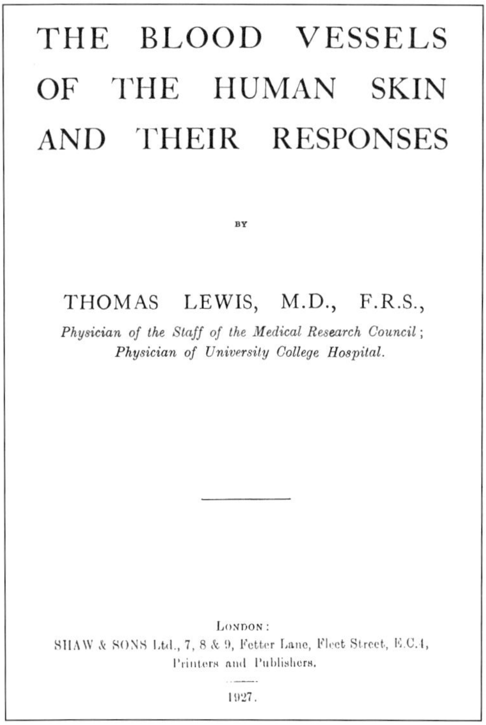

THE BLOOD VESSELS OF THE HUMAN SKIN AND THEIR RESPONSES

BY

THOMAS LEWIS, M.D., F.R.S.,

*Physician of the Staff of the Medical Research Council;*
*Physician of University College Hospital.*

LONDON:
SHAW & SONS Ltd., 7, 8 & 9, Fetter Lane, Fleet Street, E.C.4,
Printers and Publishers.

1927.

*Figure 8.4 The monograph which signalled, in 1927, the beginning of a new era of research, and the end of his work in electrocardiography.*

mous. Dale pointed out that many of the experiments, including some of the most important, used only the simplest technique and could be repeated by anyone, providing they possessed 'the only uncommon item in the equipment – a faculty of keen and accurate observation'.[44]

## The relation of physiology to medicine

In the preface Lewis says that the book has enabled him to present his work in a more connected and readable form than his articles, but adds that the chief motive for writing it was 'a desire to stimulate a wider study and teaching of human physiology; for knowledge relating to the healthy man forms the most manifest and abiding bond between Physiology and Medicine.'

Lewis pointed out that the usual method of teaching physiology by animal experiment meant that most of that knowledge had no application to the students' clinical work and therefore 'much of it rusts and is lost' Furthermore it meant that the student came to the wards with little knowledge of many phenomena manifested by normal humans. This resulted in a failure to apply scientific thought to the practice of medicine. He made a plea for the physiological teacher to use examples of human physiology because those would awaken more interest for the student than animal experiments and would be 'continuously applicable in his life's work'. Of course the response of the human skin being so readily accessible for experiment did provide an especially good example of how work on humans could replace that on animals. But it took a long time for the plea to be more widely accepted and acted upon.

Physiologists, although medically qualified, had little clinical experience and were by nature inclined towards animal studies. Furthermore, according to Dr E.E. Pochin[(2)] they were sceptical of the scientific value of clinical investigation. He said that they regarded the controlled investigation of patients as too complex and loose for reliable analysis, and a waste of the time of competent researchers who would be better occupied in reputable and simpler branches of science. Pochin added that Lewis had written the words 'A Physiological Pearl' above a framed quotation from *Nature,* which was hung on the wall of the laboratory: 'Clinical research is of course of the highest importance for only by contact with it does the clinician learn the importance of physiology'.[305] But it must be said that E.H. Starling was an exception to the remarks. In fact he was invited in 1919 to be a candidate for the new Chair of Medicine at St Thomas's Hospital and declined with some regret.

Lewis' comments in this preface were on a theme about which he had already spoken at length in 1920 to the physiological section of the British Association, at the invitation of its President, Joseph Barcroft, with an address on 'The relation of Physiology to Medicine'.[153] In this he said that physiology, originally the offspring of medicine, had come to confer great and lasting benefits on medicine as a science and also as a healing art. He considered that physiology and medicine had mutual obligations to each other but having once worked in the realm of physiology he now spoke as a clinician and, as he said, with that prejudice he placed the obligations of physiology 'well to the fore'. The first was to teach the student the normal functions of the human body and in doing so to train him as an accurate observer and thinker. 'Students in their most impressionable period would thus learn how to investigate the human body'. The second reason, and it was not a new argument, was that physiology as it was now taught was not sufficiently correlated to medical practice. Doctors did not learn the range of normality in the human being, for example they knew little about the physiology of exercise, and as a result they made errors in their clinical practice. Because physiological teaching was 'not human enough' medical men were not good at assessing the value of evidence when faced with a new problem. His strong desire to promote the teaching of human physiology never left him and 25 years later his last book was *Exercises in Human Physiology (preparatory to clinical work).*[235]

## A new edition of the *Mechanism and Graphic Registration of the Heart Beat*

Research work on the heart had almost come to an end by 1923, with just one paper in each year to 1926, and the new era of studying the vascular reactions of the skin to injury was well under way. But Lewis must have felt the need to signal the completion of a remarkably productive and innovative period of investigation which had commenced 16 years previously, and he did this by producing the third edition of *The Mechanism and Graphic Registration of the Heart Beat.*[168]

Actually the second edition of 1920 would by itself have remained a very useful reference book, but for Lewis only the best was good enough and his tremendous energy and gift for intense concentration enabled him to revise the book remarkably quickly. In August 1924 he wrote to Einthoven, 'I shall shortly have to rewrite the Mechanism book'.[317] By December, which was the date of the preface, not only was it finished but the proof sheets had already been revised by Grant. It was published in 1925, and it is clear that the revision, as with the second edition, took only three months. There were five new chapters, three being on his circus movement work, and one each on parasystole and on the refractory period. Considerable sections of the text were rewritten and it now occupied 447 pages, 62 more than before, with 41 new figures. There were 202 new references and it would be very interesting to know how he kept up with the literature. His correspondence tells us that he was a regular reader of *Archiv fur die gesamte Physiologie* and his knowledge of German and French would have enabled him to read easily the other foreign journals in the College or medical school library, or at the Royal Society of Medicine. Probably he was often sent reprints, and we know that he wrote for them, for example to Einthoven. All his reprints were bound into volumes, year by year, and they are now in the library of the Wellcome Institute for the History of Medicine and constitute a valuable source of material.

As with the previous editions the preface gave him the opportunity to explain the importance in clinical studies of using precise methods of observation. '... it was in my mind, and still is, that clinical pathology, by which I mean the study of disease in living man, suffers both from inexact observation and from hasty conclusion'. He was clearly irritated by the bedside methods which he saw other clinicians using, and teaching with dogmatic assurance, though without any understanding that their methods might be quite unreliable. 'A method depending for its success upon a supposedly unusual sensitiveness of touch or of hearing, is one the clinical scope of which is admittedly limited, the scope of which in science is almost negligible'. Clinical observers did not recognize, he said, that many methods which they regularly employed had no scientific justification. The expedients and opportunisms of the bedside worker were bolstered and preserved by 'urgency – the immediate and daily promptings of the sick' but they littered the path to real knowledge. It was not his desire to advocate the general use of costly and time-robbing laboratory methods but it was definitely his intention 'to emphasize the vital importance of precise methods in progressive studies of disease. It is from this standpoint that the example of electrocardiography is to be stressed'.

The review in *The Lancet* concluded that 'Sir Thomas Lewis' book holds a unique position in the literature of modern cardiology'.[4] And more recently the continuing value of the book has been praised by the distinguished electrocardiographer Dr Mauricio Rosenbaum. Writing in 1981 he referred to Figure 4 which shows the conducting system in the heart of a walrus, 'The first time I saw this illustration it helped me to conceive the idea of the trifascicular nature of the conduction system'. He also commented favourably on Figure 376:

> in which 'overdrive suppression' caused by runs of ventricular ectopic activity and giving rise to Adams – Stokes attacks, is beautifully depicted. This shows again how rewarding it can be to go back to Lewis' book when looking for information and ideas that may still be pertinent and valuable.[309]

## Why Lewis gave up electrocardiographic research

It is necessary to answer the question as to why Lewis stopped doing his electrocardiographic work, which had yielded such excellent results over the previous 14 years[97]. For a start it is important to note that he did not give up clinical cardiology, which he continued to practice, write about and, especially, to teach. But to label Lewis as a specialist in cardiovascular medicine (he disliked the term cardiologist) or as an electrocardiographer is to misunderstand his mission in life. His driving force was that of discovering the mechanism of disease processes by means of experimental research in the human subject. His watchword was clinical science and any aspect of human disease could be a challenge to him. Furthermore he had come to a natural end of his studies on cardiac arrhythmias. In referring to Lewis' simple but conclusive work on muscle pain and nerve paralysis during ischemia, 'using no apparatus more complicated than a blood pressure cuff and a tuning fork' his co-worker with those experiments, George W. Pickering, said, 'This was Lewis at his best, the Lewis who gave up electrocardiography because he grew tired of answering the kind of questions the instrument could answer and who longed for the adventures suggested by his own mind'.[300] However it is fair to add that his great admirer and fellow Welshman, Dr William Evans[(3)] of the London Hospital, did not see it this way. In 1970, after his own long career in studying the electrocardiogram in myocardial disease he wrote:

> Lewis turned his back on Electrocardiography and in so doing he absconded from exploration of the important and expansive field provided by affections of the myocardium. He would have gleaned even a richer harvest in the field of cardiology had he not deviated from the path he had traversed so profitably.[513]

But Dr Evans seems to have overlooked the fact that straightforward observation was not Lewis' idea of progress in medicine. Progress came from using the experimental method.

## Einthoven is awarded the Nobel Prize

During the revision of this edition it was announced that Willem Einthoven had been awarded the Nobel Prize for Physiology or Medicine. (Fig. 8.5) The award was made in recognition of his invention of a new type of string galvanometer and also on the grounds that he had elucidated the mechanism of the electrocardiogram. He was nominated for the prize by Professor H. Burger and others from Amsterdam, and also quite independently by Professor Archibald V. Hill of University College London who had been a Nobel Laureate in 1922, and Hill got Lewis to help him with the proposal. Lewis was obviously delighted with his friend's success and wrote on October 30, 1924 saying:

> The splendid news of your Nobel Prize came this morning and gave me very great pleasure . You have given so much to Physiology and to Medicine that the prize in itself is but a small return; but I rejoice, and there will be many rejoicing with me that your great work has received this public recognition. No award could have given me greater satisfaction than this one. It is very richly merited as the present generation will be quick to recognise and future generations also.[317]

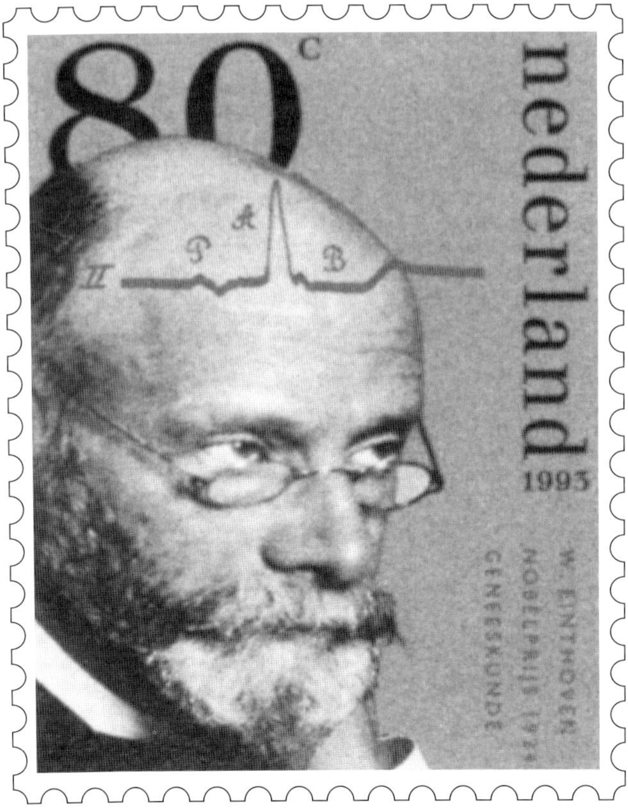


*Figure 8.5 Willem Einthoven depicted on a postage stamp issued by the Dutch Post Office in 1993 as one of three stamps to commemorate Dutch Nobel Prize winners.*

At that time Einthoven was in America (Fig. 8.6, *overleaf*) so his reply was delayed until January 2, 1925 when he wrote:

> Your words have touched me deeply. I owe so much to you. Without your steady and excellent work to which you have devoted a great part of your life there would have been in all probability no question of a Nobel Prize for me. You have given to Medicine at least as much as I have.[317]

When Hill sent in the nomination for Einthoven he combined it with one for Lewis with the intention of making it a joint award. A few weeks after the award, when he was in America he wrote to Lewis and mentioned that he had travelled to New York on the same boat as Einthoven:

> I was very disappointed that the double event didn't come off. I only wish that you could have been in too. We talked about you often on the way over, and he always regards you as 'one of his greatest benefactors'. I think that somebody else may have proposed Einthoven alone – it is only a guess. He doesn't of course know a word about my proposal, nor ever will. Nobody else must know either..[317]

Lewis' chances were probably limited by the fact that Einthoven's award was based not only on his invention of the apparatus but also on his clinical study of

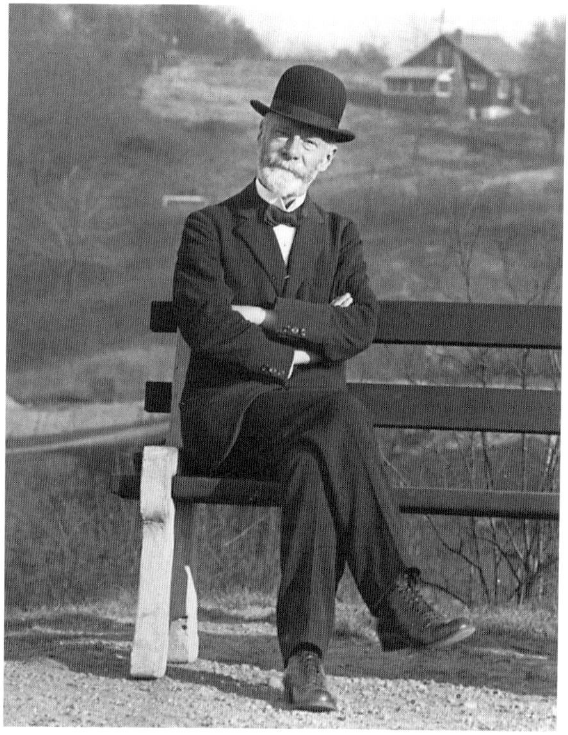

*Figure 8.6 Willem Einthoven, aged 64, photographed at Ann Arbor Michigan by Dr Frank Wilson in October 1924.*

the electrocardiogram, a study which Lewis had notably done so well. Lewis' work was commended by Einthoven in his Nobel Lecture on 'The string galvanometer and the measurement of the action currents of the heart' on December 11,1925 when he said:

> ...until now clinical work on the whole has had at its disposal only experience in electrocardiography of limited duration. The insight into the true nature of the deficiency has been given to us by later investigators. Among them the English investigator Thomas Lewis, who has played a great part in the development of electrocardiography deserves special mention. It is my conviction that the general interest in the ECG would certainly not have risen so high, nowadays, if we had had to do without his work, and I doubt whether without his valuable contributions I should have the privilege of standing before you to day.[315]

Over the next year he and Einthoven exchanged just a few letters, most notably one from Lewis sending him hearty congratulations on being elected a foreign member of the Royal Society of London. We can safely assume that it was Lewis who made the nomination and certainly Einthoven considered it a very great honour, 'I remember that our Leeuwenhoek and our Donders, the greatest physiologists we ever have had, have been proud of the same membership'.[317] There were no more technical questions from Lewis because 'It is some time now since I touched the galvanometer' and Einthoven fell ill in early 1927, dying later that year.[319] Lewis wrote a fine appreciation of Einthoven's life and work in *Heart* pointing out that the many honours he received 'were to him a smaller recompense than was the knowledge of the benefits which his long and arduous work had conferred upon his fellow men'. He would be remembered as 'a man of simple, almost humble, habits, untiring in his devotion to work'. He was greatly admired, said Lewis for 'the charming simplicity and directness of his character' and for the modesty of his thought and manner, his natural courtesy and 'by his unswerving devotion to truth in the most exacting sense'.[173]

## Death of Sir James Mackenzie and Lewis' tribute to him

The first edition of the *Mechanism* had been dedicated to James Mackenzie and Willem Einthoven, 'A token of appreciation of the services which they have rendered to the study of the clinical pathology of heart affections', and soon after the third edition had gone to press Sir James Mackenzie died at the age of 72 on January 26 1925. Lewis was much saddened by this, 'the death of my old friend Mackenzie has filled my thoughts'.[317] It had been Mackenzie who started him on analysing cardiac irregularities, who proposed him as editor of *Heart* and who established the Military Heart Hospital – three of Lewis' chief endeavours. But more than that he gave his younger colleague the inspiration to question tradition and to see where clinical knowledge ends and ignorance begins. 'He was the first authority in clinical medicine on whose lips I frequently heard the words, 'I don't know'.[166]

Mackenzie had a wider view of medicine than Lewis and his years in general practice led to his conviction that it was essential to study the life history of ill health in patients over a long course of years. This, he said, was the only way to assess the significance of symptoms, and it led him to abandon his prestigious career in London at the age of 65 and found the Institute for Clinical Research at St Andrews, Scotland.[74] At the age of 55 he had a myocardial infarction and he then got angina of effort which was severe in his last few years. He was forced to return to the warmer climate of London where he died from a second infarct which came on during the Burns' Night celebration at the Albert Hall in 1926. Acting on his instructions, Dr John Parkinson made a post-mortem examination in the bathroom of his apartment, and sent his heart to Professor David Waterston, the professor of anatomy at St Andrews. Waterston was tardy in producing a report, and six years later Lewis asked if he might examine 'his old friend's heart'.[86] He did this at UCH with R.T. Grant and their detailed study, which is said to have the earliest description of a collateral coronary circulation, formed part of Waterston's article 'Sir James Mackenzie's heart'.[325] Parkinson (later Sir John) had been Mackenzie's chief assistant at the London Hospital from 1913 to 1915 and he was to become one of the world's leading cardiologists. Mackenzie had told him at this time to buy a portable post-mortem set saying how useful such a set was for use in patients' homes, and so it proved to be on this occasion.[86] Lewis wrote a fine In Memoriam notice in *Heart* and the warmth of the wording shows clearly his high appreciation of Mackenzie's work and personality:

> The life of Mackenzie was rich, was full, it was devoted with rare singleness of purpose to his adopted profession. The patient was the lodestone of all his work. Gifted with a vigorous and impressive personality, and possessed of unusual faculties of criticism, he was intolerant of authoritative statement and of traditional

> utterance, combative in argument, yet open to conviction. In him a mind turning incessantly from the known to the unknown, in him a vision ever searching the great veil. In discriminating known from the unknown, his independent mind showed masterly power; in piercing the veil his vision was of unusual keenness. He possessed remarkably the gift of stimulating others; to know him intimately was to imbibe his spirit; his was a rare eagerness to impart knowledge. A warm-hearted man, oft touched by emotion, more often stirred by enthusiasm, cordial, a hard and tireless worker, a shrewd practitioner, whose converse with his fellows was enlightened by a bright and blunt humour he leaves behind him many friends, many admirers, many grateful patients who leaned upon his confidence and his professional skill.[167]

It has been said that much of what Lewis said about Mackenzie could equally well be said about himself, though the sentence about humour would need changing. Although Mackenzie lacked the sharpness of the scientific discipline that characterized Lewis' work he was in some ways a greater man. To have made innovative studies into pain and on the venous pulse and cardiac arrhythmias whilst working in the academic isolation of general practice were remarkable achievements, whilst his clinical experience and judgement were of a high order. He was a wise man who thought deeply about medicine and he displayed his visions of it in two well considered books, *The Basis of Vital Activity* and *The Future of Medicine.*[74,272]

## Controversy over animal experiments and the Dog's Protection Bill

The end of Lewis' electrocardiographic work also meant the end of his experimental work on the dog, which was by far the best animal for making electrocardiograms directly from the heart. These recordings, more properly called electrograms, were absolutely essential for studying the origin and spread of the heart beat. There was no substitute for them. His early experience in Starling's laboratory at University College must have influenced him to turn readily to animal work and he became an expert in experimental technique using also the cat for general haemodynamic studies. But his upbringing in the countryside obviously gave him a love of dogs as domestic friends and as we have already noted he went to great pains to ensure that the dogs in his laboratory were treated with tenderness and consideration. In any case the 1876 Cruelty to Animals Act laid down strict criteria for the regulation of experiments done by those who held an animal licence under that Act. However, as Dr Christopher Lawrence has pointed out in his comprehensive chapter in *Vivisection in Historical Perspective*,[105] 'The 1876 Act had done little to disperse opposition to animal experimentation. Indeed in the first half of the twentieth century, the issue of vivisection remained an important one, capable of mobilising powerful establishment figures or groups to pronounce on it …'. Lewis first became involved in the political issues of animal experiments in 1919 when Sir Frederick Banbury, MP introduced a Dogs' Protection Bill into the House of Commons. This bill proposed that dogs should be exempted from vivisection and when a doctors' amendment to it was defeated in Standing Committee, Lewis at once wrote a long letter to *The Times*. He emphasized that his original work with the electrocardiograph would have been impossible without using the dog, 'by painless experiment on no more than 12 London mongrels'. The complex curves from patients were 'deciphered wholly by experiments on animals: and it was the dog's heart which constituted itself our Rosetta stone'. By analogy he asked his readers to imagine how a clock-repairer would get on if he were forbidden to open the case of a defective clock or see its wheels in motion. '... discoveries are not made by superhuman faculties, but by hard work and common sense. Hinder or stop experiment and you rid the worker of a chief tool'. In Lewis' view this Bill was a retrogressive one brought forward and supported by 'a few ill-informed and prejudiced members of an antiprogressive sect'.[150] Starling also wrote to *The Times* and pointed out the incongruity of prohibiting painless experiments on a few stray dogs when each year 20 000 of them were humanely killed in the Dogs' Home at Battersea. His letter could have been better worded because it was actually illegal to use stray dogs in research. They had to be purchased from a supplier of animals. Lewis got valuable publicity for his view by inviting a journalist from the *Evening Standard* to visit his department when he explained how other animals such as the cat, rabbit, rat and guinea pig were quite unsuitable for his work whilst pigs, goats and sheep could not be housed in the laboratory in healthy conditions. He demonstrated the use of the electrocardiograph and concluded 'we do not want to experiment on animals if we could get the information in any other way. But it is the only way'. This was clearly a very useful visit, and he also wrote an article for the *Daily Mail* receiving the large fee of £52.[526]

Banbury's Bill was defeated in the House but early in 1927 a new Dogs' Protection Bill was put before Parliament which again aimed to prohibit all experiments on dogs. The Bill gained strong support but Lewis was quick to mobilize opposition to it and with others he was able to get the British Medical Association to convene a conference on Research and Animal Experimentation on April 4 at which he delivered a closely reasoned and strongly worded speech entitled 'The Practitioner's Debt to Research'. He pointed out that the dog was indispensable in gaining information about the circulation and also about other organs and systems, and emphasized that this knowledge was essential in the understanding of common symptoms such as palpitation, and in using treatments such as blood transfusion or rectal feeding. 'There is no practitioner in this land who...does not make wholesale use of knowledge won by animal experimentation'. He attacked the National Canine Defence League for their 'persistent and mischievous campaign directed against...the progress of medical science and the well being of the community'. The term 'vivisection', he said, was falsely used to suggest that dissection and cutting operations were done without anaesthesia. The leaders of the anti-vivisectionists were 'men unscrupulous... in their method of presenting a case ...who issue statements which the simplest inquiries prove grossly inaccurate (and) who pervert the meaning of plain words. The torture of animals to which reference is so free exists only in the imagination'. Their campaign, he said, satisfied in some a morbid craving for the gruesome and brought to the misanthropic a belief in the depravity of fellow beings – 'their only stimulant to self esteem'. But its worst feature was to bring mental suffering to the many right minded people who were led to believe in the false statements of cruelty, and the profession had a duty to tell them of the actual facts and to refute 'the flood of abuse'. His speech was printed by the Research Defence Society, of which he was a vice president, as a four page leaflet[522] and later reprinted by them in their journal *The Fight Against Disease.*[105] The Society had been founded in

1908 by the surgeon Stephen Paget to promote the cause of animal experiment. On April 29 the Bill had its second reading in the House of Commons and it was defeated. This was a great success for the profession in which Lewis' advocacy played an important part.

## Notes to Chapter 8

(1) Schack August Steenberg Krogh, 1874–1949, was professor of zoophysiology in the University of Copenhagen. He was awarded the Nobel Prize for physiology or medicine in 1920 for 'A contribution to the physiology of the capillaries', and his monograph, 'The anatomy and physiology of the capillaries' was published in 1922. He was also an authority on gas exchange during respiration.

(2) Eric Edward (Bill) Pochin (later Sir Edward), 1909–1990, was Lewis' house physician in 1935 and became a full time worker in Lewis' department in 1936 with a salary of £300 per year. He succeeded Lewis as the director of the department of clinical research in 1946 and undertook pioneer work in the clinical application of radioisotopes, especially in the treatment of thyroid cancer. He later became a world authority on radiation protection.

(3) William Evans, 1895–1988, was a physician in the cardiac department at the London Hospital from 1936 to 1963 where his senior colleague was Sir John Parkinson. He was also on the staff of the National Heart Hospital. He had an early and keen interest in electrocardiography especially as it related to disease of the myocardium, and he was a pioneer in describing the features of hypertrophic cardiomyopathy, and the heart in Friedrich's Ataxia. He was born in Wales, which he loved and was fluent in the Welsh language. He was proud of the fact that Thomas Lewis was also a Welshman.

# Chapter 9

## Has a myocardial infarction • The Harvey Film • Royal Medal of the Royal Society • Disagreement with W.H. Craib • Presentation volume from his associates

In April 1927 Lewis had a myocardial infarction – the first of three. Although he had very severe pain he did not recognize the nature of his illness and it was only with great difficulty that he was persuaded of the diagnosis, which Drury and Grant state was made by H.M. Marvin of Yale then working with him. (Fig. 9.1) They added, 'curiously enough he was unacquainted with the recent American

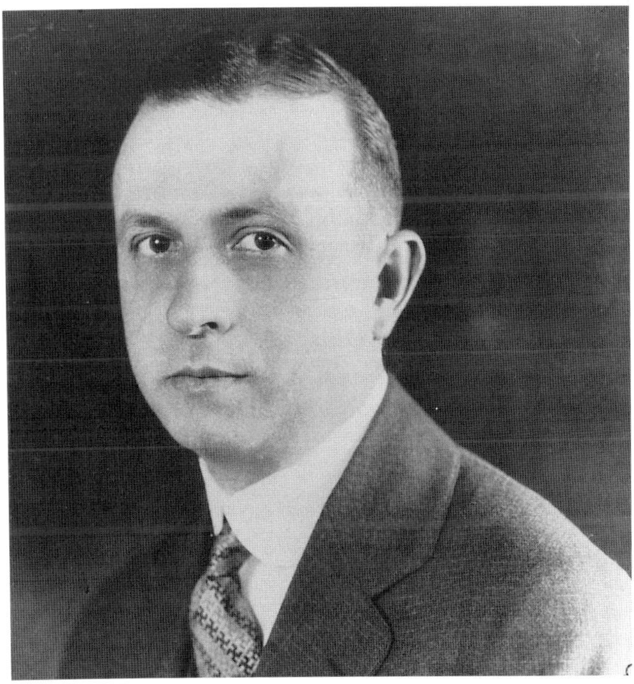

*Figure 9.1 Harold M. Marvin from New Haven did important work with Lewis on the vascular reactions of the skin to injury and was later a first class clinical investigator. He was a great admirer of Lewis and his work.*

work on the clinical diagnosis of this malady'.[50] But T.R. Elliott, who looked after him at his home, denied this in a letter to Drury in 1946:

> Grant has gone rather out of the way in stressing the diagnosis by Marvin of the coronary thrombosis in 1927. Lewis was under my care, and the diagnosis was not certain until I found pericarditis and also blood in the urine. I never had a word with Marvin about it. Then, when Lewis was unwilling to stay in bed, I allowed him to auscultate his own pericarditis. This made him at once obedient, and I assumed he had formed the obvious conclusion as to the diagnosis. To my astonishment some weeks later when convalescence was being discussed, I found that he had not done so. But this was just another example of a doctor's blind spot about his own ailment. He knew the clinical picture as I did.[362,511]

Elliott also said that when Lewis heard the pericardial friction rub he disputed its origin, saying it came from the hairs on his chest, and was only convinced when the hairs were damped down. He added that Lewis went deathly pale and nearly fainted when he did finally realize what the diagnosis was. It is indeed quite likely that Lewis would have discussed the matter with Marvin who was in a good position to give advice because it was in America that the condition had first been properly recognized in 1912 by Dr James B. Herrick.[62]

## Contemporary literature on myocardial infarction and its treatment

In 1919 Herrick wrote a paper 'Thrombosis of the coronary arteries' which contained the first published electrocardiogram of the condition.[75] Lewis has this paper in the references in his *Mechanism* book but significantly it is one of only 14 which are not referred to in the text. Dr John McNee who worked in Elliott's Medical Unit, published an article in the *Quarterly Journal of Medicine* in 1925 on coronary thrombosis describing three cases which he had seen on a visit to Johns Hopkins Hospital in Baltimore.[528] One assumes Lewis would have seen this article but maybe by then he was no longer interested in reading about cardiac conditions. In 1927 John Parkinson and D. Evan Bedford working at the London Hospital wrote a paper ' Successive changes in the electrocardiograms after cardiac infarction (coronary thrombosis)' which they submitted to Lewis for publication in *Heart*.[294] Bedford wrote an account of this:

> When I visited Lewis in 1927 to show him the work J.P. and I had been doing ... he told me that he had not been interested in the ECG lately so that he was not familiar with our records, but nevertheless he asked me some penetrating questions as I expected. He did not seem to know much about cardiac infarction clinically.[505]

Their paper was published in August 1928 so it is probable that Bedford's visit took place after Lewis had his illness. By 1929 there was enough material for S.A. Levine in Boston to write a 173 page paper on the clinical features of coronary thrombosis in which he said it was apparent that Mackenzie 'had not made the clinical diagnosis of coronary thrombosis in his practice'.[107] Even long lasting pain at rest was labelled by Mackenzie as angina pectoris, and probably Lewis did the same. It was only some years later that Lewis wrote that his father had had a coronary thrombosis, and he may well have remembered during his own illness that his symptoms were similar to those he had noted in his father.

He was treated, as was usual at the time, with bed rest for over six weeks and nurses were employed to look after him at home. This long period in bed was what he still recommended in the 1943 edition of *Diseases of the Heart* where he also added that 'the patient is to be guarded by day and night nursing, and helped in every way to avoid voluntary movement or effort'. The regime of prolonged bed rest had been introduced by Joseph Wearn of Boston in 1923, and was universally adopted.[7] It was based on the histology of the condition which indicated that the infarct took several weeks to completely heal, and it was not until 1952 that S.A. Levine introduced a more liberal regime with his advocacy of the armchair treatment of coronary thrombosis. In retrospect it is surprising that so many good physicians never challenged a form of treatment which had been dictated by pathology and not by clinical trial. One assumes that Lewis, as a patient, just went along with the current dogma, especially because it fitted in well with his belief that a damaged heart needed rest. Because he was in bed at home no electrocardiogram could have been taken then, but certainly he did have one made at some time afterwards and the episode was recounted by his technician Edward Bridger who was with him from 1925 to 1935. Bridger said that having made the recording he developed the glass plate and took it whilst still wet from the dark room. Sir Thomas at once asked to see it, held it up to the light, and then hurled it into the waste paper basket where it broke into several pieces. Later Bridger retrieved it and discerned, he thought, evidence of a coronary thrombosis.[348] It is relevant to add here that in January 1928 Marvin wrote to ask whether Lewis would put anything about the coronary T wave into the next edition of *Clinical Electrocardiography* because its absence made his students think it was not the latest edition.[453]

## Recovers well from his illness • Awarded the Royal Medal of the Royal Society

Whilst recovering, Lewis received a letter from Walter Fletcher who wrote to say he was sorry to hear about the illness which he thought was 'the direct result of your intensely hard work ... I doubt whether you ever had a truly physiological holiday ... your present visitation is no doubt intended by Providence to teach you permanent wisdom'.[487] But Lewis was not impressed. 'For heavens sake don't attribute this unfortunate illness to over work which never hurt anybody. I am only sorry that with Drury away it will smash up the output of my department for the year'.[496] That comment shows the priority that Lewis placed on work. Fletcher's reference to holidays was probably influenced by the fact that he had helped Lewis with his bird watching on a visit to the Shetland Islands, with Captain and Mrs S.R. Douglas, in July 1926 and had no doubt been impressed with Lewis' intense application to his hobby.[56] During his convalescence Lewis felt discouraged and he sought the opinion of William S. Thayer, chief of medicine at Johns Hopkins and author of a paper on coronary thrombosis who was briefly in London. Thayer, 'in his rather breezy manner', assured Lewis that he would make a good recovery, as had the 50 or so patients he had seen. Apparently Lewis was neither impressed nor convinced and he asked Thayer for the names and addresses of the patients so that he might write to them and verify Thayer's optimism. It is not known whether he did so but it is likely that the story is true because Grant told it to Edward F. Bland.[506]

He made a full recovery from his infarct but nevertheless he did, though reluctantly, recognize the need for change. He shortened his working day in the department, and considered getting a house in the country, though it was to be six years before he moved from London. He also gave up bird watching but this was largely because the children were growing up and required other hobbies to interest them, and not because of his illness. Almost certainly the best thing he did was to give up his heavy cigarette smoking. As a substitute he ate boiled sweets which he said rotted his teeth away. He also became very fond of chocolates and would beg his wife to hide any box that she had otherwise he would have been tempted to consume the whole lot. During his convalescence he received the excellent news that the Royal Society of London had awarded him their Royal Medal. This medal was instituted in 1825 and the list of distinguished medallists had included Michael Faraday, Humphrey Davy, Joseph Lister and Charles Darwin, and physiologists such as John Burdon-Sanderson, Walter H. Gaskell, Charles S. Sherrington, Archibald V. Hill and Ernest H. Starling, together with Lewis' former chief Sir Victor Horsley.

He returned to work in October, but limited his hours from 10–4. In his five months absence Grant had been in charge of the department because Drury, having been on sick leave for a year with pulmonary tuberculosis, had left to take up a post in Cambridge. In the eight years since the war Drury and Grant had been the only two full time employees of the MRC in the department apart from Lewis. But each year there were between four and six voluntary workers from abroad some of whom stayed for two years. However the most important new

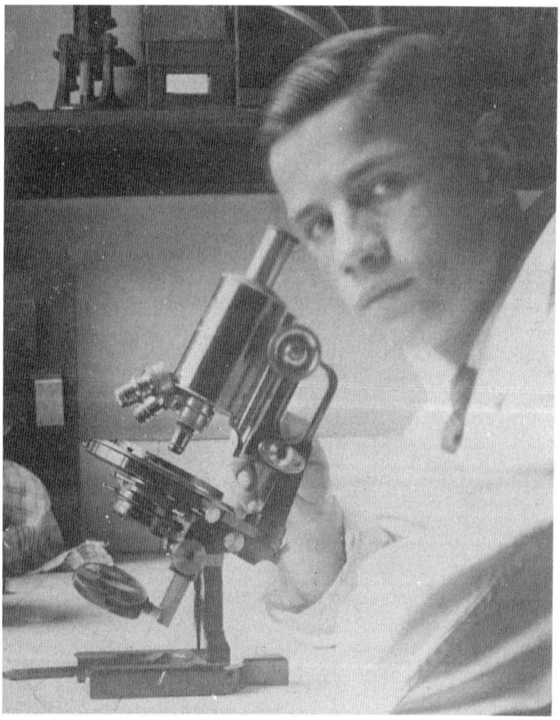

*Figure 9.2 John Honour in 1930 at the age of 18. He became Lewis' personal laboratory assistant and was an indispensable member of the department.*

members of the department during this time were not doctors. Miss Lena M. Searle became his secretary in 1925, and A. John Honour(1) was appointed as a laboratory assistant in 1926. (Fig. 9.2) They both stayed with him until his death 18 years later and became indispensable members of his staff.

Lewis' return to work after his illness did not lead to a resumption of his scientific work. As judged by his publications over the next year he was not now in an active phase of research. Work on the blood vessels of the skin had virtually ended with the publication of his monograph, and he wrote just one more paper on the subject in 1928. His own work on electrocardiography was now finished. So it was probably more an end to previous, very intensive, projects rather than his illness which led to a quiet research period which lasted for over a year.

## A film for the tercentenary of the publication of *De Motu Cordis*

However another enterprise unexpectedly came to hand at the end of 1927 which was of great interest to him. The Royal College of Physicians of London had decided to celebrate in 1928 the tercentenary of the publication of William Harvey's great work *Exercitatio Anatomica de Motu Cordis et Circulatione Sanguinis in Animalibus*. Harvey's discovery of the circulation of the blood, which he had first announced at the College in 1616 at his Lumleian Lecture, had made him their most illustrious Fellow. The president Sir John Rose Bradford, who was also Lewis' senior colleague at UCH, naturally sought his help as the Fellow best qualified to give advice on the scientific side of the project. They met on November 2 and agreed that the programme would consist of a series of demonstrations on the heart and circulation including one in which Henry Dale would repeat Harvey's experiments.[389] But by January 1928 Lewis had changed this concept to suggest that he and Dale should jointly make a cinematograph film which would show many of the experiments which Harvey had described with such originality and conviction in *De Motu Cordis*. This was a very good idea because it would have been impossible to show this wide range of experiments at a live demonstration and it presented the opportunity of providing an enduring visual account of Harvey's scientific thought. Rose Bradford warmly endorsed the project and the College gave £200 to have it made.[347] No doubt Lewis' long experience with photography gave him the stimulus for the film and the Pathé Company was employed to make it. The film, which of course was silent, was produced in an imaginative way. It opened with a portrait of Harvey and then showed his hands being replaced with the similarly dressed hands of a person, in fact Lewis, who proceeded to do the experiments giving the impression that one was seeing the experiments just as Harvey himself would have done them. (Fig. 9.3, *overleaf*) The sequences were linked with passages taken from his book, and the whole effect gave a totally convincing and very fine account of the discovery of the circulation . The Harvey Celebration took place from May 14 to 16 and was attended by an international audience including I.P. Pavlov(2) and A. Samojloff(3) from Russia.[98] It started with a reception by King George V at Buckingham Palace and ended with a banquet at Guildhall. The scientific session occupied two days and was held at University College London. There were demonstrations among others of Starling's heart lung preparation by the

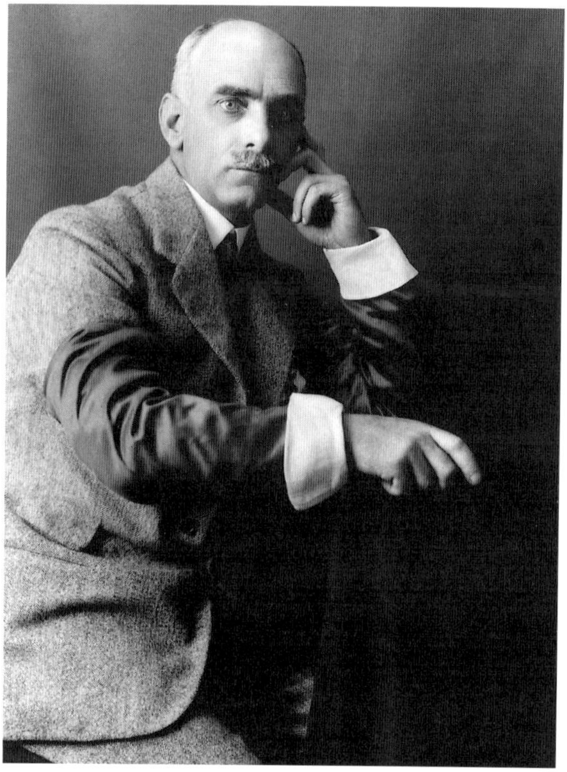

*Figure 9.3 Lewis in 1928 with 17th century type sleeves and cuffs which he wore to simulate Harvey's arms in the Harvey tercentenary film.*

physiology department, of an artificial circulation by Dale, and of reactions of the human skin by Lewis' department. But the outstanding event was Dale and Lewis' film. (Fig. 9.4) The *British Medical Journal* said, 'It was more than dramatic, it was an education in itself'[5]. Most unfortunately a brief illness prevented Lewis from attending, and he received letters of congratulation from the Royal College of Physicians.[533] Sir John Rose Bradford wrote the next day to thank him for 'making the celebration the success it was . On all sides the greatest admiration was expressed for the perfection of the film'. Dr Raymond Crawfurd, the College Registrar, also wrote as follows:

> We were all grieved that you were not present to wear your laurels. The film created a profound impression on us all: I think it may be said to be the crowning feature of an altogether successful Celebration. The foreigners have been immensely impressed by it all.

Luckily Lewis was well enough at the end of the week to attend the Harvey Luncheon of the Physiological Society at Cambridge where he met Samojloff for the first time and renewed his acquaintance with William H. Welch of Johns Hopkins who had invited him to give the Herter Lectures there in 1914.[98,102]

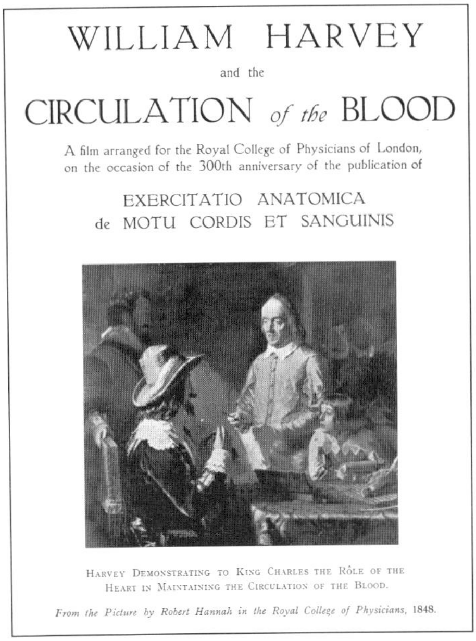
WILLIAM HARVEY

and the

CIRCULATION *of the* BLOOD

A film arranged for the Royal College of Physicians of London, on the occasion of the 300th anniversary of the publication of

EXERCITATIO ANATOMICA
de MOTU CORDIS ET SANGUINIS

HARVEY DEMONSTRATING TO KING CHARLES THE RÔLE OF THE HEART IN MAINTAINING THE CIRCULATION OF THE BLOOD.

*From the Picture by Robert Hannah in the Royal College of Physicians,* 1848.

*Figure 9.4* *The brochure which accompanied the Harvey film.*

Afterwards Lewis noted that the film was in considerable demand from medical schools having 'met with more than expected success' and it was shown too in South Africa, in the United States, and by Lewis in the Royal Palace in Brussels at the request of the Queen of the Belgians. Not surprisingly it was criticized in an antivivisection journal as being of no gain to scientific knowledge, but as Dale pointed out it was they who had suggested that medical students should be taught by film rather than by actual animal experiments.[353] The College which now owned the copyright unwisely allowed it to be shown in public and this led to a question in the House of Commons which nearly led to the discovery that Lewis had done the experiments without the appropriate animal licence. Fortunately Dale's name but not his came up and a potentially awkward affair blew over.[105]

## Appoints W.H. Craib and has a severe disagreement with him

Lewis now had two part-time research workers who had been seconded in 1927 from the Medical Unit where they were assistants to Elliott. One was Kenneth E. Harris who later became a consultant physician at UCH. The other was William H. (Don) Craib[(4)] whose work and story is more important. (Fig. 9.5, *overleaf*) Craib was a physics and mathematics graduate from Cape Town who graduated in medicine in London in 1923. He then went to Johns Hopkins Hospital where Edward P. Carter encouraged him to work with the physicist R. Canfield on

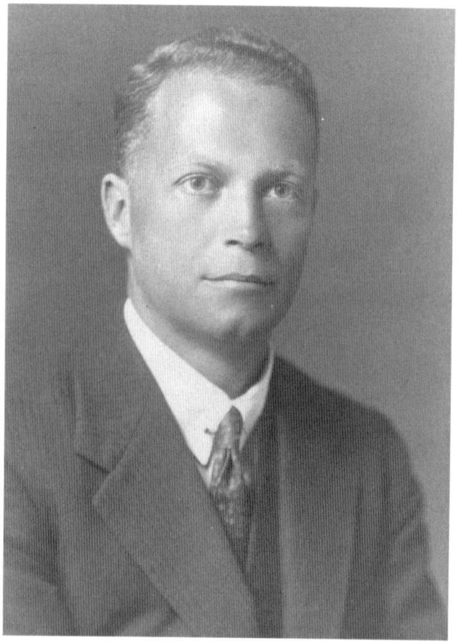

*Figure 9.5 W.H. (Don) Craib who did original work on the genesis of the electrocardiogram.*

myocardial excitation, and he presented this work at the Physiological Congress in Stockholm in 1926 with Einthoven in the chair. Lewis was impressed by Craib's work and invited him to take a post at UCH. Craib's studies showed that the active point of excitation was not a persistently negative one – the old negativity hypothesis was wrong. Instead there was movement along the muscle fibre of an electrical doublet, later to be called a dipole. This doublet hypothesis interested Lewis because it confirmed and extended his own concept of limited potential differences. Together with Einthoven he believed that the cardiac muscle segments constituted separate electrical units.[159]

Craib's experimental work in his department clearly made a deep impression because Lewis offered him a full time MRC post at £700 a year when Drury left. In getting Fletcher's agreement to this he said, 'I have met no young man engaged in medical studies of whom I have thought as highly of as Craib. His work at Johns Hopkins was of outstanding merit'.[497] This was in November 1928 and in July 1929 Craib became the chief assistant in the department. His research was concerned with recording the electrical activity of tissues immersed in a fluid medium and he showed the similarity of potential distribution in the cases of cardiac muscle, somatic muscle and nerve, but this work led to considerable disagreement between him and Lewis and early in 1931 Craib resigned and returned to South Africa, soon after his monograph *The Electrocardiogram* had been published as one of the MRC's special report series.[41]

What went wrong after such a promising start? Craib had an academic grounding in physics and electricity which Lewis lacked and it is quite possible that Lewis could not follow the technical details in Craib's reasoning. Lewis wrote nothing about this but there is anecdotal evidence available. Bridger, who was helping Craib, said that Lewis and Craib used to argue for hours at a time, sometimes every day. The point was reached when, it is said, Lewis forbade Craib to continue his experimental work, perhaps indicating that a different approach which he could more readily understand would be desirable. But Craib got round this by starting his work after Lewis had gone home and Honour remembers finding Craib asleep in the laboratory when he opened it up in the mornings. However it is likely that the friction developed soon after his appointment as chief assistant because there is a revealing comment in a testimonial which Lewis wrote in October 1929 when Craib applied for the post of Professor of Medicine in Sydney, Australia. Having written 'I have met with no senior student who has approached Craib in ability' he goes on to say 'he has been restless under conditions of work here. This restlessness has in my opinion interfered with his output of original work and it has been a source of some anxiety to me. I believe it to have been in large part due to his inability to see a definite and lifetime career suitable for his attainments and ambition in this country'.[392] Craib's own account of all his research activity, both in America and Britain, is recorded in his privately produced book *In Defence of Honour* written some 20 years later, in which he seeks to show that his work had been either neglected, misunderstood or opposed both in America and Europe.[1] Professor Edgar D. (later Lord ) Adrian,[(5)] Lewis and even Einthoven come in for criticism. It is a curious work in which he portrays himself as the defendant in an imaginary court scene with charges being levelled against him, and although written in a humorous style it has a definite streak of paranoia. Raymond Pruitt wrote a good account of the book and of Craib's disputes with Lewis and Adrian.[307] Wilson's well known 'Dipole theory' succeeded the doublet hypothesis, though it was based on a similar concept, and when Wilson was the doyen of electrocardiographers 20 years later he still praised Craib's work.[307] Lewis too had a high regard for Craib who he believed was 'one of the most, if not *the* most promising candidate for a professorship of clinical medicine and research in this country within a space of a few years'.[1] But Craib could not be dissuaded from resigning and although he became professor of medicine in Johannesburg he never returned to electrophysiological research, or did any other research. Thirty years later when aged 87 Craib wrote:

> To have been given semi independent bench space in Sir Thomas' famous laboratory for some four years provided me with the academic highlights of my life. Every step he took in dealing with me was justified, honourable, and in keeping with the dictates of an inflexible conscience; including his final rejection of me as a suitable candidate for further sponsorship by funds available from the Medical Research Council. The fact that Sir Thomas kept me on his staff for as long as he did was just another indication of the magnanimity of the man.[509]

One may well ask whether this episode had any importance. From the scientific point of view the answer might be ' not much', though we have no way of knowing what might have developed if Craib had been allowed to continue working, as he said, 'on vector-electrocardiographic problems, on Lillie's iron wire, and other forbidden projects related to the fundamentals of bioelectricity'.[510] The distinguished American cardiologist Howard Burchell wrote 'my view is that the concept was important (of the dipole) but pales markedly when on stage with the experimental work on accession of excitation in the ventricles…'[507]

Burchell is referring to Lewis' work on the spread of the excitation wave. Craib made a useful contribution to electrocardiography and although it was of less importance than he thought, his story does have its interest if only from the point of view of personal relationships. Later in his life Lewis told his wife that he much regretted his disagreement with Craib.

## Presentation volume from his former associates gives him deep pleasure

By 1929 Lewis had been engaged in full time research for 20 years and during this time a considerable number of men and women had come to work under him. On Christmas Day they presented him with a handsomely bound volume, now in the possession of the Lewis family, which contained a full page signed photograph of each of them, 38 in all. There was a letter to him at the beginning which read as follows:

> We, who address you, are those who up to the present have had the good fortune to work in personal association with you at the Cardiac Department of University College Hospital Medical School, London. We believe you must know, in some measure, how greatly the medical world values your work for the advancement of knowledge. We hope that you know also, in some measure, the great personal regard we ourselves have for you. We have tried severally to express this to you in the past and now, one with another, we unite to send our greetings. Year by year you have worked with one or another of us. You have held before us the desire for knowledge, and have not spared yourself in the search. By teaching and example you have helped us in our work. When you read our names at the end of this letter you will realise that the number of those you have guided is not small. For this guidance and for all the many kindnesses we have received from you, we wish when you look at our photographs, that you may hear us say again 'Thank you, Sir Thomas', each in his own way. We are sure that those who follow us will gladly join in what we say.

Bernard Sutro Oppenheimer, Edmund Perkins Carter, John Parkinson, Thomas F. Cotton, Marcus A. Rothschild, Paul Dudley White, Jonathan Meakins, Harold Feil, William Daniel Stroud, Alan Nigel Drury, Harold Aten Bulger, Constantin C. Iliescu, Alfred M. Wedd, Ronald Thomson Grant, William Nichols Horsfall, William Charles Munley, Antonia Sebastiani, Jaroslav J. Sumbal, Fred M. Smith, Noble Wiley Jones, Herman Blumgart, E. Cowles Andrus, George Raymond Brow, Arthur M. Master, Alfred Kendrew, Iris May Harmer, Maurice Regnier, Kenneth Edwin Harris, Yngve Zottermann, Norman C. Wetzel, James Edwin Wood Jr, Harold Myers Marvin, William Hofmeyr Craib, Thomas Duckett Jones, Imre Haynal, William John Kerr, Louis Eindred Viko, also Elizabeth Pauline Wolf Blitzsten 'Died Jan 30 1929'.

Lewis sent a letter of thanks with the heading 'University College Hospital January 1930.'

> To my associates in cardiovascular work
> on the occasion of the presentation of the album
> of your portraits.

> This gift of all your portraits came as a complete surprise on Christmas day and has given, and will continue to give, me deep pleasure. I am most grateful for the words that are written by you all in it; they are of the kindest. When I look at the pages, one after another, they bring back to me in historical sequence a flood of memories, scientific and personal, amongst the pleasantest of my life. The book makes me feel very fortunate in having been associated with so many devoted workers for medicine and in having found amongst you all, my colleagues in work, so many lasting friends. The book, in its fine binding and with its beautiful inscriptions, will always be to me a most valued possession, to which I shall turn to gather fresh courage and in gratefulness for the experiences of those years when we worked together. Very sincerely yours, Thomas Lewis.

## His associates tell of his help and kindness to them

Although Lewis was a hard taskmaster there is no doubt at all that he was regarded by his younger research associates as someone very special in their affections and respect. This is emphasized in letters he had from them. In 1918 Levine wrote from France to say, 'I can't help but thank you again for the many kindnesses and for the profit I derived by my stay with you',[373] and it is notable that the word kindness often recurs in subsequent letters from others. William Stroud of Philadelphia, writing from Paris on his way home said:[472]

> As it is impossible for me to even attempt to thank you for all your kindness towards me during the last eight months I am not going to try, but I want to be sure that you realize how very grateful I am and that I appreciate with all my heart what you have done for me.
> Ever your sincere and grateful friend William Stroud

In referring to the presentation volume Marvin wrote that he felt the preface to it, 'did not precisely err of the side of warmth and appreciation and graciousness. My own feelings toward you and your great kindness could never be expressed in words so cool and formal'.[454] William J. Kerr from San Francisco wrote on returning home in 1929:

> I was tremendously impressed by your directness and simplicity of approach in the solution of the problem at hand and by the manner in which you cast away the non-essentials and the care with which you persevered in the search for truth.[371]

After a brief visit in 1927 Soma Weiss from Boston wrote, 'In your ideas of medicine I have found a crystallized concept of things of which I have had independently a vague suspicion only. If therefore I should ever be able to act accordingly I will be thankful to you for the stimulus'.[480] In 1930 Eugene Landis spoke of 'my gratitude for the extremely instructive and enjoyable year spent in your laboratory'.[372]

## Notes to Chapter 9

(1) Alfred John Honour, MA, D Phil, 1911–, is an important figure in the history of cardiology. He was Lewis' chief laboratory technician for nearly twenty years and was an indispensable member of the department. Although he was only 15 years old when

appointed he soon learnt how to use the electrocardiograph apparatus, then not an easy task. He assisted Lewis with all his experiments and drew the diagrams and figures for Lewis' papers. He also assisted with the proofs of *Heart* and *Clinical Science.* John Honour was a great help to the research workers in the department, some of whom such as Eugene Landis, Myron Prinzmetal and George Pickering became important figures in medical science. After Lewis' death he worked in Oxford with Sir George Pickering and gained the degree of Doctor of Philosophy for work on arterial thrombi.

(2) Ivan Petrovich Pavlov, 1849–1936, was a world famous Russian physiologist who had done early work on the circulation. His main research was concerned with the physiology of digestion and he is especially remembered for his work on the conditioned reflex.

(3) Alexander Filipovich Samojloff, 1867–1930, was a Russian physiologist working in the University of Kazan. He wrote the first book on electrocardiography, *Electrokardiogramme,* in 1909, and was a close friend of Willem Einthoven.

(4) William (Don) Hofmeyr Craib, 1895–1982, was born in South Africa where he took a degree in mathematics and physics. He served in the British army from 1914–1918 and was awarded the Military Cross and Bar. After graduating in medicine at Guy's Hospital he gained a Rockefeller Scholarship and went to Johns Hopkins Hospital where he studied electrocardiography. His work with Thomas Lewis is recorded in the text. In his later years he was a much respected physician and teacher in South Africa where he received several honorary degrees.

(5) Edgar Douglas Adrian, FRS, later Lord Adrian, 1889–1977, was a distinguished neurophysiologist working in Cambridge. He shared the Nobel Prize for physiology or medicine with CS Sherrington in 1932 for his work on the mechanism of nervous action.

# Chapter 10

## Clinical Science

FROM THE beginning of his earliest research work Lewis had shown a strong attachment to applying the experimental method to clinical problems. This is well shown in work he did in 1906–7 just two years after qualifying when he used a laboratory model and also animal experiments to supplement clinical observations. In a study of the dicrotic pulse he devised a mechanical system with an artificial 'pulse' to show the influence of factors that could not be altered in a human subject.[113] In another study the changes in the pulse in patients with pericardial effusion were reproduced in cats which allowed the haemodynamic features to be more closely analysed.[115] He developed and refined this approach with his work on cardiac arrhythmias where he always strove to show the similarity of a clinical arrhythmia to its experimental counterpart in the dog. One gets the impression that experimental medicine, that is to say the application of scientific methods to medical problems, was something that came naturally to him, though he was the first to acknowledge the inspiration he gained from his teachers Ernest H. Starling and Victor Horsley in this respect.

### Origin and definition of the term Clinical Science

He especially admired the views on clinical research of that fine surgeon Sir James Paget, FRS (1814–1899). In his presidential address to the Clinical Society of London in 1870 Paget had urged its members to show faith in the power of clinical research. He thought there was too great a readiness to reject results which did not accord with beliefs in physiology or pathological anatomy. Some seemed to think, he said, that all knowledge of diseases and their remedies could be deduced from physiology and other sciences. He stated his own view in these words:

> I feel sure that clinical science has as good a claim to the name and rights and self-subsistence of a science as any other department of biology; and that in it are the best means of increasing the knowledge of diseases and their treatment...I am anxious to urge that all our work should be really clinical; all our chief studies among the living; our final appeal in all doubts to what in clinical researches can be discerned...let us still hold that, within our range of study, that alone is true which is proved clinically, and that which is clinically proved needs no other evidence.[292]

Lewis first proposed the adoption from Paget of the name 'clinical science' in an important article, 'Observations on research in medicine: its position and its needs' which he wrote in 1930.[176] In a footnote to this article when it was reprinted in his book *Research in Medicine and other Addresses* he said:

> For twenty-five years ...I have had what is perhaps a unique first-hand experience of the ways of medical research within the walls of a teaching hospital, from the time when there were no facilities or aids worth the name, to more recent times when these have come. Out of this experience, and out of an unusual association with younger workers, there should be something that can usefully be said to help these on their way. What is said is not put down hastily, but is the outcome of long years of experience, thought and discussion; the views are in fact developed from those expressed (*Morning Post*, April 25th, 1914) by myself sixteen years ago.[212]

In the article he emphasized that 'the final use...of almost all medical science is to maintain health and combat disease in mankind'. To this end, he said, it should be recognized 'that there is a fertile science that deals primarily with patients'. To call it experimental medicine would, he thought, link it too strongly with animal experiments, whilst the term 'clinical pathology' – which he had favoured in the past – was now used in connection with laboratory tests and was 'too narrowly fenced around by test tube and needle'. Therefore, he declared, 'It may be termed Clinical Science'.

## The development of clinical research in Britain

By 1929 Lewis' MRC funded department had been in existence for ten years after the war and he had been engaged for nearly 20 years almost wholly in research work arising directly or indirectly out of contact with patients. He had created a branch of medical science unique in Britain and his success was applauded by Sir Walter Morley Fletcher (Fig. 10.1) in the MRC Annual Report for 1926–27 who wrote, 'It is not an exaggeration to say that the output of valuable work from this Centre has constituted the central stream of progress made in this subject anywhere'.[21] But his department was still the only one with a clear commitment to clinical research, in spite of the creation in 1920 of academic professorial units. This was a situation which began to worry Lewis at that time and there can be little doubt that his anxiety was largely the result of his illness. He knew that if he died in the near future there would be no one to carry the banner of Clinical Science which he had hoisted 15 years ago and carried with such determination. His two main collaborators were possible successors, but although Drury was a good leader his interest was more in physiology than medicine, whilst Grant was more an individual worker than a departmental head, and was not an innovator.

Lewis had several conversations with Fletcher about his department and about the position of clinical research in general and he set out his views in a letter to Fletcher on May 31 1929 which are worth quoting at length. His conclusions were as follows:

> 1. That the lack of progress on the clinical side of Medicine (and Surgery) is due chiefly, not to inherent difficulties presented by the subject, but to what has become a traditionally low standard of work and thought from a scientific standpoint.
> 2. This low standard is the direct or indirect outcome of the almost constant association between clinical research work and the opportunistic atmosphere of practical or curative medicine.

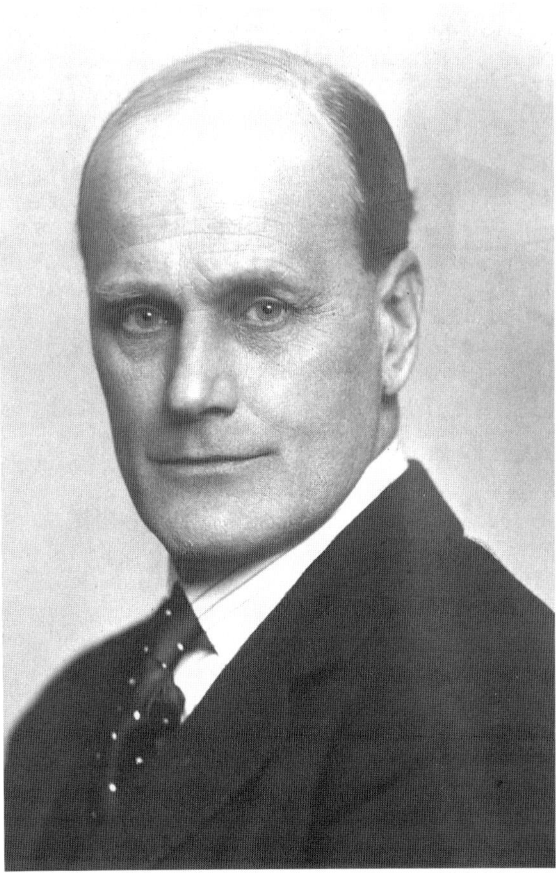

*Figure 10.1 Sir Walter Morley Fletcher, the first Secretary of the Medical Research Council, an outstanding organizer who gave great support to young research workers.*

> 3. To remedy this defect and to create stable conditions for progressive work I believe that it will be necessary for the Medical Research Council sooner or later to develop a department or departments of clinical and experimental work on a broader and sounder basis than at present exists. I have in mind an institute, the atmosphere within which shall not be influenced by the immediate needs of consulting Medicine or Surgery, but shall be derived from the purer sources from which the atmosphere in other institutes (in which the natural sciences are studied) is derived. An institute in which the workers may be free from the distractions presented by the petty and mainly diagnostic problems of diverse and obscure cases, and in which they can settle down to a more profound and uninterrupted study of the natural history of selected diseases.[498]

This was a remarkable exposition of how Lewis viewed the future development of clinical science and being a private letter he was able to indicate very clearly his low opinion of medical practice at the time, at any rate as far as a scientific approach was concerned.

## A research hospital at Cambridge is proposed

It was early in 1929 that The Cambridge Scheme, as Lewis called it, began to develop. Drury was now working in Cambridge under the MRC and had accommodation in the department of pathology whose head was Professor Henry R. Dean. Drury told Lewis it was possible that a department of clinical research might be opened up at Cambridge and, in Lewis' words 'He said that he had related to Professor Dean the dissatisfaction I had long felt with the contemporary position of clinical research and told him that I was prepared to consider a move if it offered a prospect of successful work.'[393] It looks as if Lewis had been thinking about the scheme for some while because on March 26 he wrote to Dean saying that he had come to a definite decision 'that the team would need to be associated with a general hospital and that a separate institute would not do'.[393] The idea was to build research wards on a university site close to Addenbrooke's Hospital so that it would be easy to transfer patients to and from the hospital and the institute. The hospital would contain 'a large selection of clinical material' and its proximity, Dean pointed out, would make it easy to return patients to it if they required treatment for an acute condition such as appendicitis. One can readily understand that the staff of Addenbrooke's might not be too keen to be used as a source of patients for an elite research institute and it seems that there was opposition from them. He was nevertheless offered the Regius Chair of Medicine and the proposal went far enough for him to go to 10 Downing Street to see Mr Stanley Baldwin who was the Chancellor of Cambridge University, as well as being Prime Minister. He told Mr Baldwin of his objections. The facilities were inadequate, the university and examination functions were burdensome, it was not a post for progressive medicine, and the salary of £1200 was too small – it should be not less than £2000. Fletcher was closely involved from the start and it was probably his influence that persuaded Dr Alan Gregg of the Rockefeller Foundation to provide the necessary finance for a new department. It was even envisaged at some stage that Lewis could occupy the Downing Chair of Medicine but the snag was that it was still held, as it had been for 36 years, by Professor John B. Bradbury now in his 90th year. But his death on June 4 removed that obstacle and Fletcher wrote to Lewis, 'Bradbury has died at last'. But the idea of a Cambridge clinical research institute never came to fruition. However it is not difficult to see that it was reborn with the opening of the Clinical Research Centre at Northwick Park Hospital[(1)] in 1970, where the research departments were adjacent to the clinical units of a general hospital. The Centre was originated by Sir Harold Himsworth[(2)] when he was secretary of the MRC. Himsworth had worked in Lewis' department whilst still a medical student in 1931 and became his colleague when he was appointed Professor of Medicine at UCH in 1939 in succession to T.R. Elliott. (Fig. 10.2) Himsworth told me that he had never heard of the Cambridge Scheme, but clearly he was well acquainted with Lewis' ideas.[515]

## The MRC and the promotion of clinical research

Lewis did not get his institute, but his memorandum had the useful effect of getting the Medical Research Council to set up a subcommittee on the 'Future

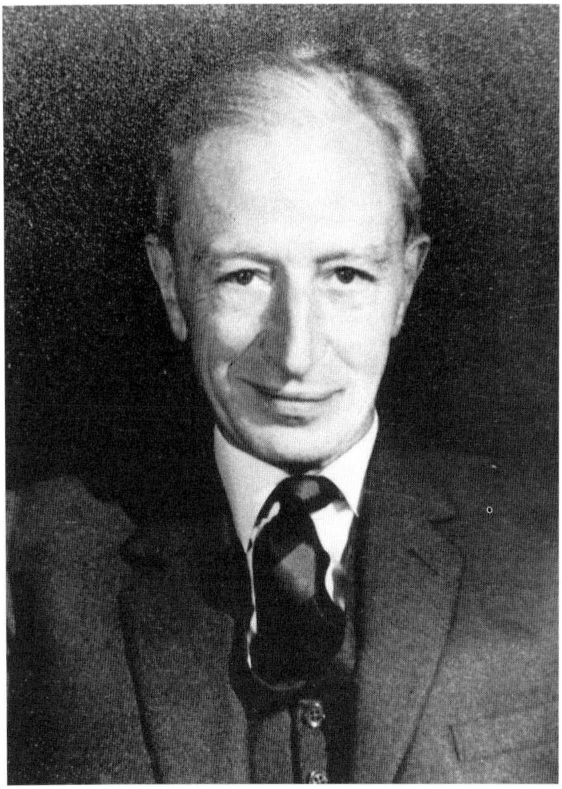

*Figure 10.2* *Sir Harold Himsworth, a pupil of Lewis, who was professor of medicine at UCH, and then the third Secretary of the Medical Research Council.*

Policy for the Promotion of Clinical Research'.[402] Its members, all Fellows of the Royal Society, were T.R. Elliott, Wilfred Trotter, John Parsons and Lewis, and by November 1929 Fletcher had incorporated their views in a long draft which he wrote for inclusion in his next Annual Report. One of the problems they addressed was that of getting able young men to pursue a lifelong career in clinical investigation in 'the present absence of stable positions in which the work may be pursued with proper facilities and with reasonable remuneration'. They did not see that the University clinical units were currently providing 'a field in which original research can be most effectively pursued or recruits to its service be most effectively trained'. But in spite of having limited financial resources it was their hope 'to be able in the near future to provide more than one purely research unit of the kind they now support under Sir Thomas Lewis'.[22] Among other important points the report raised the question as to whether there actually was a science of experimental medicine with research work done on patients, or whether scientific work by clinicians was just the application by them of scientific results worked out elsewhere in the laboratory and delivered to them for use.[320]

## Fletcher angered over an article by Lewis

*The Lancet* gave a warm welcome to the Council's 'masterly report' in a three column editorial on March 15 1930.[8] But on the same day, the *British Medical Journal* gave less than a column to the MRC report.[6] Most of its editorial was taken up with discussing an article by Lewis in that same issue of the journal on 'Observations on research in medicine: its position and its needs'[176] which of course covered much the same ground as the MRC report. Fletcher was angry that his Council's report had been largely upstaged by Lewis' article and he was even more upset that Lewis, in his article, had not even mentioned the MRC which had supported him and his department for the previous 14 years. Fletcher wrote a letter to Elliott, which he actually never sent, complaining of 'Lewis' touchiness and manners' adding that 'he has the discourtesy of carefully avoiding any reference to his service under the Council'.[488] This episode probably reminded Fletcher of the similar one in 1919 when he had complained that the MRC had not been properly acknowledged in *The Soldier's Heart and the Effort Syndrome*. But it turned out that it was an error on the part of the *Journal's* editor Dr Norman G. Horner that had led to the article being published on that day. Lewis had written three months previously saying it was undesirable from the MRC's point of view for his paper to appear before their Report had been commented on. Horner apologized saying, 'I was horrified when you telephoned me on Friday as the last thing in the world I wanted to do was to let you down'.[369]

## Research in medicine • Lewis' article and the views of others

Lewis' paper generated a good correspondence which is still of value for those studying the earlier history of clinical research.[31] Dr John A. Ryle agreed with Lewis' main thesis that it was impossible to successfully combine the practice of curative medicine with experimental clinical research but he took Lewis to task for saying that the research physician must be largely relieved of the onus of diagnosis and treatment. 'Without considerable and constant solicitude for the patient there can be no deep understanding of disease'. He also doubted whether Lewis' approach 'of study by a precise physical method' could be applied to other systems in the body, 'At the moment there is little indication that other morbid functions can be approached in so separate a manner and by methods so precise as those which have been employed in the study of normal and abnormal cardiac rhythm'.[311] Ryle, who was then a physician at Guy's Hospital, later became professor of physic at Cambridge and afterwards was professor of social medicine at Oxford; but in 1930 his view of the applicability of clinical science was too pessimistic.

Dr Robert Hutchison welcomed the experimental method of investigation, but he spoke up for the observational method of the clinician who was, he said, 'the field naturalist of medicine'. Like Ryle he was unhappy about Lewis' comment that the research physician should not allow 'solicitude for his patients to preoccupy his mind', and hoped that he would in fact do just that. 'We cannot really treat patients in a ward as the physiologist does rabbits in a laboratory'.[90] But the opposite and interesting point had been made by Ryle, whose letter appeared in the same issue, when he quoted Ivan Pavlov's work on conditioned reflexes saying that the experiments would have been useless had not Pavlov exercised the greatest solicitude in the handling of his dogs, treating them with care and affection. Dr Helen M.M. Mackay, a clinical research worker, asked Lewis whether he really meant to imply that a training in research rendered a man less fitted for diagnosis and treatment, 'for no hospital would appoint a 'research physician' in such circumstances'.[263] She went on to emphasize, as Lewis himself often did, that the financial barricades which at present closed the road to clinical research to all but the very few must be removed by the provision of adequately paid posts with security of tenure. The danger of using Lewis' 'exact methods', wrote Dr I. Harris from Liverpool, was that only a fraction of a complicated problem might be worked out, leaving great gaps to be filled by arbitrary assumptions. To illustrate his point he criticized the circus theory which did, he said, explain the excitation waves, 'but as soon as an attempt is made to fit in this theory to the broad clinical features of fibrillation it becomes an absurdity'.[72] Lewis drafted a reply to this correspondence on which there is a hand written note, 'Idea of replying abandoned when correspondence ended. Used in part in the Huxley lecture.'[394] In the draft reply it was probably typical of him not to yield to any of the criticisms, though he did offer an explanation of the most serious one, concerning solicitude for the patient. He said that by this he meant that the research worker need not feel he had to deal with a patient's problem which was unconnected with the disease being studied. Nor need he for example hesitate to withhold a drug in order to study its effects. But withholding a possibly useful drug 'is not easily defensible' and this meant that the researcher was not therefore preoccupied by solicitude for his patient. He also denied he had said that the research physician must be relieved of responsibility for diagnosis and treatment. He meant, he said, *general* diagnosis and *general* treatment 'a wholly different matter'. It has to be said that the replies in his draft are not too convincing.

## The scope of clinical science • The Harveian Oration and the Huxley Lecture

The scope and content of Clinical Science was further developed and explained by Lewis in his Harveian Oration at the Royal College of Physicians in October 1933 (183) and in his Huxley Lecture at Birmingham in March 1935.[203] He defined clinical science as:

> the branch of knowledge that centres upon diseased human beings, but which also includes directly relevant parts of the allied sciences. The central field of work is the human patient; and this will remain the field peculiar to the science. But work will often extend to more distant boundaries; these will include human physiology, because the normal is the control to the diseased man; will include the morbid anatomy and the bacteriology of man; and will include 'experimental medicine', which has come especially to mean such experiment upon the lower animals as is inspired by clinical problems.[203]

Lewis stated that clinical science was not the same thing as the clinical practice of medicine and surgery and he maintained that there was a distinction between the science and art of medicine which should be kept 'as separate directions of human endeavour, in working to practical ends'.[203] He conceded however that the science and the art could be practised by the same person. Our knowledge of medicine, according to him, rested on a tripod the three limbs of which were each essential to the stability of the superstructure. These limbs comprised studies of living men in health and disease, studies of dead men, and studies on animals, and clinical science embraced all three but 'its central and unique province concerns living men'. Clinical science he maintained 'has also the long established right to wander unimpeded into any branch of medical science in search of information directly relevant to the problems of human disease'.[192] So, for example, it was in his view essential that the clinician should undertake pathological studies and not leave them to a 'skilled deputy' who lacked the opportunity and inspiration to correlate function and structure. Similarly the necessary information from animal studies should not be left to the physiologist. He identified the scope of clinical science as follows, 'Work belonging to it exclusively is any such relating to the identification of disease, to its cause, mechanism, diagnosis or management, which is undertaken on man himself'.[192] Looking ahead, he envisaged that there would be university departments of clinical science with a professor in charge who would be appointed primarily for his distinction in his science, rather than for his expertise as a practising doctor, but he made it clear that the patients on whom investigations were undertaken must be the full clinical responsibility of the research worker 'experience has shown that this policy is alone practicable'.

## The Medical Research Society is founded

All this was very much for the future and in 1930 there was first of all the need to get clinical science off the ground and widely established as a going concern. The most important initial step was to gather together the few full time research workers in Britain and provide them with a forum for discussion. Lewis did this by founding the Medical Research Society. The objects of the Society in his view were to provide regular meetings whose business was to promote progressive medicine especially on humans or else directly related to disease in man. It would enable the members to get to know each other and each others work and unite in a common purpose of lifting work in medicine to a higher plane. The Society would be able to encourage original work by informal, critical and helpful discussion. It was, he said, most important that the ideal of truly original and new work should be steadily maintained. Communications that were not original would be quietly but steadily discouraged, but this would take time and patience was required. However there was no doubt in his mind that if the right atmosphere was created the Society would come to be the place where new work was assessed and would have the same relation to medicine as did the Physiological Society to physiology. The formal decision was taken by himself with Professors Thomas R. Elliott, Francis R. Fraser, Edward Mellanby and Ernest Verney when they met at his house on May 18 1930. They invited a further 20 to become members and Lewis chaired the first scientific meeting which was held at UCH Medical School on October 24, and at which Pickering gave the first Demonstration. Membership was open to anyone who engaged in or directed research, but if the person was in private practice he was permitted only associate membership. This reflected

Lewis' belief that it was only full time workers namely those 'who are prepared to devote their lives to the study of disease without forethought of practice' who could build up and maintain the prestige of clinical science which 'those engaged in the busy routine of daily practice cannot hope to accomplish'.[182] There had been a problem over the name of the society when Fletcher, having been asked his opinion, consulted the Treasury Solicitor who said that the name was too similar to that of the MRC. A possible alternative was 'Clinical Research Society' but Fletcher said that clinical research was a phrase 'prostituted by custom' to routine work of a kind done typically by the Clinical Research Association. Eventually Lewis wrote to Fletcher with the appeal, 'the very suggestion of altering the name awakens in me a feeling of consternation and I sincerely hope you will not press the matter'.[397] The Society became invaluable for the younger research workers to present their work and to have it properly understood and discussed. (Fig. 10.3) In 1932 it had 28 members and nine associate members, and Grant was the secretary. By 1940 it had grown to 55 members with 15 associates. Lewis was naturally always looked up to with respect and admiration as the father figure of the Society, and indeed his concept of it was a vital contribution to the progress and development of scientific medicine in Britain. At its 50th anniversary the Society had about 1000 members and its history was recalled by Professor Raymond Hoffenberg,[77] Sir Edward Pochin,[306] and Sir Robert Aitken.[2]

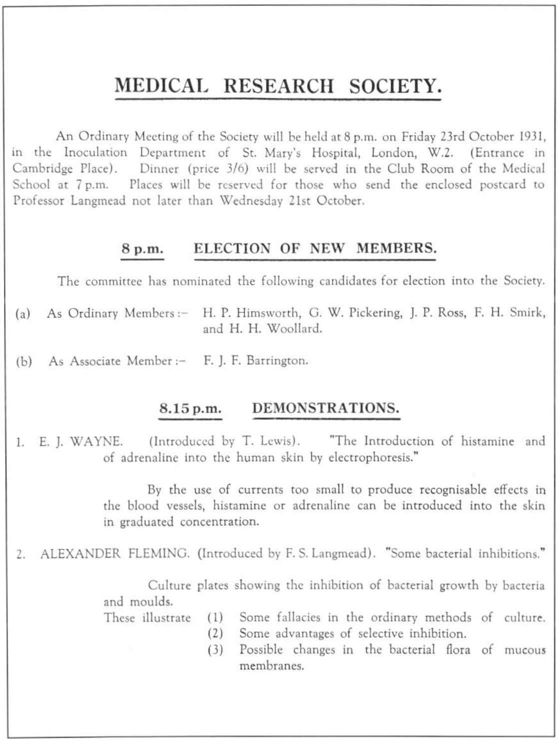

**MEDICAL RESEARCH SOCIETY.**

An Ordinary Meeting of the Society will be held at 8 p.m. on Friday 23rd October 1931, in the Inoculation Department of St. Mary's Hospital, London, W.2. (Entrance in Cambridge Place). Dinner (price 3/6) will be served in the Club Room of the Medical School at 7 p.m. Places will be reserved for those who send the enclosed postcard to Professor Langmead not later than Wednesday 21st October.

**8 p.m. ELECTION OF NEW MEMBERS.**

The committee has nominated the following candidates for election into the Society.

(a) As Ordinary Members :– H. P. Himsworth, G. W. Pickering, J. P. Ross, F. H. Smirk, and H. H. Woollard.

(b) As Associate Member :– F. J. F. Barrington.

**8.15 p.m. DEMONSTRATIONS.**

1. E. J. WAYNE. (Introduced by T. Lewis). "The Introduction of histamine and of adrenaline into the human skin by electrophoresis."

   By the use of currents too small to produce recognisable effects in the blood vessels, histamine or adrenaline can be introduced into the skin in graduated concentration.

2. ALEXANDER FLEMING. (Introduced by F. S. Langmead). "Some bacterial inhibitions."

   Culture plates showing the inhibition of bacterial growth by bacteria and moulds.
   These illustrate (1) Some fallacies in the ordinary methods of culture.
   (2) Some advantages of selective inhibition.
   (3) Possible changes in the bacterial flora of mucous membranes.

*Figure 10.3 The notice of the third meeting of the Medical Research Society. Having discovered penicillin three years before, Fleming was now using it as an aid to isolating some strains of bacteria in the laboratory.*

## Posts for young research workers

In 1930 there were in fact few young men or women in medical research, though the professorial units did provide a limited number of posts. So Lewis recommended to the MRC that it should create up to three posts in his department with a duration of one year for young workers to have, so to speak, an apprenticeship in full time research. However this idea seems not to have been implemented until 1936 when ten such posts, tenable anywhere in Britain for one to two years, were established. Oddly this met with opposition from one of Lewis' own students, Hugh Sinclair, later a noted nutritionist, who wrote to *The Lancet* over the pseudonym 'Peter Shaw' saying that the £3000 a year would be better spent on creating a few full time posts for workers of high merit who were currently unable to find such a post.[313]

## The journal *Clinical Science* is founded

There was yet another move by Lewis to promote clinical science and have it treated 'on precisely the same basis as the allied sciences physiology and pathology are treated', and this was to provide it with a journal of its own. In America the *Journal of Experimental Medicine* had been published for over 30 years and the *Journal of Clinical Investigation* for six years but there was still no British

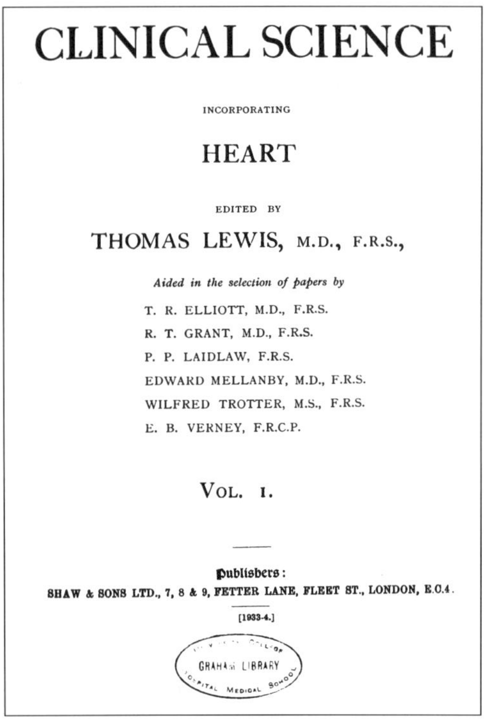
CLINICAL SCIENCE

INCORPORATING

HEART

EDITED BY

THOMAS LEWIS, M.D., F.R.S.,

*Aided in the selection of papers by*

T. R. ELLIOTT, M.D., F.R.S.
R. T. GRANT, M.D., F.R.S.
P. P. LAIDLAW, F.R.S.
EDWARD MELLANBY, M.D., F.R.S.
WILFRED TROTTER, M.S., F.R.S.
E. B. VERNEY, F.R.C.P.

VOL. I.

Publishers:
SHAW & SONS LTD., 7, 8 & 9, FETTER LANE, FLEET ST., LONDON, E.C.4.

[1933-4.]

*Figure 10.4 Title page of the first volume, in 1933, of* Clinical Science.

journal primarily concerned with clinical research. Lewis solved the problem in 1932 by the simple expedient of changing his journal *Heart* into *Clinical Science*, with the subtitle '*incorporating Heart*', and he continued as its editor for the next 13 years. (Fig. 10.4) The journal was owned and published by Shaw and Sons, and their admiration for Lewis and his work no doubt made the transition an easy one in spite of their financial responsibility. Eventually in 1947, after a transition period, ownership of *Clinical Science* passed into the hands of the Medical Research Society with the assistance of the Faust Fund and the Nuffield Foundation. The authority to appoint the editor changed in 1938 from the MRC to the Society.

## The Rockefeller Foundation funds Lewis' post

Yet another change was made now and this concerned the future of Lewis' department which was situated at University College Hospital and its Medical School because of the fact that Lewis was on their staff. He obviously wanted the department to continue there after he retired or died and in 1930 the hospital proposed to the MRC that the department should be permanently associated with them and the school. This was achieved by a generous donation of £48 000 from the Rockefeller Foundation in 1932 which endowed the post of director and freed it from MRC funding.[357] Lewis resigned from his hospital posts as consulting physician and physician in charge of the Cardiographic Department and became their first director of the hospital's Department of Clinical Research. It became in fact a joint department with the MRC because the Council still funded the assistants, laboratory attendants and the running costs.

## Lewis praises the MRC and Fletcher's skill as secretary

On June 10 1932 Lewis sent a letter to Fletcher some of which is worth quoting in full because he expresses in it his admiration of the Council's work. It will be remembered that Lewis never knew of Fletcher's acid comments in the letter to Elliott two years before, so this letter is in no sense a reply to them:

> Dear Fletcher,
>
> In replying to your kind letter of June 8th, I would like to avail myself of this opportunity of more formally expressing my gratitude to the Council for the opportunities it has provided me with during the 16 years of my full time service, and of repeating what I said to you in conversation, that it has been for me a time of happy relations with the Council and with all my colleagues. The Council will also I trust welcome from me a brief statement conveying my appreciation of what, so it seems to me, it has done for its workers.
>
> May I say that in my view the Council (or Committee as it then was) within a short time of its institution, and remarkably, established in the minds of its workers a feeling of real security that they were free to pursue their work without other cares. With many of my colleagues I have felt it an inestimable advantage to know that during our working years the Council has been constantly alive to, and endeavouring to guard, our personal interests, and has encouraged us to pursue in our own way such investigations as we have felt moved to pursue. I know of no

> other public service in which such security is felt or in which such freedom from direction and restraint is enjoyed. I regard the acute foresight which from the start recognised this security and freedom to be essential, as having been a main factor that has brought conspicuous success to the work of the Council's many departments. At the same time it has been impossible to work for the Council without knowing that it has its workers' efforts under constant, sympathetic, and encouraging survey; thus creating a most desirable atmosphere and cordial relationships.[500]

Fletcher wrote to say that the Council were gratified by his letter which had been read out to them. Much of the credit was due to Fletcher himself and Lewis made this known in a further letter to him:

> In speaking of the happy relations I have always enjoyed with the Council and of the conditions of work under the Council I fully appreciate that you have been chiefly responsible for both these relations and conditions and that with other workers I not only feel personally grateful but recognise that it is to your foresight and skill in guiding the Council that the conditions and opportunities for research in Medicine in this country have come to be what they are.[501]

## Sir Walter Morley Fletcher dies in 1933

It was a happy chance that Lewis' resignation came at this time because it enabled him to give warm thanks and appreciation to Fletcher who tragically died the following year from a cerebral abscess at the age of 60. Whilst the two men had had their differences these letters show the high regard that Lewis had for Fletcher's work, whilst Fletcher was certainly a great admirer of Lewis' research. Henry Dale wrote a splendidly warm tribute to Fletcher in *The Lancet* which ended 'To every worker in medical research he was a friend and a champion'.[45] The obituary in *Munk's Roll* was a bit more critical. 'In Fletcher, a rare blend of administrative skill and scientific foresight enabled missionary fervour for the cause of medical research to achieve the best possible results. This same fervour was responsible, too, for the less attractive aspects of his character – ruthlessness towards opponents and the bestowal of unsought advice on associates'.[13] Fletcher was succeeded by Professor (later Sir Edward) Mellanby, with whom, as judged by the files of the MRC, Lewis had much less correspondence. The development of clinical science in Britain, and of clinical research in general, have been excellently reviewed by Sir Christopher Booth.[(3),20–22]

## Notes to Chapter 10

(1) The Clinical Research Centre of the Medical Research Council was established so that an adequate concentration of clinical and para-clinical research groups could be together on one site. It was decided to place it in the new district general hospital at Northwick Park on the outskirts of London, in order to further the aim that it should largely study diseases which occurred in a community hospital and not to serve as a tertiary referral centre. The centre opened in 1970. Much of the early planning was done by the director-designate, Professor John Squire, a former house physician to Sir Thomas Lewis who died at the age of 52 in 1966.

(2) Harold Percival Himsworth, (later Sir Harold) FRS, 1905–1993, succeeded TR Elliott in 1939 as professor of medicine and director of the medical unit at UCH. He had a brilliant research career, with especial interests in diabetes and liver disease. At the age of 44 he became secretary to the Medical Research Council which he served with conspicuous success for 19 years. The inspiration for founding the Clinical Research Centre came from himself.

(3) Sir Christopher Charles Booth, 1924– , is Harveian Librarian at the Royal College of Physicians of London. He is an acclaimed medical historian and has written widely on the history of clinical research. Formerly he was professor of medicine at the Royal Postgraduate Medical School, London, and director of the Clinical Research Centre at Northwick Park.

# Chapter 11

## Cold and the skin • Cold urticaria and haemoglobinuria • Acrocyanosis • Raynaud's disease

QUITE OFTEN Lewis would get started on a line of research by making a chance observation on a patient, or sometimes on himself as happened for example when he noticed his hands became swollen after pulling weeds out of a stream. He recommended this approach to the junior members of the Medical Research Society. Take, he said, an interesting looking sign or symptom; find out how you can elicit it at will, especially under varying conditions and then consider what this tells you about the physiological mechanism of its production. Then pursue this mechanism as far as you can by human experiments and if need be on animals.[2]

This seems to have been the way, or at any rate one of the ways, in which he became interested in the effect of cold on the skin. His work on the triple response had naturally led his colleagues to refer patients with similar problems to him, and in this instance it was a girl aged 11 who got urticaria in the cold. She also had episodes of haemoglobinuria.[73] By injecting the patient's serum into the skin of other subjects he showed that there was a circulating dermolysin. The dermolysin increased the permeability of the cells in the skin causing urticaria whilst a circulating haemolysin did the same thing to the red cells causing them to discharge their contents. Lewis was pleased at being able to demonstrate the same mechanism both in the blood and in the skin. It was appropriate that his research assistant in the study was Dr J.M. Vaughan (later Dame Janet) who subsequently had a distinguished career as a haematologist. His testimonial for her when she applied for another post said, 'In some work we undertook together I was greatly impressed by the admirable caution of her conclusions. She is a lady in every sense of the word and most tactful and kind in her relations with patients and colleagues'.[395]

## Mechanism of acrocyanosis identified

Another patient, this time a woman of 45, was referred to him by T.R. Elliott because she had noticed with the onset of winter that her hands became deeply blue in colour when exposed to the cold. She had acrocyanosis and Lewis set about investigating the vascular mechanism of this condition, about which practically nothing was known at the time. He did this with Dr Eugene M. Landis

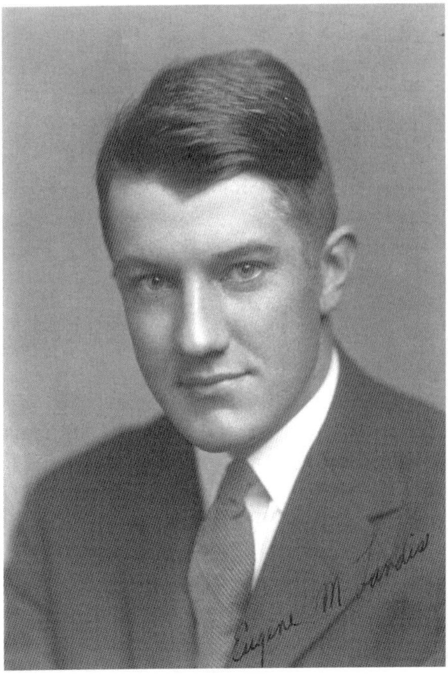

*Figure 11.1 Eugene M. Landis of Boston worked with Lewis in 1930–31 and the two men kept up a friendly correspondence for the next twelve years.*

(Fig. 11.1) from Boston who was later an authority on renal disease and on the physiology of the circulation especially the blood capillaries, being like Lewis both a clinician and a physiologist. The possibility that the cyanosis was due to venous spasm was very simply disposed of by showing that the hand became pale when it was elevated. Blood had drained out of the capillaries and this could not have happened if the venules were obstructed. Arteriolar spasm was likely because a local area of cyanotic skin could be made red by friction or heat, and especially by pricking histamine into the skin. Landis made a very elegant contribution using his technique of measuring capillary pressure with a micropipette. With this method he was able to show that blood flowed into the capillaries much slower in the patient than in a normal control. Together they were able to conclude that acrocyanosis was due to spasm of the arterioles leading to diminished blood flow in the skin. It is of note that Lewis felt confident enough from this study of only one patient to define the vascular abnormality in acrocyanosis – though he did say 'assuming the present case to be representative of this malady'.[244]

## Standard colours for use in vascular reactions of the skin

For several years Lewis had used a series of standard colours in order to allow a given skin colour to be recorded so that it might be compared with ones seen later, and he now published an account of them, chiefly with the idea of telling other workers how to make their own series. The method consisted of matching a skin colour with an oil paint, and it was essential to place this directly on the subject's skin. First a basal colour was made which was that of the bloodless skin and the problem of varying skin pigment was overcome by using only blue-eyed individuals. Then a bright red colour and an extreme cyanotic colour were matched and used as the end colours of the series. These were obtained from warm hands, with the flush of reactive hyperaemia and with venous congestion respectively. By mixing the end colours in different proportions, nine intermediate colours were obtained, giving eleven in the full series, and these were placed on celluloid strips where they remained unaltered and serviceable for years. Lewis was a good artist who knew his pigments well. To get the eleven colours he used varying amounts of scarlet, vermilion, crimson lake, indian red and Leitch's blue mixed with the basal colour which was flake white with raw umber, yellow ochre and Naples yellow. The article had a colour plate which 'after repeated attempts have brought the tints close to the originals', but even so he found that the reds were not quite right and the plate was not recommended for use in practice.[175]

## Dr George Pickering joins the department

It was around this time, in fact in December 1929, that George W. Pickering[(1)] then aged 25 joined the department. He was to become one of the best known figures in British medicine, a torch bearer for clinical science, and a world authority on hypertension. (Fig. 11.2) It was an appointment that was to be almost as import-

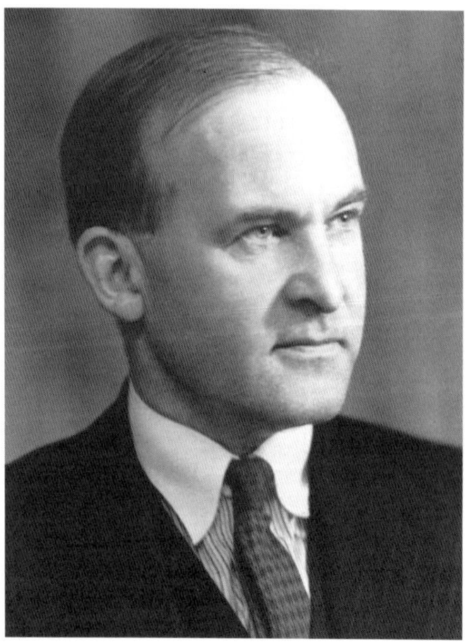

*Figure 11.2 G.W. Pickering (later Sir George) worked with Lewis for 11 years and became his closest friend.*

ant to Lewis as it was to himself, because Pickering became not only a close associate but also one of his few close friends. Pickering recounted how it happened in an issue of the *UCH Magazine* in 1955 for which I obtained personal reminiscences, on the tenth anniversary of Lewis' death, from several of his co-workers. Whilst a physiology student at Cambridge he had come to admire Lewis' work on the heart and then learnt with surprise that he was also the author of a classic paper on the haemolymph glands. Then whilst he was a clinical student in London he heard first hand accounts of 'this fascinating man' from his fiancée Carola Seward, one of Lewis' own clerks, who took him onto a ward round. His teacher at Cambridge, Joseph Barcroft, later Sir Joseph – who had worked on the effort syndrome – arranged an introduction. Lewis asked him how he liked medicine. 'I told him that I found it fascinating but disturbing because I did not understand what I was doing. I have always suspected that it was this reply that won me a place in Lewis' esteem. At any rate he offered me a job on the spot and I came to him after I had taken six weeks off to take my MRCP and get married'.[300] Lewis wrote 'he comes to test his capacity for original work but with the definite idea of his entering upon a career of full time work...he is averse to practice'.[499] The testing period was short because only six months later he was given a full time appointment at a salary of £600 a year. It is interesting that he had the training of only a house physician job before going into a post where he had clinical responsibility for patient care – but he had, with typical acumen, obtained the passport to do that by succeeding in the Membership examination of the Royal College of Physicians – at his first attempt too.

## Raynaud's disease

The next and obvious problem to be tackled in the context of cold and the skin was that of Raynaud's disease and Pickering succeeded Landis and Kerr in studying this malady in which the skin, especially of the hands, becomes white and numb in response to external cold. Maurice Raynaud had separated this syndrome from that of obstructive arterial disease in 1862 and his view that it was due to irritability of the vasomotor centres had become widely accepted. Lewis challenged this view and the first reason for doubting it was one of simple observation. The pallor started in the tips of the fingers and then spread to their bases. If this were due to abnormal sympathetic vaso-constriction then it should have affected the whole finger at the same time. This led him to consider the possibility that the abnormality lay in the digital arteries themselves and he proceeded to investigate this by trying to induce attacks in patients. This method of study, that of provoking symptoms and signs whilst under careful observation, was a favourite one with him because it enjoyed 'the full advantages of the experimental method (and) promises to develop into a fertile branch of clinical science'.[193] But attempts to induce attacks by putting the hands in cold water turned out to be very disappointing until he realized, from measuring the finger temperature in spontaneous episodes, that he was making the fingers too cold. This actually prevented attacks by producing vasodilatation, but work proceeded well after an optimal provoking temperature of 15°C was found.

## A local fault in the digital arteries

Lewis showed that the fault in Raynaud's disease was purely a local one of the digital arteries, and his series of simple but conclusive experiments to show this is one of the classics of clinical science. But although the fault was a local one, the calibre of the digital arteries was also influenced by the vasomotor tone and this had to be taken into account too, even though it was normal. So, as he pointed out, the problem was not a simple one. In summary the proof came, among others, from the following observations. With the subject in a warm room vasomotor tone is normal and equal in both hands, but an attack develops only in the hand which is placed in cool water – or only in the one finger which is selectively cooled at its base: the fault must be a local one. The subject is taken into a room at 15°C and the right hand is placed in water at 30°C. Although vasomotor tone is raised in both hands in response to cooling of the body only the left hand develops an attack. The right hand is protected from local cold and because the increase in vasomotor tone is not itself abnormal it fails to produce spasm in it. In another experiment one ulnar nerve is paralysed with a local anaesthetic after an attack has developed in a cold room The attack continues because removal of normal vasomotor tone is insufficient to release spasm in arteries that are closed owing to a local abnormality. These and other studies showed beyond doubt that it was a local fault in the digital arteries which made them unusually susceptible to cold, causing them to go into spasm. But he recognized that closure of the arteries and arterioles could not account for the dead whiteness of the skin which is so obvious in an attack, and proposed that there must in addition be an active and strong spasm of the minute vessels themselves.[180] Recent work has shown that the microvasculature of the skin is itself abnormal in Raynaud's and it may be that the 'local fault' lies in a failure of a protective vasodilatory mechanism in the skin, rather than in the arteries.[24] He emphasized that just because an increase in vasomotor tone could bring on an attack this did not mean that the tone was abnormal. An artery which was narrowed by local cold could be completely closed by a natural increase in vasomotor tone due to cooling of the whole body, or sometimes due even to sudden pain or an emotional disturbance. Whether frequent spasm of arteries could lead to structural changes within them remained for him an unsolved question.

## Histology of the digital arteries

A few patients had very severe and prolonged attacks and in them there was atrophy of the fingers with painful necrotic areas at the tips. They had permanent organic changes in the digital arteries and this situation demanded a different type of investigation – namely a pathological one, but biopsy of the affected vessels was of course inadmissible, so how did he study the histology? He was able to do this in five of his patients who died of other diseases but in order to interpret the changes it was necessary to look at normal arteries. He could have used routine post-mortem examinations but with typical insistence on proof he decided that the subjects must be shown not to have Raynaud's disease. There was only one way to do this and together with Dr B.B. Gelfand of New York he carried out a remarkable study. This consisted of asking a large number of ward

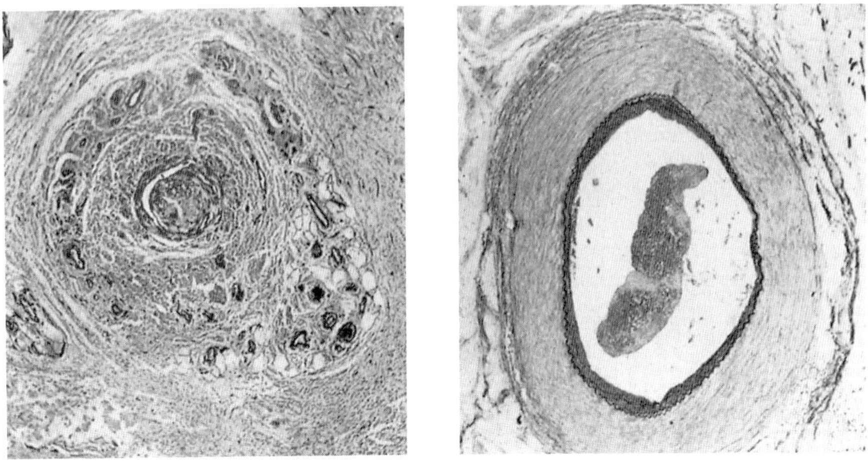

*Figure 11.3 Photomicrographs of the digital arteries in Raynaud's disease showing (left) the most severe form with only a tiny lumen and (right) the mildest form with just slight intimal thickening. (From reference 213.)*

patients who had incurable diseases about the warmth and colour of their hands. Of the 20 who died and were examined post mortem, 18 had normal hands and provided the controls. But two had slight Raynaud's and they gave a unique opportunity to study the changes in the mildest form of the disease.[213] Histological study showed that severe cases had intimal hyperplasia with thrombosis whilst the mild cases had normal digital arteries. (Fig. 11.3) A.J. Honour helped in this work and recalls that the long stay patients in the wards got to realize the significance of Dr Gelfand's enquiries!

Treatment in the mild cases consisted of avoiding the cold and wearing warm clothing with thick gloves, but this was not sufficient in the severe cases and for them he strongly advised cervical sympathectomy. He found that vasodilatation was not fully maintained after the operation but even so the patients still had a useful result. However it gave rise to the curious paradox that when both hands were placed in cool water whilst the patient was kept warm, an attack developed only on the sympathectomized side. This was because natural vasodilatation on the normal side was greater than the now limited dilatation on the operated side.

Together with Pickering he studied all the conditions in which there was intermittent spasm of the digital arteries, and having placed them in nine categories he proposed that the term Raynaud's disease should be abandoned.[249] But later he changed his mind and retained this term for the common type, the type that had no obvious cause, apart from a familial tendency.[205] For those in whom the condition was associated with scleroderma, the use of vibrating tools, or cold haemagglutination he used the term Raynaud's phenomenon. Lewis developed a special interest in scleroderma and this led in 1932 to his election as an honorary member of the British Association of Dermatology and Syphilology of which his colleague Dr A.M.H. (later Sir Archibald) Gray was a distinguished member.

# The jugular venous pressure is the best sign of heart failure

Lewis' last research paper on a cardiac problem had appeared in 1926, but this did not signal the end of his interest in heart disease. In 1928 he wrote an article on 'Early signs of cardiac failure of the congestive type', which was based on a lecture he gave at a British Medical Association meeting in Portsmouth. He emphasized that the earliest and indeed the best way of diagnosing congestive failure was to measure the jugular venous pressure, because the usually taught features such as oedema, ascites and enlarged liver were late signs.[177] Lewis' important contribution and one in which he was the pioneer was to devise a way of measuring the pressure by a simple bedside test, instead of using a fluid filled manometer connected to a vein in the arm. It was easy to see the height of the pressure from the upper level of filling in the external jugular vein, but it was more difficult to find a reference point. He found that the manubrium – the sternal angle – was the best because it represented zero or atmospheric pressure whether the body was horizontal or vertical, and he emphasized the importance of placing the patient in a position that showed the jugular vein filling most clearly. (Fig. 11.4) His method became universally adopted. And still on the

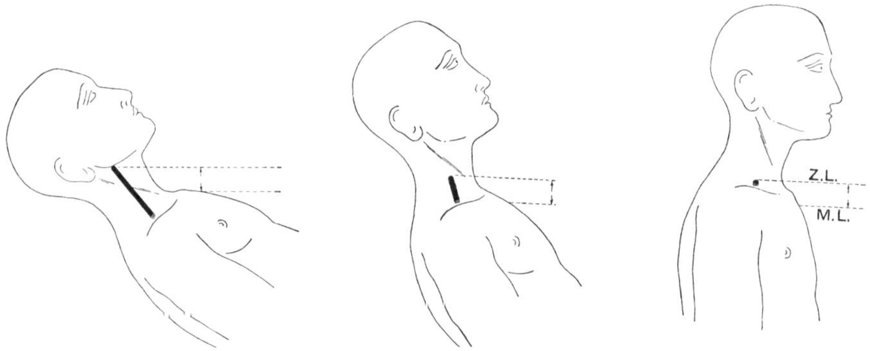


*Figure 11.4 A diagram showing how to measure the height of the jugular venous pressure from the sternal angle; in this case about +8 cm. ZL, zero level; ML manubrial line. (From reference 177.)*

subject of cardiac failure he devised a special bedstead for treating patients with congestive failure. It was hinged in two places so that the head of the bed could be raised to about 70 degrees and the foot lowered a similar amount. (Fig. 11.5, *overleaf*) This prevented orthopnoeic patients slipping off their pillows during the night 'an accident usually occasioning distress and loss of sleep', and which also enabled oedema fluid to drain into the legs prior to removal with an incision or a tube. The bed position was changed with a handle and it freed the nurses from the heavy work of lifting a patient up into the sitting position. This invention is evidence of his concern for the comfort and welfare of his patients.[174]

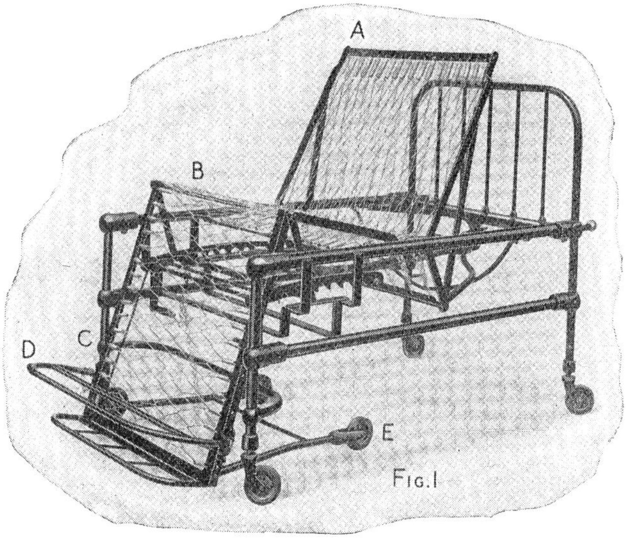


*Figure 11.5 A bedstead for treating patients with cardiac failure. The patient was supported in an upright position to relieve dyspnoea whilst the legs were dependent to drain oedema fluid. (From reference 174.)*

## Note to Chapter 11

(1) George White Pickering, FRS, (later Sir George), 1904–1980, joined Lewis' department a year after qualifying in medicine and stayed in it for ten years. He became Lewis' closest research associate and later was an intimate friend. In 1939 he became professor of medicine at St Mary's Hospital London, and was finally the Regius Professor of Medicine in Oxford. He was a world authority on hypertension. He achieved much for medical education in Britain, helping to plan two new medical schools. He was a strong advocate of integrating the scientific method with the practical training of a medical student, holding that education was much more important than instruction based on memorization.

# Chapter 12

## Intermittent claudication • Factor P. Angina pectoris • Erythralgia • A visit to the United States of America in 1931 • R.T. Grant's 1000 patient follow up study

THE SYNDROME of pain in the leg brought on by exertion and associated with arterial disease had been recognized in man since its description by Jean M. Charcot, the French neurologist, the term intermittent claudication having been used by J.-F. Bouley in 1831 to describe a similar condition in the horse characterized by lameness. Charcot thought the pain was due to muscle cramp, but a muscular origin was discarded by others in favour of pain arising in an artery and caused by spasm.

Lewis became interested in the mechanism of claudication following his study of Raynaud's disease but although both conditions were concerned with the limbs the stimulus to investigate it arose quite separately. The idea came about because he had seen a series of patients with the condition, and as we have already noticed it was often the case with Lewis that a clinical situation led him to a line of profitable research. He did this study with Pickering who recalled:

> Lewis used to ask my wife and I round to his home in Chesterford Gardens. One evening we began discussing intermittent claudication and its mechanism. The next morning, we began work. In contrast to the last problem this went with a swing and, in three months, we had the problem finished. Lewis used to come in in the morning with a list of experiments to do and he, (Rothschild who soon joined us) and I used to do them on ourselves in rotation from 10 to 12.30 and from 2 to 4, day in and day out. Towards the end, Lewis began writing it up and in the last month Rothschild and I were often performing the experiments while he sat in the laboratory and wrote the text.[300]

It had long been known that pain can be produced in a healthy limb by exercising the muscles with the circulation arrested and that was their first experiment.[260] But having reliably produced this pain it was then important to show that it was identical to that which occurred in patients. Such an identity could not be assumed; it had to be demonstrated. The opportunity to do this came when a patient presented with claudication in only one leg. When this leg was exercised he developed intolerable pain at 95 seconds. When the circulation to the healthy leg was arrested with a pneumatic cuff exercise was halted by pain at 92 seconds. This striking similarity of the times provided evidence that the pain had the same origin in both the healthy and diseased limbs, and this evidence was supported by the patient's statement that the pain had exactly the same characteristics in both legs. This evidence gave them the necessary security to draw conclusions from observations done only on healthy limbs. The symptom could be provoked in normal men who were trained observers, and repeated many times under constant conditions giving precise and reliable results.[199]

The theory that the pain was due to arterial spasm was neatly disposed of by inducing pain in a forearm with the circulation arrested and measuring the volume of the limb when the cuff was released. The volume increased immediately indicating a rapid inflow of blood through a widely patent artery. Muscle cramp was easily shown to be absent because exercised muscles, although tender, were flaccid. What then was the pain due to?

## Muscle pain is caused by Factor P

From the experiments on themselves they found that once the forearm pain had been induced by exercise it persisted for as long as the circulation was arrested, but that it disappeared within 3 seconds of releasing the cuff. They were led 'by this simple but striking observation' to conclude that the pain is determined by a chemical stimulus which was developed in the muscle during exercise. It was assumed that this stimulus, in the form probably of metabolites, diffused out of the ischaemic muscle fibres into the tissue spaces between them where it acted on the sensory nerve endings. This action they felt should be kept separate from the changes within the fibre, and they achieved this by labelling it 'factor P'.[199] A series of ingenious experiments were then undertaken to show that the pain factor acted in the tissue space and not in the muscle fibre. For example if exercise were done first and the circulation then stopped, the pain came on after a latent period of 30 seconds. This latency was not due to a delay in the development of 'factor P' for other observations denied this possibility. It was due to the time taken for the factor to diffuse out into the tissue space.[178,179]

This work illustrated very well the experimental method of clinical science. A manifestation originally observed in a patient was provoked in normal subjects and it was ensured that their reaction really was equivalent to that induced in the patient by disease. With that assurance the experiments on normal people provided a clearer understanding of the way in which pain arises in intermittent claudication and of its behaviour in different circumstances of everyday life. The study provided the material for his St Cyres Lecture at the National Heart Hospital on May 14 1931 entitled 'Pain in muscular ischaemia'.

## Complaint to the editor of *The Lancet*

*The Lancet* published an account of the lecture written by a staff reporter. At that time it was a well established custom of medical journals to send one of their staff to report on a public lecture. However, quite naturally, this annoyed Lewis and he complained to the Editor that it had been done without his knowledge and was full of errors. He pointed out that he would spend many hours getting the wording of a manuscript just right and that it was the manuscript, not a verbatim report, that should be published. A lecture, he said, might be heard by 100 people, whereas a paper could be read and also re-read by say 10 000 and therefore much more care should be given to the written than the spoken word. He ended by drawing the analogy of having a painting hung at an exhibition, 'I go to the show on varnishing day and find that a fake of my own picture has been accepted.'[398]

## Mechanism of angina pectoris, a study by E.J. Wayne

Having established the mechanism of pain in ischaemic leg muscles it was natural to extend the concept to explain the pain of angina pectoris and coronary occlusion. With angina, as with claudication, it was reasoned that the heart's increased energy expenditure on effort outpaces the limited blood supply and that an accumulation of factor P produces pain which resolves with rest. With a myocardial infarction however the heart continues to work producing factor P continuously, and so the pain is long lasting and severe. The idea that anginal pain was due to coronary disease and that it was brought about by relative ischaemia of cardiac muscle had been proposed as far back as 1799 by the Welsh physician Caleb Hillier Parry for whom Lewis had a high regard.[224] But other hypotheses had sprung up since then including a recent one from Sir Clifford Allbutt that the pain was due to tension in the wall of the aorta, occasioned by the increase of blood pressure with exercise. Lewis found that surprisingly few clinical measurements had been made in angina in spite of much discussion about its origin and he set about remedying this defect. He gave the task to Dr Edward J. Wayne[(1)] from Leeds who had become a full time worker in the department in April 1931. (Fig. 12.1) The problem was attacked by the method which Lewis had by now made very much his own, namely that of making frequent measurements whilst the symptom under study was produced under controlled conditions. Another hallmark of his investigations was that of emphasising the need to justify any experiment which provoked a patient's symptom. In this instance he said that 'we ask him to do no more, while under our close control, than he is in the habit of doing several or many times a day without supervision, when he walks until pain comes: such tests, undertaken with scrupulous care, are justified by the information they give us about our patients individually'.[200] They used the simple test of having the patient walk up and down two steps at a fixed rate and recording the pulse and blood pressure before and after effort. As with claudication it was found that even if the effort did not produce angina it did lead to its earlier appearance when a second period of effort was made without adequate rest in between. In other words factor P had accumulated during the first though painless period and had not dispersed fully before the second test. This alone was a good argument against some of the other hypotheses. It was soon shown that pain could come on without a rise in blood pressure, but equally it became clear that an elevated heart rate was a constant association – provoking pain by increase of energy expenditure. It was confirmed that a meal hastened the onset of pain, whilst simple distension of the stomach did not. Nitroglycerine given before effort increased the time before pain came on and shortened its duration, and it was concluded that its effect was mainly produced through dilatation of the coronary vessels. But it was also shown to lower the blood pressure both before and during effort so it is difficult to see how Lewis and his colleagues could have been confident in excluding at least some action on the periphery. Nevertheless it was a good study which placed the role of myocardial ischaemia on a secure

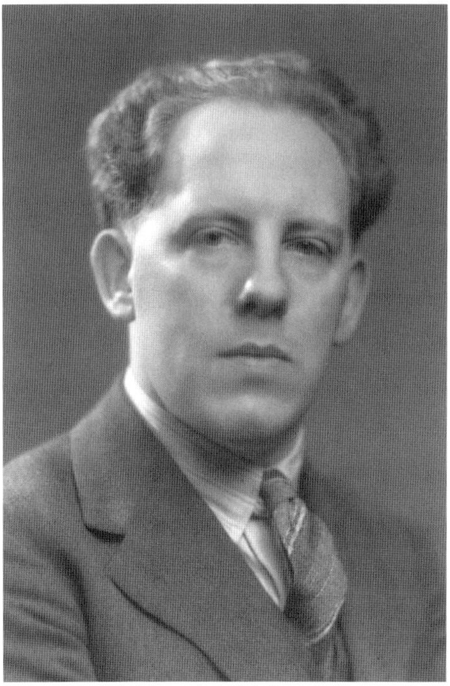

*Figure 12.1* *E.J. (later Sir Edward) Wayne, worked on angina pectoris with Lewis who said he had a highly critical mind and was much liked by his co-workers.*

footing.[327,328] Wayne has stated that he wanted to record the electrocardiogram during the episodes of pain. This would, he said, have meant using a continuous recording camera and when Lewis was approached be replied that no funds were available to get one.[479] So the opportunity was lost for Wayne to develop, in 1932, an electrocardiographic effort test. In fact the standard machine would probably have served quite well and one wonders if Lewis was just distancing himself from using what he still regarded as a specialist piece of apparatus to study a common problem. However in the previous year Francis C. Wood, who had worked under Lewis in 1920, had published a paper in the United States which contained the first account of using exercise to provoke electrocardiographic changes in angina.[25]

## Angina in aortic incompetence and Nothnagel's syndrome

Lewis' interest in the relation of angina to the blood pressure led him to record and study attacks of angina, often nocturnal, in patients with severe aortic regurgitation which were preceded by a rise in blood pressure and readily relieved by amyl nitrite. It was just such a patient that led Dr Thomas Lauder Brunton(2) in 1867 to introduce nitrites for the treatment of angina, and happily although these patients had normal coronary arteries, the therapy turned out to work just as well on the vast majority who did have coronary disease.[79] Lewis also referred to Nothnagel's syndrome, in which it had been claimed that vasoconstriction preceded an attack of angina.[181] This curious and now long forgotten condition had been described in 1867 under the term 'angina pectoris vasomotoria' as comprising attacks in otherwise healthy men of pallor, fear, palpitation and chest pain brought on by cold or inebriation. Lewis dismissed it with the comment that it was so rare that no similar cases had been described since then, another way of saying there was no such entity. But he was careful to mention separately the somewhat similar symptoms of the recently recognized condition phaeochromocytoma, a comment which shows that he was up to date with advances in medicine.

## The pain of injured skin • Erythralgia

Yet a third condition was studied as a result of proving that pain can arise from a natural chemical or physico-chemical stimulus. This was the burning type of pain that occurs in some patients who have a painful redness of the extremities, a condition labelled 'erythromelalgia' in 1872 by Weir Mitchell and attributed by him to a 'vasomotor neurosis'. Emphasis had been laid by him and others on vasodilatation as a primary feature of this malady, but there was little evidence to support this idea and Lewis decided to investigate the matter.[186] He employed his well tried and favourite method of inducing a similar condition in normals, and found that various forms of injury to the skin such as ultraviolet light, freezing, and abrasion would all reproduce the clinical syndrome of tender red skin with a burning pain made worse by heat. It was notable that the tenderness spread beyond the injured area and sometimes spread distinctly up nearby veins. This suggested that the injury, such as an abrasion, brought a substance into the tissue spaces which caused the nerve endings to discharge pain impulses after the initial pain of the abrasion had passed off. The matter was tested by abrading the skin on a limb with the circulation to the limb either free or arrested. In both cases the initial pain was the same, but when the artery was occluded the second pain was indefinitely prolonged and intensified, as would be expected if a pain producing substance had been liberated from the injured area. He termed it a 'susceptible state of the skin' and for brevity named it 'erythralgia', from the red painful skin.[186] Erythralgia as it occurred in patients was found usually in association with inflammation. This could occur acutely with infection and injuries such as sunburn. In a chronic form it was found after hard usage, frost bite, immersion foot, chronic chilblains and incipient gangrene, but sometimes the aetiology was obscure. His investigation had shown he said the danger of labelling diseases upon loose grouping of symptoms without attempting to investigate their pathogenetic basis. The term erythromelalgia had 'acted as an anaesthetic rendering medicine unresponsive to the idea that there is no such special malady and incurious to the meaning of a number of phenomena...which at once yield up much of their meaning when probed by simple and commonplace enquiry conducted in an atmosphere free from the prejudice of nomenclature.[201]

CHAPTER 12

# His third visit to the United States

In the autumn of 1931 he made his third, and as it happened, his last visit to the United States. This came about in an unusual way which is worth recounting. Each year the New York Academy of Medicine held a postgraduate fortnight and the organizer for that year's session on Disorders of the Circulation was Dr Emanuel Libman, a leading physician noted for his work on endocarditis. It was his ambition to get Lewis as the guest lecturer but he knew of Lewis' reluctance to accept invitations especially during the working part of the year. So he decided that the best way of ensuring acceptance would be to talk to Lewis on the telephone. In those days a trans-Atlantic phone call was a rarity except for those in commerce and the like, and it was also very expensive. But Libman was rich and the combination of the novelty, and perhaps the flattery, of such a call succeeded![466] During the fortnight in October Lewis gave four lectures on the subjects of cutaneous reaction to cold, intermittent claudication, tests of cutaneous innervation and Raynaud's disease. Word obviously got around that Sir Thomas was making this visit and other invitations came in. But he declined to give the Thayer Lectures in Baltimore or to talk in Cincinnati, Richmond or Toronto, whilst the famous Mayo Clinic (fee only $50) and the humble Lackawanna Medical Society were both turned down. He gave the Janeway lecture and demonstration at the Mount Sinai Hospital in New York on paralysis with ischaemia, assisted by his former associate B.S. Oppenheimer who was chief of the medical service at the hospital. Lewis had written to him some weeks beforehand with the request to provide a large reservoir to put a subjects legs in. Lewis was a careful planner. Then followed the Frank Billings lecture in Chicago and the Mary Scott Newbold lecture in Philadelphia. This last one was on vasovagal syncope and the carotid sinus mechanism, and he pointed out that it had been Parry who first described pulse slowing with carotid pressure.[181] In 1933 Dr Soma Weiss of Boston published his seminal paper on carotid sinus syncope and we can speculate that Lewis must admired Weiss's very fine experimental observations.[330] The Chicago lecture enabled him to go to Ann Arbor and spend two days with Frank Wilson and his wife, the last time they were to meet. No doubt they watched birds but as was always the case with Lewis' personal diary that visit is irritatingly silent on detail. His crowded trip continued with a visit to Boston and a welcome in the editorial page of *The New England Journal of Medicine* for November 5. This recalled his visit there as a young man 17 years before and praised his books which 'have been invaluable aids to thousands of physicians the world over in their study of cardiovascular disorders'. The editorial, probably written by Paul White, ended by saying 'To meet Sir Thomas Lewis is a happy and stimulating event. We hope that we in Boston may have this privilege soon again'.[9] Lewis was obviously touched by this tribute because he kept that editorial among his private papers. As we shall see he would, but for illness, have returned five years later. He sailed from New York in the Cunard ship *Laconia* on November 14th and was home on the 23rd after six weeks away.

Whilst Lewis and his associates had been pursuing this work on ischaemia in skeletal and cardiac muscle and the skin, other studies had been in progress in his department under the direction of R.T. Grant aided by Edward F. Bland from Virginia and Paul D. Camp from Boston. Grant was interested in the reaction of arteries to various mechanical and chemical stimuli and by using the rabbit's ear, where the vessels can be directly observed, he made pioneer observations on the function of arteriovenous anastomoses noting that they are important factors in regulating body temperature. He then showed too that there are many anastomoses in the hands and feet of man which need to be considered in considering the action of drugs on peripheral blood flow.

## A ten year follow up study of 1000 cardiac patients

R.T. Grant (Fig. 12.2) was now concluding his study on the follow up, conducted for ten years, on 1000 ex service men with organic heart disease. This study had been conceived and organized by Lewis at the end of the war when he realized that there was a unique opportunity to get objective evidence on which to base prognosis in these war pensioners. Thanks to the diligence of the department's secretary Miss Lena M. Searle only 13 of the group remained untraced, a splendidly complete follow up. Grant's massive paper (Fig. 12.3) occupied 207 pages of *Heart*, comprising 59 pages of text and 148 pages of tables.[68] 51% of the men were alive at 10 years and in one half of them Grant was impressed by observing no change in either their symptoms or physical signs over this period. Furthermore in those who died there was in the majority 'no steady progression towards a fatal termination'. The original condition, he said, remained stationary until auricular fibrillation, intercurrent infection or an unknown cause led to congestive failure and death within a short time. His conclusion that it was only the complications

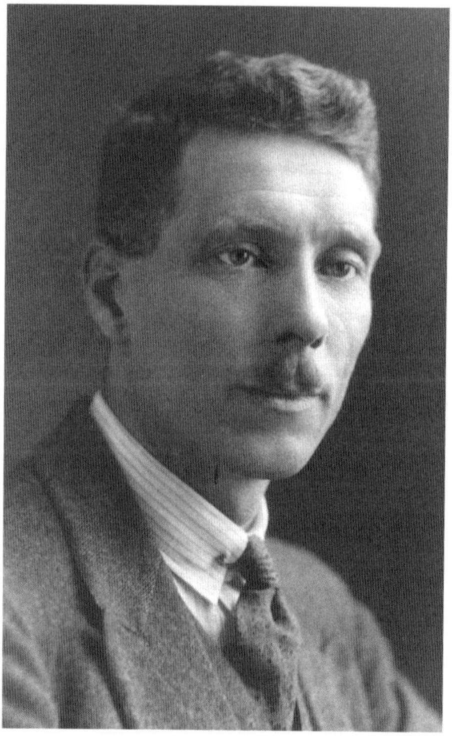

*Figure 12.2 Ronald T. Grant, aged 35, was Lewis' senior research worker for 15 years.*

AFTER HISTORIES FOR TEN YEARS OF A THOUSAND MEN SUFFERING FROM HEART DISEASE.

A STUDY IN PROGNOSIS.*

By R. T. GRANT.

*(From the Department of Clinical Research, University College Hospital Medical School).*

CONTENTS.



* Work undertaken on behalf of the Medical Research Council.

*Figure 12.3 Title page of Grant's paper on the huge and pioneer follow up study of 1000 ex-soldiers with heart disease. This was a milestone in the assessment of prognosis. (From reference 68.)*

that determined the outcome would now be judged wrong, but they must have given Lewis strong support for his belief that valve lesions as such were secondary in importance to myocardial disease in determining outcome. However it is notable that of the 31 patients coming to autopsy with mitral stenosis, about 80% had severe stenosis and none had mild stenosis, a finding which Lewis either overlooked or ignored when he wrote 'Prognosis is most satisfactory when based on cardiac enlargement and cardiac failure'.[285] Lewis always played down the importance of valve lesions in the genesis of heart failure. However it is likely at that time that there was only a limited understanding of how to assess the severity of stenosis of the mitral and aortic valves. Aortic regurgitation was easier to quantify, from the water hammer pulse and cardiac enlargement. Speaking of that lesion reminds one of the investigation which Grant did during this study into the treatment of 175 patients with syphilitic aortic incompetence. They were placed into three groups and followed for ten years or until death. The group given arsenic, mercury and iodides did better than those having either iodides alone, or no treatment, having a mortality of 48% compared with 64% and 67%, and having also twice as many cases with no deterioration. It was an early and good example of a therapeutic trial.[68]

## Scheme for a modern cardiac rehabilitation institute

Lewis' work with disabled soldiers soon after the War had led him to urge at that time for a sympathetic understanding of their need for conditions of work which were appropriate for their physical ability. This pioneering belief in the need for organized rehabilitation did not leave him and he returned to it in 1927 when he persuaded the General Committee of UCH to support a scheme which he had formulated for the after care of patients.[390] He contended that many patients were not fit to return to work on their discharge from hospital, and that if they did return at once the beneficial effect of treatment was soon lost. He regarded this as a very serious defect in the current hospital system. 'We have in mind', he wrote, 'the complete remedying of this defect by means of a really modern and properly equipped and staffed institute in the country'. He thought that the capital cost would be about £50 000 with running costs of around £2,500 a year. His scheme was worthwhile, imaginative and innovative, but not surprisingly at that time the large amount of money required was not available and nothing came of it.

## Pickering's own research work

In the 1930's Pickering was beginning to undertake work on his own and he extended the department's long involvement with histamine into studying its mechanism in producing headache. By arresting the circulation to the scalp he showed that the pain did not arise in this structure. In patients having diagnostic lumbar puncture it was shown that histamine produced a rise in intracranial pressure due to cerebral vasodilatation. Patients who had had their trigeminal nerve divided got pain only on the normal side showing that the headache probably arose in the dura mater.[298] These experiments were virtually the first scientific investigation of this common symptom, and they showed how a patient's illness could be utilized with propriety to advance knowledge in a field outside their own disease.

## Research in the Medical Unit

There was good investigative work too in T.R. Elliott's Medical Unit where three of his research assistants held Beit Memorial Fellowships, and as it happened were all to be associated in one way or another with Lewis in their later careers. Harold P. (Harry) Himsworth who had uniquely won a Gold Medal in both the MB and MD London was starting a brilliant career with his work on diabetes. John McMichael[(3)] studied the function of the spleen and liver with J.W. McNee, and then returned to Edinburgh where he started his important work on the cardiac output. This led to his notable work on cardiac catheterization at Hammersmith Hospital and to a disagreement about it, with Lewis, which we shall come to later. F. Horace Smirk[(4)] had come from Liverpool to work on renal function and later was a professor of medicine in New Zealand, and a world authority on hypertension. UCH Medical School had become the leading centre in the country for clinical research. There was also excellent research work in other departments of the medical school, for example the synthesis of thyroxine by Professor Charles R. Harington.

## The scope of the Department of Clinical Research is widened

As already mentioned, Lewis resigned from the Medical Research Council in July 1932 when he became the first Physician in Charge of the hospital's Department of Clinical Research, which served in effect both the hospital and the council. The title 'Cardiographic Department' was no longer used, and in his Annual Report for the year 1931–32 Lewis was keen to point out that 'The Department is not to be regarded as a cardiac department or as studying only cardiac and vascular diseases: its scope has been deliberately widened.'[284] As examples of this change he mentioned studies of renal disease, hypertension, and headache and also work on muscle pain, on nerve function after limb ischaemia and on the sympathetic nervous system. These illustrated, he said, the natural extensions from one field of clinical work to another, and he stated that such extensions would be encouraged in his department so long as they remained within its capacity. He added, 'It seems desirable, moreover, to show by illustrative experience that a scientific method of work, which has proved applicable to the cardiovascular system, can be applied quickly, by those trained in it, to problems concerned with other systems'.[284] This was his reply to the criticism by some scientific workers, such as J.A. Ryle,[311] that clinical research had been shown to effective only on what they perceived as simple circulatory problems.

## Notes to Chapter 12

(1) Edward Johnson Wayne, (later Sir Edward), 1902–1990, worked first in Lewis' department and later became an important figure in British medicine. He held the chair of pharmacology and therapeutics in Sheffield, and then became the Regius Professor of Medicine in Glasgow. He was a pioneer in the clinical use of isotopes and in the use of computers in diagnosis, and he was an excellent teacher. His skilful chairmanship of the Alcohol and Road Accidents Committee of the British Medical Association led to government action on introducing a blood alcohol limit for drivers which saved many thousands of lives.

(2) Thomas Lauder Brunton, FRS, (later Sir Lauder), 1844–1916, was a house physician in Edinburgh when he showed in 1867 that the newly discovered chemical, amyl nitrite, was a very effective treatment for angina pectoris. His patient's angina was due to aortic regurgitation but happily the treatment proved equally effective in coronary heart disease. Brunton pioneered the scientific approach to therapeutics and wrote many important papers on clinical pharmacology. He suggested in 1904 that mitral stenosis might be treated surgically.

(3) John McMichael, FRS, (later Sir John), 1904–1993, did highly acclaimed research work on the cardiovascular system and in 1942 he was the first in Britain, with E.P. Sharpey-Schafer, to perform cardiac catheterization in man. He was professor of medicine at the Royal Postgraduate Medical School, London and due to his great abilities the department of medicine there achieved world wide fame.

(4) Frederick Horace Smirk, FRS, (later Sir Horace), 1902–1991, did important research work on the cardiovascular system. After working in the Medical Unit at UCH under the tenure of a Beit Fellowship he first held a chair in Cairo and then from 1940 to 1968 he was professor of medicine in the University of Otago, New Zealand. He achieved wide recognition for his work on the use of ganglion blocking drugs in hypertension. Smirk was a fine academic research worker, and from one of his investigations into blood pressure came his pioneer identification of the R on T phenomenon in the electrocardiogram as a premonitory feature of ventricular fibrillation.

# Chapter 13

## *Diseases of the Heart* • The Harveian Oration • Completion of eight years' work on the peripheral circulation • The last volume of *Heart* • *Vascular Disorders of the Limbs* • A second myocardial infarction

THE LONG visit to the United States and the necessary preliminary work occupied the autumn term of Lewis' academic working year in 1931. With typical efficiency and foresight he had arranged for the publication of his lectures before he had delivered them, and so early in 1932 there was nothing to impede the continuation of his research work, but illness soon overtook this plan. Early in February he developed a severe attack of neuritis in the left arm for which he consulted his neurological colleague, Francis M.R. Walshe(1) who later recounted the episode in a talk on neuritis given to the students, 'I advised Sir Thomas to rest in bed for eight weeks and to my great surprise he agreed to do so. Whilst there he wrote his textbook, with his left arm resting on a pillow. At the end of the time his neuritis was better and his book completed'. The ailment had in fact troubled Lewis during his American tour, so it was not a new condition and today it would be called a cervical disc problem, and not managed by the prolonged bed rest apparently then thought essential for a possibly infective condition. Nevertheless it turned out very well because the book *Diseases of the Heart described for practitioners and students* (Fig. 13.1) became widely acclaimed.[188] It was published, in 1933, by Macmillan and Co of London and not by his usual publishers, Shaw and Sons. The reason for the change is not known. He explained in the preface, dated July 1932, that whilst it had been his desire to write an outline of the clinical teaching given to his own students, 'the impulse to write a work of reference has not stirred me'. His teaching, he said, had always been guided by two ideals. Firstly that it was based on what he had seen himself and proved to be true and secondly that he was convinced of the need for simplicity, and would therefore lay emphasis on physical signs but not on electrocardiography.

### A new approach with emphasis on function, not structure

He was keen to point out that the arrangement of the subject matter was an unusual one in that it rejected the traditional way of classifying heart disease on

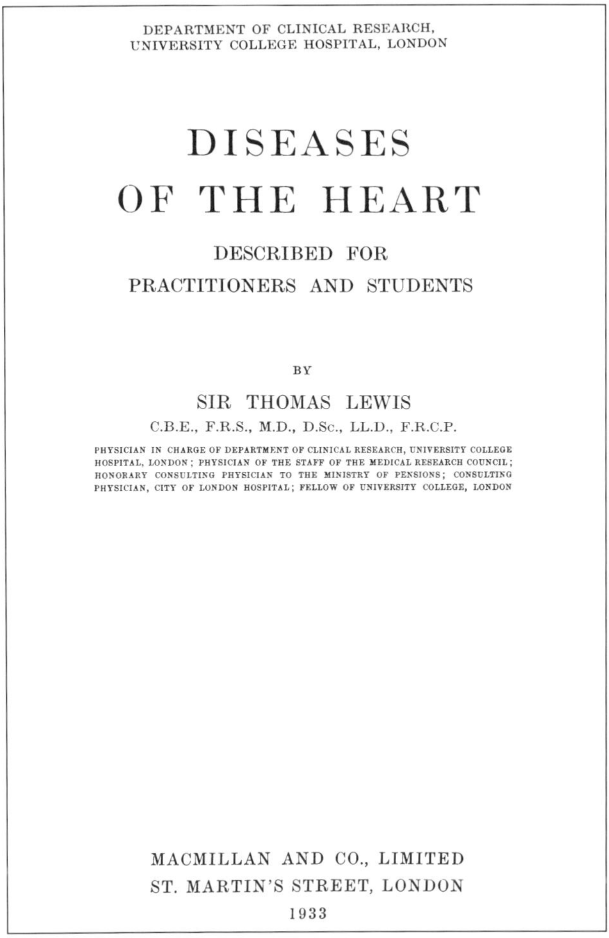

DEPARTMENT OF CLINICAL RESEARCH,
UNIVERSITY COLLEGE HOSPITAL, LONDON

DISEASES
OF THE HEART

DESCRIBED FOR
PRACTITIONERS AND STUDENTS

BY

SIR THOMAS LEWIS
C.B.E., F.R.S., M.D., D.Sc., LL.D., F.R.C.P.

PHYSICIAN IN CHARGE OF DEPARTMENT OF CLINICAL RESEARCH, UNIVERSITY COLLEGE HOSPITAL, LONDON; PHYSICIAN OF THE STAFF OF THE MEDICAL RESEARCH COUNCIL; HONORARY CONSULTING PHYSICIAN TO THE MINISTRY OF PENSIONS; CONSULTING PHYSICIAN, CITY OF LONDON HOSPITAL; FELLOW OF UNIVERSITY COLLEGE, LONDON

MACMILLAN AND CO., LIMITED
ST. MARTIN'S STREET, LONDON
1933

*Figure 13.1 Title page of his very successful 1933 textbook* Diseases of the Heart. *(From reference 188.)*

an anatomical basis. 'Models of heart disease cannot be cast in anatomical moulds'. It was the symptoms of disease that held the attention of the patient and usually the doctor too, and symptoms were derived from faults in function. 'Therefore, in managing our patients, our thoughts must be chiefly set in terms of function and not of structure. To whom I fail to teach this first simple, but essential lesson, I have nought to teach'.

So the first eight chapters dealt with cardiac failure and angina pectoris, the two most important things to understand, he said, in managing heart cases. He emphasized the value of measuring the venous pressure as the best index of congestive failure and taught exactly how to do this from examination of the jugular veins – a study of which, he said, still suffered from a most unfortunate neglect. Some physical signs, notably cardiac murmurs, had of course to be described under anatomical headings but he managed to dilute that arrangement by giving separate chapters to cardiac enlargement and to the manifestations in general of rheumatic heart disease. Arrhythmias, endocarditis and the effort syndrome were

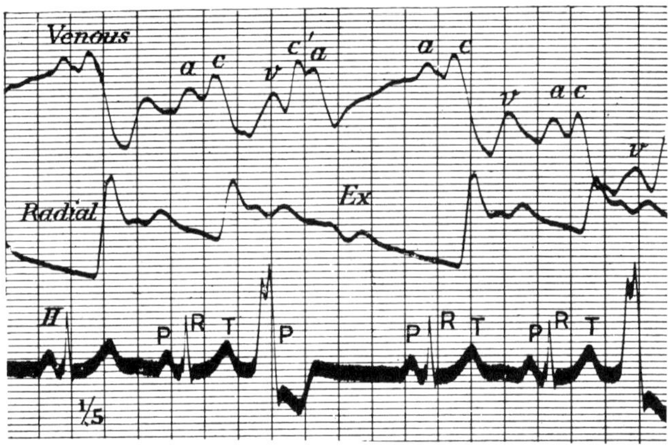


*Figure 13.2 A fine illustration with venous and arterial pulses and electrocardiogram showing two ventricular extrasystoles, and also normal beats. (From reference 188.)*

all expertly handled as one would expect, whilst he acknowledged the help of S.A. Levine in describing the effects of anaesthesia in heart cases. Auscultation of the heart was dealt with thoroughly and there were lengthy accounts of cardiac murmurs. There was good practical guidance in auscultation as for example with the murmur of mitral stenosis:

> It is erroneous to believe that the murmur is usually recognised by timing it, although this is steadily taught. Most people, though capable of recognising the chief murmurs readily, cannot and never will time murmurs reliably. They recognise this murmur of mitral stenosis the instant it is heard, as I do myself in routine work, by its low-pitched abruptly ending noise. Much labour is lost and many ultimately fail to know this murmur through persisting in the effort to time, instead of learning to know it as one learns to know a dog's bark.

The analogy with a dog's bark became a frequently quoted phrase. The book was very well illustrated with 45 figures showing arterial and venous pulses, X-rays of the heart, phonocardiograms, and electrocardiograms. (Fig. 13.2) The radiology of the heart was not the usual chest X-ray. It was an orthodiagram whereby a beam from the X-ray tube is carried round the heart's margin and traced out on a sheet of paper. (Fig. 13.3) This gave a more accurate estimate of heart size, but of course it had the drawback that the lung fields were not examined. This could have limited Lewis' appreciation of left heart failure.

## Guidelines for prognosis and treatment

The final chapter was on 'Diagnosis, prognosis, and treatment' and is worthy of comment. It starts off with a good analysis of the problems encountered in naming disease, and especially of how short terms such as mitral stenosis or aortic disease, although convenient, fail to convey much about the state of the patient. On the other hand no system of diagnostic terms had been devised to summarize cardiac patients because the many defects of structure and of function

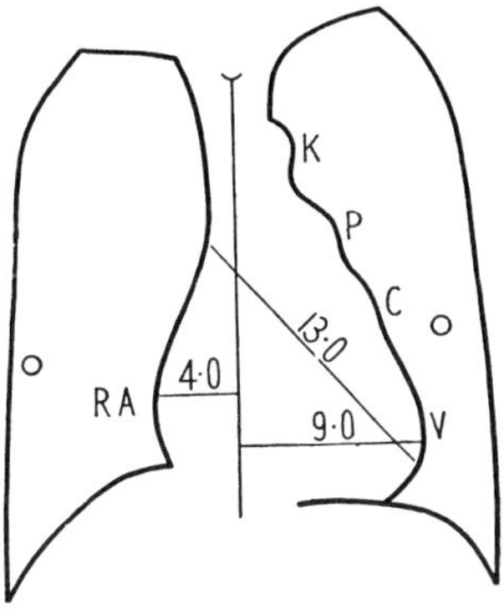


FIG. 30.—Orthodiagram. Man aged 24; weight 113 lb. Mitral stenosis (developed). Below the aortic knob ($K$) appear the projection of $P$, the dilated pulmonary artery; of $C$, the enlarged conus; and the outline of the ventricle ($V$), the apex of which is unusually round. The right auricular shadow ($RA$) is enlarged.

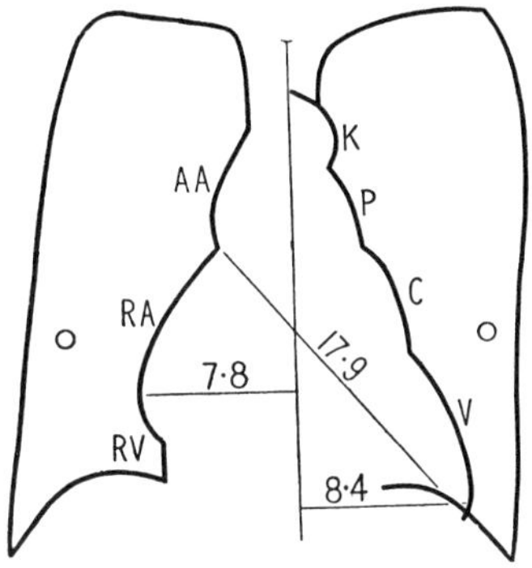


FIG. 31.—Orthodiagram. Man aged 29. Mitral stenosis (developed), aortic regurgitation (slight), and great enlargement of the heart. The right border is composed of ascending aorta ($AA$), which is displaced, an enlarged right auricle ($RA$), and the beginning of the enlarged right ventricle ($RV$). The left border consists of aortic knob ($K$), dilated pulmonary artery ($P$), greatly enlarged conus ($C$), and ventricle ($V$).

*Figure 13.3 An illustration to show the value of radiography. The cardiac silhouette is accurately outlined by orthodiagrams in two cases of mitral stenosis. (From reference 188.)*

'combine in an endless variety of ways'. His own system which he had used for a long time and found to be adequate was a simple one which briefly recorded all the essential features which were required for prognosis or for treatment. It was one, which as I can personally remember, had to be written down as a routine on every outpatient. There were eight headings, as follows: exercise tolerance, congestion, enlargement, rhythm, valves, infection, vessels (including blood pressure) and aetiology. The first entry under the heading of prognosis was certainly an unusual one for any book because it told the practitioner is some detail how to decide whether a patient's heart was normal. He said that a normal exercise tolerance was a valuable indicator, whilst an isolated systolic murmur or an abnormal electrocardiogram might be disregarded. Then there were good guidelines for assessing whether life expectancy was in one of six categories ranging from normal to imminent danger though he emphasized that no enquiry 'would carry our prophetic powers to such a pitch that we could state definitely how long a patient has to live'. There must have been many doctors, especially those in general practice, who found this advice invaluable and not obtainable elsewhere.

## Talking to the patient

There was another section too which was quite remarkable for a textbook. It was entitled 'Conversing with the patient and his friends'. In two pages Lewis told the doctor how to manage his patient, what to tell him and his family, how to answer his questions and also what not to tell him. The doctor's visit – the chief event of the day to a sick man – should convey comfort and encouragement; 'A countenance of gloom is as out of place in a sick-room as is a coffin'. Truth of statement was a first essential and whilst the whole truth need not be volunteered, answers should be given to direct questions because evasions usually defeated their purpose. It was rarely necessary or desirable to tell a patient that he was dying but if he asked – and few did – then he should be told and the answer could be conveyed with compassion. The words disease, malignant and dropsy should never be used and the not uncommon phrase 'may drop dead at any minute' categorized the doctor who used it as being 'guilty both of cruelty and folly'. The final section on treatment also has good practical advice on the amount of exercise and types of employment suitable for cardiac cases. It contains too some well phrased comments on healthy habits of living. People who followed these habits 'welcome the freshness of abundant air and open spaces, delighting in the feelings of invigoration that accompany active exercise; they love the warmth of sunlight playing on their skins, and the sleepiness of healthy fatigue'. Writing of that quality ensured the book of widespread and well deserved acceptance. But it is necessary critically to examine some other features, namely those of heart failure and valve disease.

## His views on heart failure

Lewis defined heart failure as an inability of the heart to discharge its contents adequately, resulting in pulmonary and systemic venous congestion. The symptom of breathlessness was the earliest manifestation of failure and systemic congestion was the late one, but he was reluctant to accept that left or right heart failure could occur independently. It was his view that when the heart failed it usually failed as a whole. If we look ahead for ten years or more to later editions of the book we find that although Lewis accepted, as he said, that first the left or the right heart may fail he emphasized that 'in the great majority both right and left weakness are present simultaneously'. He was still not willing to accept that left ventricular failure occurred by itself, but others had shown it to be a definite entity and he rather grudgingly admitted that the idea had value providing it was recognized as being still hypothetical. In fact as Bedford pointed out the syndrome of left ventricular failure had been described in Britain in 1839 by Dr James Hope(2) – with whose work Lewis was acquainted – and confirmed in at least ten articles from France and America between 1889 and 1935.[16]

## The myocardium is more important than the valve

When it came to valve disease he made two remarkably erroneous statements in his book. 'There are no symptoms of aortic stenosis', and 'Although many symptoms may be complained of by patients suffering from mitral stenosis, there are none that can be ascribed properly and usefully to this deformity of the valve.' Well, if it was not the stenosis that caused the symptoms, what was it? A damaged myocardium, was the answer which Lewis gave and which had been given before him by Mackenzie who wrote 'In chronic valvular affections the subjective symptoms of heart failure only arise when exhaustion of the heart muscle sets in'.[271] There seem to have been two main reasons for this belief. Both men were impressed by noticing that in some cases of mitral stenosis there were no symptoms until the narrowing was extreme, whilst others died with only moderate stenosis – and in them the muscle wall was always found, they said, to have been damaged. Lewis did concede that cardiac failure in valvular disease was partly due 'to the unusual burden of work that the heart has to bear', but asserted that 'the chief factor nevertheless must be inherent in the muscle itself for failure can occur without the increased burden'. However he had to admit that histological examination showed no changes, 'for the most part the fibres seem sound'. This did not deter him from stating that in mitral stenosis there was a rheumatic inflammation, past or present, affecting all parts of the heart and that with this lesion 'the muscle should be suspect before the examination has proceeded further'. Mackenzie and Lewis were also influenced by their quite proper belief that doctors had paid far too much attention to cardiac murmurs and far too little to the functional capacity of the heart. Mackenzie wrote 'it can now be seen that auscultation can throw but little light upon the essential problem of heart failure' and Lewis pointed out that undue attention to cardiac valves was unsatisfactory for prognosis adding that 'This over emphasis resulted largely from an exaggerated notion of the extent to which valve defects burden the heart mechanically'.

## Why his views on mitral stenosis were wrong

To illustrate his point he squeezed water out of a tennis ball which had a hole cut in it and noted that reducing the size of the hole by one quarter from 4 to 2 cm had little effect, the water was still easily ejected. This was close to being a misleading comment because the valve size in critical mitral stenosis is 1 cm or less. So how and where did Lewis go wrong? In the first place he paid too little attention to the effects of a high pulmonary venous pressure or pulmonary congestion as it was often called. He states that this congestion arises because the narrowed valve raises the left atrial pressure, and he knew that mitral stenosis causes pulmonary oedema, but he chose to disregard these aspects. Why was this? His emphasis was on cardiac failure and because the elevated pulmonary venous pressure could not be measured, and believing anyway that the heart failed as a whole, the systemic venous pressure came to be his index of failure. And he explained the breathlessness of cardiac failure as being due to a deficiency of oxygenated blood going to the head and neck, when a pulmonary cause might have seemed the obvious explanation. In the second place he did not accept that right heart failure, failure with congestion, was due to the stenosis. He knew that pulmonary hypertension was present having noted the dilated and atheromatous pulmonary artery and the right ventricular hypertrophy, features indicating its severity, but he rejected this as the cause of the failure. He supported this idea by comparison with pulmonary stenosis where failure was less and came later – the muscle being healthy he pointed out in this congenital lesion. But the comparison is not valid because the outflow tract resistance is much higher with pulmonary hypertension with its elevated diastolic as well as systolic pressure. It is fair to point out that knowledge of pulmonary vascular disease was then in its infancy, but even so his reasoning seems to have been dictated by a requirement to prove that myocardial disease was the main problem in valve disease. Two years beforehand, in 1931, his former pupil Paul D. White had written in his textbook – a copy of which he sent to Lewis – 'it is the valve lesion, if well marked, and not myocardial disease that eventually causes failure and death. In recent years there has been much too great a tendency to blame the heart muscle and exonerate the valve lesion. This is a wrong point of view…'.[332]

## The surgery of mitral stenosis

The proof came in 1948 with the introduction of mitral valvotomy which gave impressive symptomatic benefit, prevented complications and prolonged life. But this operation had been done in Britain 23 years previously in 1925 by Mr (later Sir Henry) Souttar at the London Hospital. Souttar performed what was to become the accepted procedure of freeing the commissural fusion by dilating the mitral valve with a finger inserted through the left atrium. His patient, 15 year old Lilian Hine, survived and lived for several years until she died with a cerebral embolus. This was a surgical triumph but as Souttar explained, 'I did not repeat the operation because I could not get another case. Although my patient made an uninterrupted recovery the Physicians declared that it was all nonsense and in fact that the operation was unjustifiable.'[321] This was certainly Lewis' view. 'Surgical attempts to relieve cases of mitral stenosis…will continue to fail..because the attempt is based upon what, usually at all events, is an erroneous idea, namely that the valve is the chief source of the trouble'.[188] Physicians continued to deny the importance of the anatomical lesion right up to 1948 when Charles P. Bailey and Dwight E. Harken in the United States and Russell C. Brock in Britain started to undertake mitral valvotomy, or commissurotomy as it was also known, with tremendous benefit to their patients. The attitude of physicians led Brock(3) to sarcastically declare, 'I can only conclude it is something in the very nature or atmosphere of the Royal College of Physicians – perhaps a cloud of some special canonising dust falls upon its habituees'.[82] Souttar's patient had significant mitral regurgitation as well as stenosis. He said that when he put his finger into the left auricle there was a jet like a fire hose coming through the mitral valve. This leads us onto another aspect of Lewis' views on valvular disease, for it was his opinion that the diagnosis of mitral regurgitation was of very limited importance. He based this on the difficulty of being certain, even at post mortem, as to whether regurgitation was actually present and of being unable to assess its degree if it was there. No doubt too the uncritical acceptance of apical systolic murmurs as indicating heart disease, when some were certainly innocent, also quite rightly coloured his views. As we know it is not always easy to tell whether an apical systolic murmur has the pansystolic quality of mitral regurgitation and it is a pity that Lewis did not employ the phonocardiogram to help in the differentiation, especially since he had previously been skilful in using this technique. I remember him teaching that the main value of a mitral systolic murmur was that it directed ones attention more closely to diastole where a previously unnoticed diastolic murmur led to a diagnosis of mitral stenosis!

CHAPTER 13

# Wide acclaim for *Diseases of the Heart*

*Diseases of the Heart* was an immediate success both with undergraduate students and with doctors. The subject matter was presented in a clear and logical fashion and the descriptions of disease were written in a style that held the readers attention throughout. The first edition came out in January 1933, and was reprinted six months later and again the next year. It sold nearly 6000 copies and a new edition was needed four years later. The American edition, published by the Macmillan Company of New York, was remarkably successful too and sold over 11 000 copies in spite of competing with Levine's *Clinical Heart Disease,* and to some extent with White's *Heart Disease* though this was a much larger reference volume. Its outstanding merit was soon appreciated in Europe and it was translated into the Dutch, German, Italian, Portuguese, Spanish, and Polish languages. *The Lancet* reviewed the book favourably and followed it with an entertaining editorial on 'The New Cardiology'. Lewis, it said, was one of the ablest critics of this day:

> He exposed, with logical and forceful argument, the fallacy of many beliefs which have been handed down from generation to generation. Had medicine not claimed his services, Sir Thomas Lewis might well have made a reputation at the Bar. One can visualise his righteous wrath when confronted by a criminal accused of being an accessory to the theory of 'compensation'. When a 'plain observation is garnished with an assumption and served up in an unrecognisable form', a heavy sentence would obviously be asked for, since he protests against the prevalence of this pernicious habit. A number of outwardly respectable clinicians who read this book will know themselves to be guilty of this crime. Some will be prepared to put up a spirited defence...They may even argue that...if one interpretation is discredited it is necessary quickly to invent another, before confidence is irretrievably lost. But beneath an unruffled surface the seed of a more scientific conception of medicine will have taken root, and Sir Thomas Lewis will not have laboured in vain.[11]

The *British Medical Journal* reviewed the book in a 1600 word editorial called 'Progress in Cardiology', saying that 'The ghosts of many erstwhile cardiological fancies have been laid, it is hoped for all time, by Sir Thomas Lewis (who) has provided English cardiologists and clinicians with a work for which many must have been waiting'. Commenting on the future of cardiology it said prophetically that the prevention of coronary sclerosis was an urgent need which awaited a full understanding of the normal and pathological metabolism of the heart.[10] Lewis would no doubt have regarded this as speculation, but it is true to say that biochemistry was not one of his strong points. Neither of these reviews commented especially on the book's value to undergraduate students but its attraction for them is testified by the fact that it soon became the book on heart disease which was owned by nearly every medical student in Britain. The phrase 'new cardiology' was probably first used in print by Dr Alexander Morison in a letter to *The Lancet* in 1917 when he described Mackenzie as 'The protagonist of the Newer Thought himself' and in which he criticized the Lumleian Lectures of Dr George A. Sutherland.[290] Mackenzie himself certainly used it then, or perhaps even earlier.[447]

## The department's work during 1932 to 1933

From 1932 to 1933, Grant, Pickering and Wayne continued as the whole time members of the staff whilst the visiting workers were Paul Rothschild and Werner Hess from Frankfurt, Paul D. Camp and Ashton Graybiel from Boston, and Louis B. Laplace from Philadelphia. Hess worked with Lewis on skin pain and with Pickering on vasodilatation in response to warming the body. Graybiel assisted Wayne with further work on angina pectoris, and he then joined Grant, as did Camp and Rothschild in his work on the vessels and nerves of the rabbit's ear. Grant's work was concerned with the problem as to why vascular tone returns after denervation of blood vessels and was undertaken to obtain a better understanding of vascular surgery in man.[285]

## The content and editing of *Heart*

In June 1933 the last two issues of *Heart* were published and in July the first issue of its successor *Clinical Science incorporating Heart* came out. It was now 24 years since Mackenzie and Lewis had founded *Heart* and it had run to 16 volumes. Lewis had never accepted any need to publish the individual issues at regular intervals and they came out when there was enough material to fill them. Four issues formed one volume. Sometimes the issues were only one or two months apart. It must have been the number of pages per volume that ultimately governed the timing, and this ranged between 273 and 405 with an average of 347 pages. With the exception of the war years there had been about one volume per year up to 1926, but in the final six years of *Heart* there was only one volume every two years. Papers from Lewis and his department naturally dominated the scene and accounted for 152 of the total of 326 papers, namely 46%. Of the remainder about a quarter each were from elsewhere in Britain, and from the United States. Other British papers actually outnumbered those of Lewis in the first six years but in the last six years there were only four compared with his 39. Workers in Europe had their own good journals in France, Austria and Germany and they contributed all told only ten papers. There were even fewer from other countries with just one each from Japan and Australia and two from Canada. The United States had been an important source of material with 31 papers in the first six years, and 25 in the six years after the war, but after the *American Heart Journal* was founded in 1926 only eight appeared. The title page of *Heart* listed those who 'aided in the selection of papers', or assistant editors as they would probably now be called. Professor George N. Stewart from Cleveland served nearly the whole time, from 1909 until 1927. He was joined in 1920 by Frank N. Wilson from Ann Arbor and there are several letters of interest between him and Lewis.[483] It is clear that American papers were sent first to Wilson, and these included ones from Paul S. Barker, Alfred E. Cohn and Harold M. Marvin. Wilson's letters contain personal remarks too. In 1925 having told Lewis about the problems in his department he wrote, 'I am buying new lenses and cameras every year. Small motion picture outfit, Bell and Howell, results are very good. It is a great sport. Good pictures at 40 feet.' In a letter about the effect of iced water on T waves, he also mentions that he has found a woodcock's nest. In a later letter in 1928 he says that although his health is still troubling him he is getting better, 'I have recently bought a place in the country which includes a small lake. I feel much better when I am out of doors getting some exercise in the fresh air'.[481] In 1933 Lewis sent a copy of *Diseases of the Heart* to Wilson who replied with the comment that he could not have afforded to buy it 'times are unusually hard' and adding 'I am sorry I have not been of more help to you in the selection of papers for *Heart*'. Wilson was now at the peak of his career and he is revered as one of the finest workers in the development of modern electrocardiography.[26] Grant gave Lewis a good deal of help, and there were 38 collaborators on the title page, but although Lewis often asked others for their opinion on submitted papers, he read and judged every one himself. It is surprising to find that Lewis made handwritten copies of letters which had been sent to authors.[380] Whether the letters were themselves in type or by hand is not known but either way it seems a remarkably inefficient way of conducting business. He went to great pains in editing as is shown by a letter to Professor Carl Wiggers in Chicago who had sent an article by his then young associate, later a famous electrocardiographer, Dr Louis N. Katz. Lewis took four pages to explain the deficiencies in an article by Katz on aortic stenosis and ends with a typically abrasive comment, 'until Katz has mastered the art of writing he should publish in American journals where there will be closer contact between the author and the editor'.[391] In referring to the change of title to *Clinical Science incorporating Heart* Lewis explained in a letter to Wilson that for some years it had been apparent 'that the continued publication of *Heart* on the old lines depends upon my laboratory turning out a large volume of cardiovascular work' and mentioning that the United States now had its own journal.[401] In his 'Final Editorial Note' in the last issue of Volume 16 of *Heart* Lewis wrote as follows:

> The first number of this Journal, '*Heart*', was issued in July 1909. At that time, 24 years ago, cardiac problems were being studied with unusual intensity, and a journal specially designed to publish original work dealing with the physiology and pathology of the cardiovascular system had become a necessity to workers in this field. It served this purpose. It was understood, however, even at its conception, that such a journal might not always be required.[185]

He went on to say that the rate of publication was declining and that this decline could be halted in one of two ways. The first was to admit articles 'of a different character, by breaking the rule that has been rigidly maintained, namely, that all matter published shall be based on original observation and experiment'. The second was to widen the scope of the journal whilst maintaining the standard. He chose the second course, which of course fitted in well anyway with his wish to have a journal for the Medical Research Society. Lewis' editorial comment has been interpreted by some as indicating that he thought there was no future for further progress in cardiology. In fact he was indicating that there was, at that time, not enough good material from British sources to fill the journal. The Americans had their own specialist journal and his own department was no longer working on cardiac problems. Lewis also commented that articles now had to be shorter, 'workers have really no time to plough through it'. This was a criticism that could certainly be levelled against his own papers which were of considerable length. They ranged from six to 76 pages, with an average of 30 pages – about 9000 words.

The journal was largely unprofitable to the publishers, Shaw and Sons, whose chief interest was in legal work, but Mr Henry Morten Bond and his brothers who owned the firm continued to do it because they liked Lewis as a man and admired his work. At one point, in 1924, Lewis got concerned about the financial position and asked Mackenzie for his help and advice. The journal, he explained, cost £700 a year to produce and with 400 subscribers that meant selling each volume at thirty eight shillings and sixpence, which he thought was too high. He was looking for someone to give an endowment of £5000 to reduce the cost of publication – did Mackenzie know anyone who could be approached from that point of view?[88] Presumably he thought that Mackenzie, even though he had left London some years before, might have a wealthy patient or friend who could oblige. Nothing came of this approach, but he also suggested that the editor should be appointed by a body such as the Royal Society. This idea did come to fruition later on when *Clinical Science* was transferred to the control of the Medical Research Society. *Heart* had been one of the most prestigious medical journals of its time, and Lewis certainly earned and deserved much of the credit for its high standard and great success.

## The Harveian Oration

In October 1933 Lewis gave the Harveian Oration at the Royal College of Physicians of London and selected 'Clinical Science' as his title.[183] The post of Harveian Orator is an honour which is conferred only upon distinguished Fellows of the College. This gave him his first opportunity to proclaim to a wide audience the importance of clinical science with its emphasis on the experimental method, a subject which he had made very much his own. It also gave him the occasion to point out that the outstanding quality of Harvey's discovery of the circulation was not so much the actual discovery but rather the exact observation and experiment which furnished the convincing proof of it. Harvey, he said, had been termed the father of physiology, 'he was much more than that, for his child was Clinical Science, out of which physiology and pathology were later born.' Lewis was at his most lyrical in the Oration:

> His book is a romantic example of scientific exposition, unsurpassed at his time and since his time. *De Motu Cordis* holds its reader entranced, while each stretch of the path brings a surer promise of the approaching vista; and when the path ends it ends on the hill-top, and there is unfolded to our gaze a land that is ours with certainty, ours for all time. This culmination brings with it a sense of security and accomplishment that fills us with profound and lasting emotion; and we go forward to hold what he has given us with a great thankfulness to this pioneer, who has not only led us to a new country, but has inspired us and taught us how farther to explore.

The nomination of a Harveian Orator was in the gift of the president of the College and several months beforehand Lewis thoughtfully called on Lord Dawson[(4)] in order to tell him that the proposed content was 'not entirely uncontroversial'. Dawson consented to the title of clinical science providing, he said, that it was given 'with urbanity' on the subject. He then launched into a tirade against Fletcher, 'and gave me a full view of the gulf between them'.[403] The gulf had arisen because it was the view of Dawson, who was a member of the MRC, that Fletcher took a superior attitude towards clinical doctors who he regarded as being unsuitable to guide research and that he minimized the value of clinicians' work in comparison with that of the research worker. Lewis wrote that he warned Elliott of the position – Fletcher was too frequent in his criticism of Lord Dawson. There is a good letter in reply from Elliott who said that Fletcher had definitely sought to humiliate Dawson again and he agreed that Fletcher should now receive a sharp lesson. Apparently Lewis must have written a critical letter to Fletcher for which he asked Elliott's approval, because Elliott said that for personal reasons he strongly desired that Fletcher 'should escape humiliation' adding 'I did not post your letter. You left the decision to me'.[403]

## Changes in the Department of Clinical Research

Lewis' crusade for clinical science envisaged the creation of departments similar to his own at other hospitals and in 1934 Grant left UCH after 14 years to become director of the newly established MRC Clinical Research Unit at Guy's Hospital. Money for the new post had become available because of Lewis' salary being funded by the Rockefeller Foundation. By this time Wayne too had left, to become Professor of Pharmacology and Therapeutics at Sheffield. Pickering had now turned his attention to hypertension – a subject on which he was later to become a world authority. He showed that patients with malignant hypertension had elevated cerebrospinal fluid pressures, due to the high diastolic blood pressure, and indicated that this was the cause of the changes in the retina.[280,296] Lewis' own research papers comprised three in 1933, one on coarctation and two on the mechanism of skin pain, whilst in 1934 there was just one paper, though an important one written jointly with Pickering on Raynaud's disease. He was now 52 and although excellent work on pain was still to come there seems to have been a lull in his research efforts. However as Dale later said, 'to suppose that at any moment of his waking life his brain was ever idle, relaxed, or inattentive is just impossible to anybody who knew him'. He went on to point out that as the years went by the centre of Lewis' thoughts and interest were more and more occupied by his mission in clinical research, 'The sword must not sleep in his hand till he had built here a temple for the service of medicine by the direct experimental investigation of disease in man, with proper careers and prospects open to its priesthood and its votaries'.[46]

## Clinical science, a students' course and a book

This was what Lewis was now about. He created a course for senior medical students into aspects of clinical science and then, in 1934, he wrote an outstanding book (Fig. 13.4, *overleaf*) based on this course with the title *Clinical Science illustrated by personal experiences.*[190] In the preface he explained that 'This book has been written in the hope of encouraging some young men, whom curiosity impels, to contemplate Clinical Science as a field of fruitful and interesting life work'. Using a military analogy he went on to state that it had been his faith that the normal advance of clinical science came not from 'mass attacks on

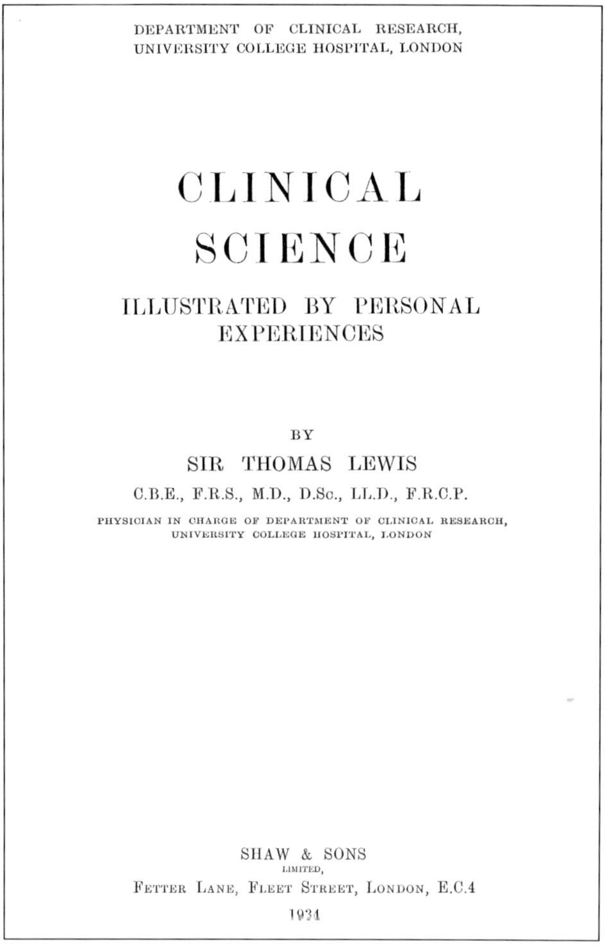

DEPARTMENT OF CLINICAL RESEARCH,
UNIVERSITY COLLEGE HOSPITAL, LONDON

CLINICAL
SCIENCE

ILLUSTRATED BY PERSONAL
EXPERIENCES

BY

SIR THOMAS LEWIS

C.B.E., F.R.S., M.D., D.Sc., LL.D., F.R.C.P.

PHYSICIAN IN CHARGE OF DEPARTMENT OF CLINICAL RESEARCH,
UNIVERSITY COLLEGE HOSPITAL, LONDON

SHAW & SONS
LIMITED,
FETTER LANE, FLEET STREET, LONDON, E.C.4
1934

*Figure 13.4 Title page of the book which is an invaluable source for his own account of his discoveries in clinical research. (From reference 190.)*

strongholds' but by pressing against the whole line of defence. One should search for vulnerable points, breaking in here and there, and consolidating each advance. 'Thus every small patch of new territory won becomes a permanent gain, and takes an essential part in the gradual disintegration of the defence'.[191] The first 14 chapters recount his own research work ranging from auricular fibrillation to erythralgia. The remaining three are thoughtful accounts of Diagnosis, Prognosis and Therapeutics, with the last one being especially interesting. It has a section on 'Testing the curative properties of remedies' which contains what may be one of the earliest accounts of how to conduct a controlled trial. He indicates the importance of making sure that the patients in the treated and control groups are composed as similarly as possible, and also warns that one should not compare the treatment of an earlier series with another one treated later. The whole book is well worth reading because it is an excellent account of much of Lewis' scientific career.

## F.G. Banting and others tell him of their discoveries

Another section in the last chapter was headed 'Discovery of new remedies' and among his personal papers there are several letters, dated around January 1935, which indicate that he probably had in mind writing a fuller account of this topic.[524] Frederick G. Banting wrote to say that he had not been interested in diabetes prior to his work on insulin, had no relatives with the disease and saw only one case of it whilst an undergraduate: 'the original experiments were planned simply to satisfy scientific curiosity. I am very glad that you are interested in the manner in which important discoveries in medicine are made.' Another Nobel Prize winner, George R. Minot who had discovered liver treatment for pernicious anaemia, wrote a 600 word letter telling how even as a house officer in Boston he had come to believe that 'what the pernicious anaemia patient needed was the right kind of food'. He also mentioned that he had been very ill with diabetes for two years before Banting's discovery restored him to health and enabled him to write his seminal paper with William P. Murphy three years later. Dr Mary B. Walker,[(5)] a London physician, had just discovered the physostigmine treatment of myasthenia gravis and Lewis asked if she had been influenced by Dale and Feldberg's work on acetylcholine, 'I should be ever so grateful if you would tell me; and allow me simultaneously to congratulate you on your success'. The answer was no, her observation came first.[474] It was good that he wrote warmly to Dr Walker because a letter from E.A. Carmichael in the MRC unit at the National Hospital for Nervous Diseases shows a lack of enthusiasm for her discovery which she had made single handed in a nonteaching hospital. Lewis' interest in how important discoveries are made continued a year later with a letter to Dr Chassar Moir, about his discovery of the new ergot alkaloid ergotamine, and the file also contains the obituary notice of Sir Frederick Banting in 1941. So it is surprising that he did not gather more information on the subject because his renown made it easy to get replies from other eminent medical scientists. And his wide knowledge of research, combined with his fluent pen, could have produced a fascinating book.

## Peripheral vascular disease

The year 1935 saw the conclusion of eight years work on the peripheral circulation with the publication in the second volume of *Clinical Science* of a paper, written with the collaboration of B. Gelfand of New York, on 'The manner in which necrosis arises in the fowl's comb under ergot poisoning'. The start of this long period of almost uninterrupted research had been signalled by his monograph in 1927 on *The Blood Vessels of the Human Skin and their Responses*[172] and the subsequent work was chiefly concerned with problems whose approach had been opened by studies described in that book. Prior to his work little attention had been paid to peripheral vascular disease apart from its morbid anatomy and, for example, reliable tests of limb circulation were scarcely known. Now there was an impressive amount of information on the way in which vascular disorders originate, of how disturbances of circulation produce their symptoms, and of means of testing the blood supply to the limbs. Clinical science had contributed much to the physiology of the circulation, and had gone on to make equally valuable advances in the understanding and treatment of its disorders. In his annual report Lewis wrote:

> There has followed a close revision of nomenclature and important changes; in particular, the attitude towards states formerly regarded as disturbances of the vasomotor system has been altered profoundly. There has been a large growth of accurate observations of fact, and the gradual welding of these together by new conceptions to form simpler and truer systems of thought; a type of work fundamental to the progress of clinical science.[286]

He distilled the essence of this research into a 109-page book, in which, judging the time to be opportune, he outlined conceptions of some peripheral disorders of the circulation for those engaged not in research but in practice.

It was called *Vascular Disorders of the Limbs* with the sub-title *described for practitioners and students.*[205] (Fig. 13.5) The first two chapters on testing the circulation in the limb and on the effects of circulatory arrest were especially valuable, giving precise information on practical points such as how to test blood flow rate and the patency of vessels. He emphasized that the most reliable method of gauging the state of blood flow in a resting limb was to estimate its surface temperature, whilst the colour of skin needed to be carefully assessed in relation to its

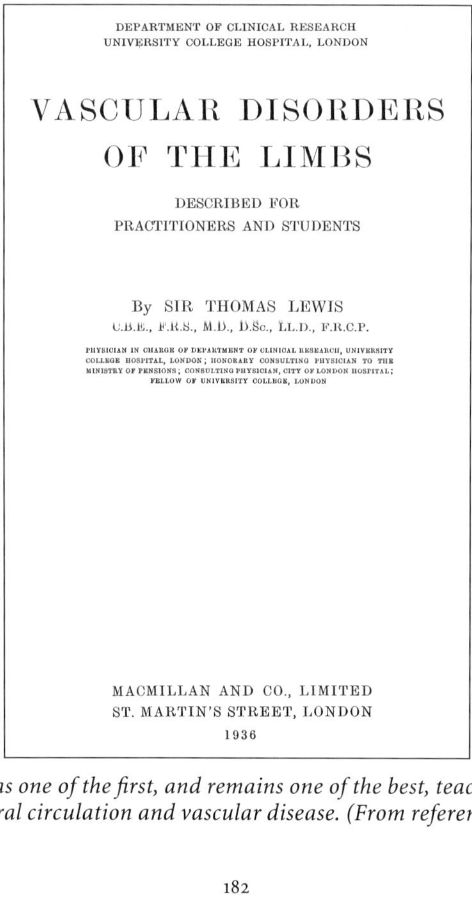
DEPARTMENT OF CLINICAL RESEARCH
UNIVERSITY COLLEGE HOSPITAL, LONDON

VASCULAR DISORDERS
OF THE LIMBS

DESCRIBED FOR
PRACTITIONERS AND STUDENTS

By SIR THOMAS LEWIS
C.B.E., F.R.S., M.D., D.Sc., LL.D., F.R.C.P.

PHYSICIAN IN CHARGE OF DEPARTMENT OF CLINICAL RESEARCH, UNIVERSITY COLLEGE HOSPITAL, LONDON; HONORARY CONSULTING PHYSICIAN TO THE MINISTRY OF PENSIONS; CONSULTING PHYSICIAN, CITY OF LONDON HOSPITAL; FELLOW OF UNIVERSITY COLLEGE, LONDON

MACMILLAN AND CO., LIMITED
ST. MARTIN'S STREET, LONDON
1936

*Figure 13.5 This was one of the first, and remains one of the best, teaching books about the peripheral circulation and vascular disease. (From reference 205.)*

temperature. For example skin with a good blood flow was pale, not red, because small vessel tone was high. The following nine chapters dealt with the conditions such as Raynaud's disease, intermittent claudication, and vascular disorders in diseases of the nervous system, which he had studied himself. He chose he said not to write a comprehensive account and so he excluded conditions such a varicose veins and aneurysm on which he had nothing to add to available accounts. In writing this book he was following the pattern he had set with his earlier teaching books on disorders of the heart beat, electrocardiography and on the effort syndrome. Speaking of this, Drury and Grant wrote

> Yet, as he knew, he was suspected of vanity and self seeking, a suspicion fed by the success of his small books for clinical use, by his emphasis on his own work in *Clinical science illustrated by personal experiences,* and by his apparent hardness in dealing with those who worked with him and those who could or would not further the mission which inspired his own life. But Lewis did not write these books for money or display. He grudged the time spent on them, feeling that this should be given rather to his proper work of gathering new and important knowledge; but he felt also that he ought to write these books to spread the gospel, knowing that few would read his closely reasoned scientific papers and fewer still appreciate them. For the emphasis on his own work he offered no apology; an author should write mainly on that which had passed within the range of his own experience, the basis of his teaching should be that which he himself had seen and proved to be true.[50]

A second revised edition of *Vascular Disorders of the Limbs* came out in 1946 and to this day it remains an excellent practical guide to the subject, and valued by vascular surgeons as well as by physicians. Surprisingly few other short books have been written on this topic, in marked contrast to the plethora of handbooks on electrocardiography. A review of the book in *Nature* led Lewis to object vigorously to its editor Sir Richard Gregory. The reviewer had used the occasion to criticize clinical science and Lewis complained that 'highly controversial matter is put into a review of a book intended for students. Your reviewer fails to play fair either to my book which I mind little enough, or to clinical science which I greatly resent'.[405] Later Paul Rothschild, now a general practitioner in Blaengarw, Glamorgan, Wales, wrote to say that Professor Werner Hess (Fig. 13.6, *overleaf*) would translate the book and that Professor Franz Volhard had accepted Lewis' request to supervise production of the German edition.[465] Volhard was professor of medicine in Frankfurt and a leading authority on renal disease and hypertension. Lewis had corresponded with him back in 1910 and on his visits to London would meet him off the boat train at Liverpool Street station. Once he took Volhard into the refectory and all the students, knowing of the visitor's eminence, stood up as he walked through. Rothschild and Hess were the only two German doctors who worked with Lewis and they were both from Volhard's department. Luckily the manuscript (Fig. 13.7, *overleaf*) has survived of the first handwritten draft of chapter 8 and the frequent deletions, even of whole paragraphs, and re-written sentences show how much revision Lewis required to achieve the clarity of his final text.[523] For example, 'It is probable that…' is replaced by 'It is supposed, though unproved, that…'. In another example, 'The pathological interest lies in the fact that…' is replaced by 'It is of interest that…' Drury and Grant were correct to say 'His clinical books are masterly in their directness and simplicity of statement and ease of comprehension', but they may have been thinking rather of the way he wrote papers rather than books when

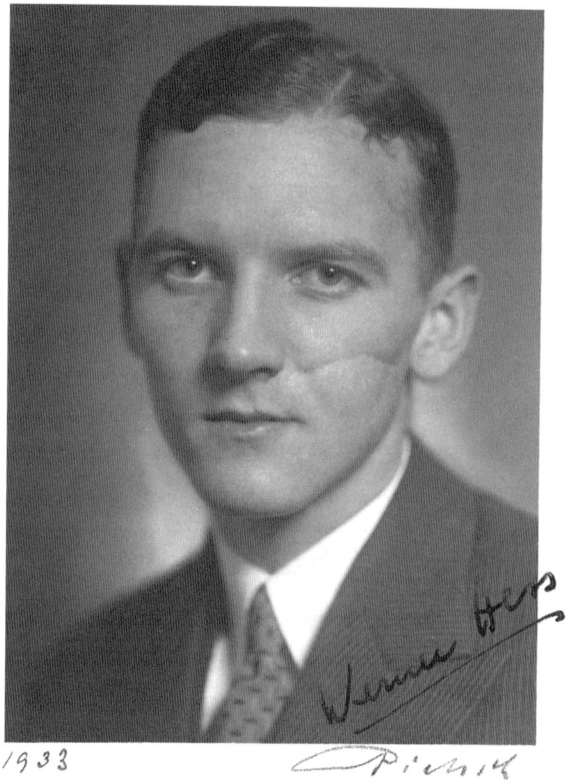


*Figure 13.6* *Werner Hess from Frankfurt am Main (1908– ) worked in 1932 on the mechanism of skin pain. He was one of two research workers from Germany with Lewis. Note the duelling scar on his left cheek.*

they state 'He so schooled himself to see clearly what to say before putting pen to paper that he could write swiftly and often almost without erasure.'[50]

## A second myocardial infarction

Whatever plans he may have had for starting a new line of research towards the end of 1935 were halted, as they had been on two previous occasions, by illness. On November 16, having returned home from what he described in his diary as a 'stupid meeting' of the Physiological Society, he sustained that evening his second attack of coronary thrombosis. He still preferred this term, even though Parkinson and Bedfords's 1927 paper in *Heart* had used the more precise term myocardial infarction. He chose Dr John Parkinson, who had worked with him at the Military Heart Hospital as his physician. (Fig. 13.8) It is said that this attack was less severe than the first, but even so he was kept in bed at home, as we can tell from his diary, for nearly six weeks. His electrocardiogram taken on November 18 (Fig. 13.9), is the first to have been kept and it shows just minor ST

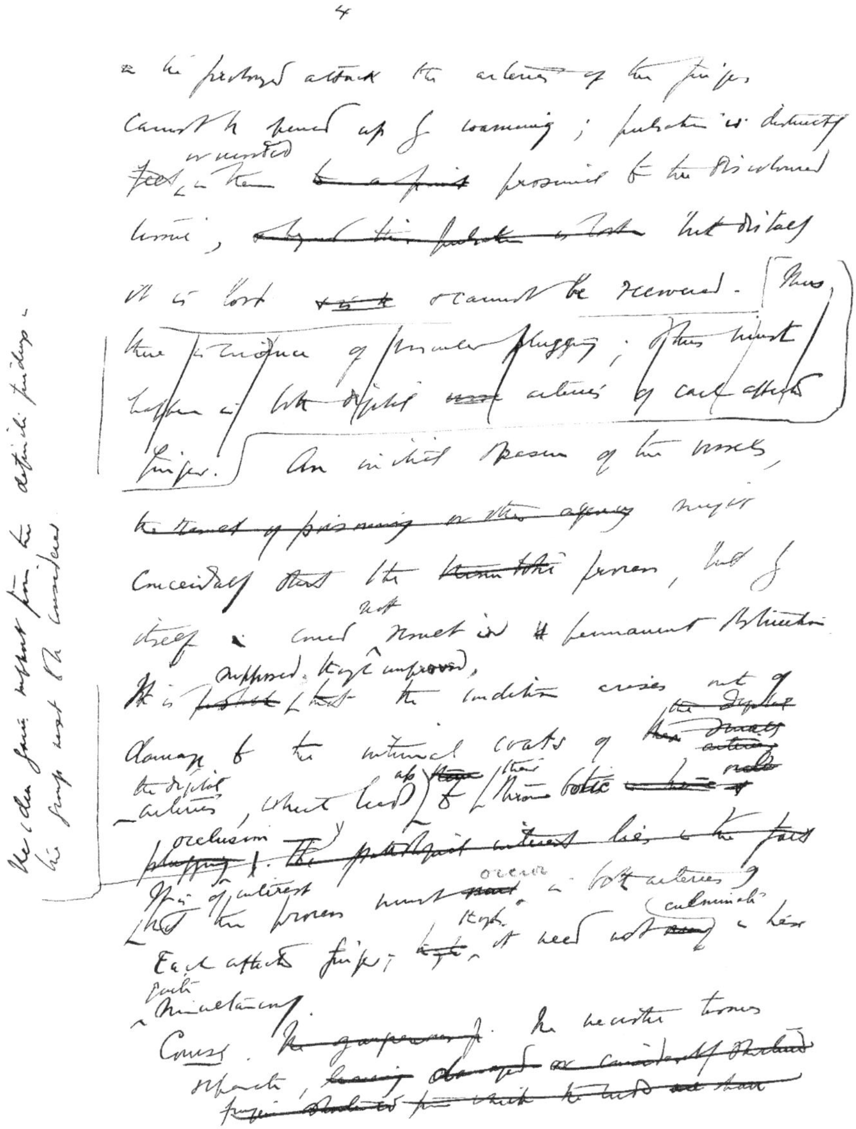

*Figure 13.7 Manuscript of part of pp 77–78 of* Vascular Disorders of the Limbs.

segment depression, with possibly an abnormal Q wave in lead I due to the earlier episode. It gives the impression of being a substandard tracing, and there is no millivolt deflection to check on the response time or calibration. On January 18 1936 he and his wife went to the Canary Islands and arrived back in England on board the *Garth Castle* liner on February 13. He made a good recovery from this illness but in addition to interrupting his research programme it had another adverse effect. He explained this soon afterwards in a letter to B.S. Oppenheimer in New York, saying that he had planned to visit the United States with Lady Lewis and lecture in Cleveland, in Richmond (fee $350), and at Harvard but that

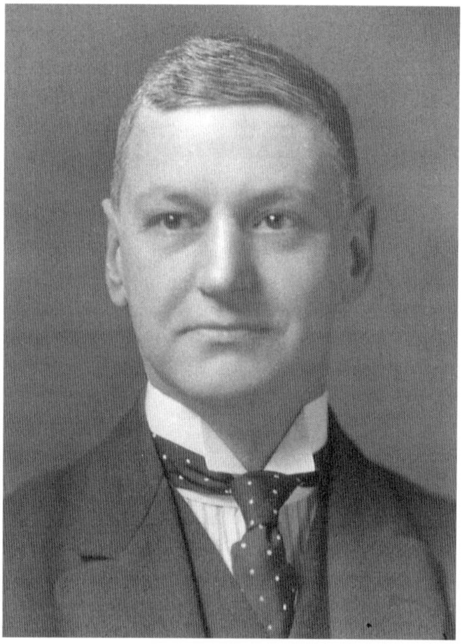

*Figure 13.8* *Dr J. (later Sir John) Parkinson in 1929 aged 44. He was Lewis' personal cardiologist.*

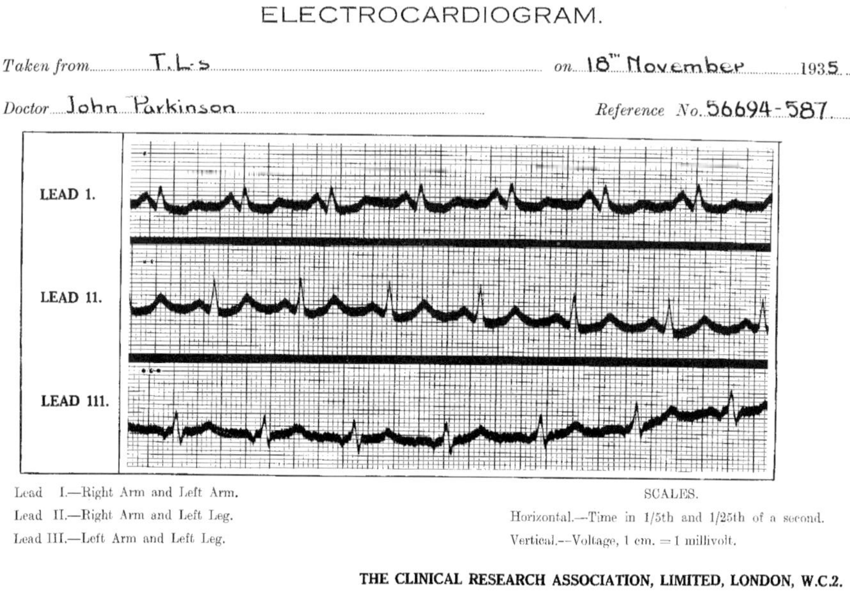


*Figure 13.9* *Lewis' electrocardiogram taken three days after his second myocardial infarction in 1935. See text for description.*

this visit was now cancelled.[409] He never had another opportunity to visit North America.

## Notes to Chapter 13

(1) Francis Martin Rouse Walshe, FRS, (later Sir Francis), 1885–1973, was a distinguished neurologist who was on the staff of the National Hospital for Nervous Diseases at Queen Square London, and also at UCH. He was a gifted writer and was noted as a witty and incisive speaker. He edited the journal *Brain* and wrote a popular textbook on *Diseases of the Nervous System.*

(2) James Hope, FRS, 1801–1841, was a great pioneer of cardiology. After graduating in Edinburgh in 1824 he studied in Paris and then became physician to the Marylebone Infirmary in London and also to St George's Hospital. He investigated the origin of heart sounds and murmurs, recently described by Laennec when he invented the stethoscope, by auscultating the exposed heart of unconscious animals. He wrote a classic book, *Treatise on the diseases of the heart and great vessels,* in 1831 and was the first to identify left ventricular failure as an entity. He also published a fine illustrated work on Morbid Anatomy for which he made the coloured lithographs himself.

(3) Russell Claude Brock, (later Lord Brock), 1903–1980, was a most distinguished cardiac surgeon. In 1948 he was among the first in the world to operate on mitral stenosis and he later pioneered an operation to relieve congenital pulmonary stenosis. He had a deep interest in the history of surgery. He became president of the Royal College of Surgeons of England.

(4) Bertrand Edward Dawson, (later Lord Dawson), 1864–1945, was appointed physician to the London Hospital in 1906 and did good work on infective endocarditis. He was physician to King George V, and was president of the Royal College of Physicians of London from 1931–1938. He was a medical statesman and played an important part in planning the Ministry of Health.

(5) Mary Broadfoot Walker, 1881–1974, qualified in Edinburgh in 1913. She worked largely in the 'Poor Law' hospitals of the London County Council, and whilst at St Alfege's Hospital, Greenwich she had a patient with myasthenia gravis, a then untreatable disease. She asked the visiting neurologist what kind of disease it was and when he replied that it was like curare poisoning, she decided to treat her patient with the curare antagonist physostigmine. The patient improved and this perceptive discovery by Dr Walker initiated effective treatment for the disease. She was a modest person, with a lowly position in the medical hierarchy, who never got proper recognition for her important work which she published by only a letter to *The Lancet.* But it clearly impressed Sir Thomas Lewis who wrote a warm letter of congratulation.

# Chapter 14

## Studies of pain • The nocifensor system of nerves • Double pain response in the skin • Referred pain and tenderness

ALTHOUGH HIS research on vascular problems in the skin had now finished there was one aspect of it which led Lewis on to what became one of his most interesting though controversial studies. It concerned the finding that many subjects develop soreness of the skin around a small area of injury. He had first noticed it on his own arm after stimulating it locally with a faradic current during his work on erythralgia, and he thought that investigation of this diffuse hyperalgesia 'might possibly throw light on the long disputed origin of referred tenderness'.[204] Lewis was commenting here on the fact, known for decades, that visceral disease caused skin tenderness and muscular rigidity too, at a distance from the affected organ such as a diseased gall bladder. It is likely that the problem had been in his mind ever since Mackenzie had discussed it at length in his book on *Symptoms and their Interpretation* which was written at about the time they first met.[267] He started work on this topic in 1936 with the assistance of Professor R. Hussey from New Haven and with A.J. Honour who Lewis knew was good at making accurate observations.[204]

### Skin hyperalgesia following injury

They injured a small area of skin on their forearms either by faradic current, by crushing with forceps or by freezing and showed that a large area of soreness, up to 18 cm by 7 cm, appeared around that point, reaching a maximum in one hour and lasting for several hours. The same area was involved when the injury was repeated several days later. A needle prick in the area gave intense pain, but heat and touch sensations were not changed. What was the origin of this hyperalgesia? Lewis devised some simple and ingenious experiments with local anaesthesia to try to answer the question. If a cutaneous nerve was blocked and the anaesthetic skin injured, the hyperalgesia appeared as the nerve block wore off, showing that it was not dependent on impulses reaching the central nervous system. When local anaesthetic was injected intradermally and that area injured, then the soreness did not appear until the injured area itself had recovered from the anaesthetic. This showed that the soreness was produced through the nerves that had been anaesthetized, and incidentally not by spread of a substance through the skin. Furthermore if the anaesthetic area was injured eccentrically with a tiny

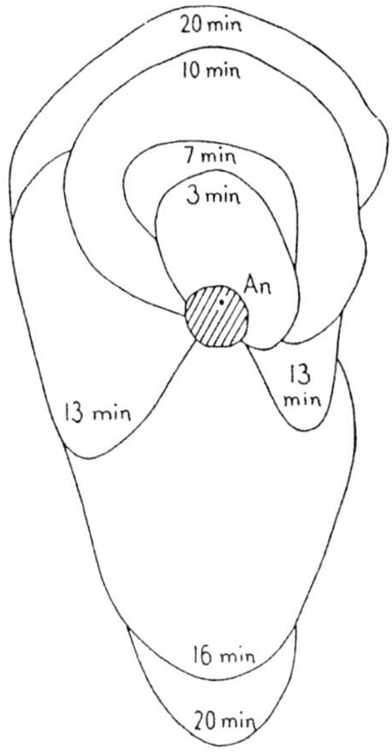


Fig. 11. (× 2/3). Crush placed eccentrically over anæsthetised skin. A.J.H., July the 18th. A circular area of skin (*An*) is anæsthetised by intradermal injection of 1% novocaine. The area of analgesia is mapped out and it is noted that there is no surrounding hyperalgesic skin 2 min. later.

*Figure 14.1 The nocifensor reaction. Areas of hyperalgesia are shown at the times they appear after crushing the skin eccentrically within a circle of local anaesthetic. Hyperalgesia appears first where the crush is near to edge of the anaesthetised circle. See text. (From reference 204.)*

crush, the hyperalgesia appeared first only on the side of the crush. (Fig. 14.1) These experiments showed that the nerves responsible for the phenomenon lay in the skin itself and were in the form of arborisations rather than of a network.[204] He also showed that mucous membrane, too, could produce cutaneous tenderness in an experiment, done in fact on himself, which is a good example of his ability to exploit a disease process for research.[210] After an operation on his maxillary sinus he had been left with a permanent hole between the antrum and nose, through which an electrode could be passed. He stimulated his antrum with a faradic current and produced hyperalgesia of the face. (Fig. 14.2, *overleaf*)

## The nocifensor system of nerves; a hypothesis

From these studies and others Lewis decided that the nervous pathways involved in hyperalgesia could not be the usual pain or sensory nerve fibres, nor the sympathetic fibres, and he concluded that there must be a hitherto unknown system of richly arborising nerve fibres to explain his findings. He called it the 'nocifensor' system, having invented the word as meaning to defend from injury, and by December 1936 the work, which must have gone well, was published in *Clinical Science* under the title 'Experiments relating to cutaneous hyperalgesia and its

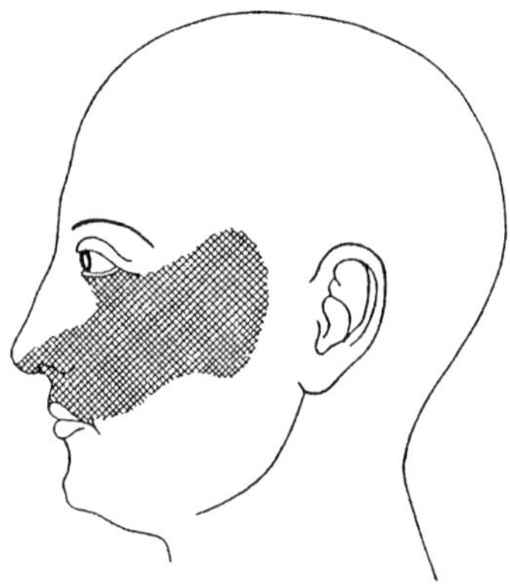

Fig. 10. A diagram of the face showing the area of hyperalgesia developing on stimulating the mucous membrane or dental nerves within the left maxillary antrum.

*Figure 14.2 Hyperalgesia of the face produced by stimulating the maxillary antrum with a faradic current showing that injured mucous membrane could give cutaneous hyperalgesia. See text. (From reference 204.)*

spread through somatic nerves'.[204] He then wrote a definitive account of the work in a paper in the *British Medical Journal*, 'The nocifensor system of nerves and its reactions'.[210] This followed his usual policy of placing his research work before a general audience in a nonspecialist journal. The paper was a summary of his two George Halliburton Hume lectures given in Newcastle-upon-Tyne in February 1937. As we have already noted Lewis was reluctant to give lectures outside his own medical school and the attraction here was doubtless because they were named after the father of Dr (later Sir William) Hume, a pioneer cardiologist and member of the Cardiac Club, who had been his colleague at the Military Heart Hospital. In spite of the novelty of the subject there was no correspondence in the *British Medical Journal* following his paper.

## The hypothesis attacked

The obvious objection to the concept of a nocifensor system lay in the fact that no such nerves could be shown anatomically to exist. F.M.R Walshe thought the hypothesis was untenable in the absence of such nerves.[324] Pickering, too, was sceptical of the idea because he could not reproduce on himself the same results that Lewis obtained and decided that he could not continue to work with Lewis on pain. In fact they seem to have had quite a row about it. But Lewis was sure of his observations and wrote, 'The fact that a system of nerves which I conclude to be present has previously escaped recognition is no argument against its existence'.[232] His final remarks came in a paper on the vascular axon reflex when he said, 'Committed permanently to this nocifensor hypothesis I naturally am not...the hypothesis is serving its purpose...Whether, as new evidence comes, it continues to stand, or like most hypotheses falls I am content to think that (my) observations will remain as contributions to knowledge whatever interpretations may come ultimately to be put upon them'.[227]

## Lewis shown to be correct

Nearly 50 years later new evidence did come and it showed that Lewis was right.[106] His nocifensor nerves are now known to be primary afferent neurones (C fibres). These fibres convey the modalities of pain to the central nervous system, but they also contain, and can release, large amounts of neuropeptides at their peripheral endings by an axon reflex mechanism. Thus the C fibres can rightly be described as 'noci-' since they convey information about noxious stimuli, and '-fensor' because they generate a local inflammatory response to aid in counteracting the noxious stimulus. Modern research has thus amply confirmed his hypothesis and a recent worker has described as truly prophetic the way in which he regarded 'the nerves as liberating potent substances from cellular elements of the skin into surrounding space thus controlling partly or wholly within the skin important elements of defence, including inflammation'.[106] The nocifensor work came from the observation that there was tenderness around an area of injury. This was known to many, but it was he who took up the challenge of explaining it. His experiments were simple but conclusive, and gave him the authority to state a bold but logical interpretation of them. This work was intellectually better even than that on the excitatory process in the dog's heart which had won such acclaim, and it shows him as scientific worker of the highest calibre.

## The double pain response of the skin

Edward Eric (Bill) Pochin was selected by Lewis as his house physician in 1935 and became a full time worker in March 1936 with a salary of £300 a year, at which time Lewis told Mellanby 'he is a man I have had under close supervision for four years...Pochin has unusual ability and a strong desire to enter the field of Clinical Science'.[502] He succeeded Lewis as director of the department in 1946. Pochin joined a project which Lewis had been pursuing for five years on the altered pain response to asphyxia. It had begun as a by-product of his work in the 1920's on the skin circulation when numbness of the skin was often noticed after depriving a limb of its bloodflow for several minutes. This phenomenon had been investigated in 1933 by Lewis, Pickering and Rothschild who found that ischaemia first eliminated the sense of touch and then produced a delay in the perception of pain.[261] For a start Pochin and Lewis carefully studied the pain of a needle prick in normal fingers. To their surprise they found that there was a double pain response from the skin, an immediate slight pain being followed by a longer and more intense one. Asphyxia abolished the first response – hence the delay in perception. The explanation of their findings was facilitated by recent animal work in New York by Herbert S Gasser and Joseph Erlanger which showed that there are faster and slower conducting fibres in peripheral nerve trunks.[65] Their use of cocaine, and Lewis' use of asphyxia, together gave weight to the idea that the two pain responses are carried by fibres with different conduction rates. To test this view Lewis devised an experiment of characteristic simplicity. He reasoned that the longer the nerve, the greater would be the delay of the second response, and when he measured it the delay was nil in the trunk, 0.9 seconds at the thigh and 1.9 seconds at the toe. 'Those expectations,' he wrote, 'proved easy to demonstrate'.[231]

## Itching studied by a medical student

Another aspect of cutaneous sensation was investigated soon afterwards, and again the research worker was a man who had attracted Lewis' attention whilst a medical student. This was Reginald G. (Reggie) Bickford who was recommended to Mellanby for a grant with the comment 'he has insatiable curiosity', having been a voluntary worker in the department before qualifying. Bickford's project started, as several of Lewis' had done, when his interest was aroused by a chance personal observation. He had been bitten by a gnat and noticed that whilst the subsequent itching came directly from the bite itself, the surrounding skin itched only when it was rubbed. By using histamine to produce itching he showed that nerve asphyxia abolished the itchy skin but not the spontaneous itching, and therefore reasoned that the two sensations were carried by separate types of nerve.[19] Lewis must have been pleased that one of his own students had been attracted to a problem in clinical science in just the way he liked to do himself.

## Study of referred pain

The work on pain continued with a study of structures deep to the skin, and attention was directed especially to the question of referred pain, a problem which had fascinated so many previous workers. Mackenzie had studied it closely, in 1893 whilst in general practice, and this alone would have been an attraction for Lewis who greatly respected Mackenzie's work. Somatic pain was the first aspect to be tackled and in 1937 Lewis was joined in this by Jonas Henrik (Yonki) Kellgren,[(1)] who had been his house physician. (Fig. 14.3) Kellgren's Swedish grandfather had set up an institute in London for treatment

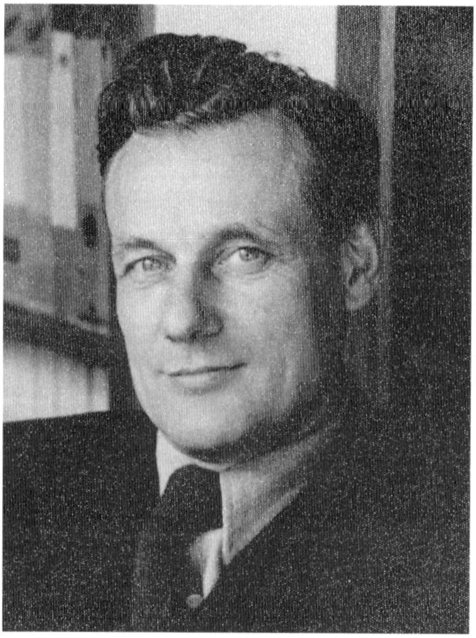

*Figure 14.3 Jonas H. ('Yonki') Kellgren who did important and original work on referred pain.*

by massage and exercises, in which he was followed by Kellgren's father who graduated from St George's Hospital. So musculoskeletal problems were very much in the family. He got the idea that muscle pain was not always arising from the place where it was felt, and discussed this with Lewis. Actually Lewis wrote that he had himself been impressed by the way in which pain from a muscle is often referred to a distance and that he had been fortunate in interesting Kellgren in these reactions, but it is Kellgren's belief that it was he who initiated the investigation.[518] Whoever it was who first started things off, the fact is that Kellgren did nearly all the investigations himself with Lewis coming into the laboratory each day to discuss the results and to jointly plan the progress of the study.

## Experiments on referred pain by Kellgren

It was found that muscle pain was most reliably produced by injecting a small amount of 5% saline. The pain so induced was felt over a definite area which had a segmental distribution and Kellgren concluded that this area was determined by the nerve roots which supplied the corresponding muscles. Thus different muscles supplied by a common root source gave a common field of pain distribution. For example pain from the first intercostal muscle was referred down the inside of the arm – a feature of obvious clinical significance. Kellgren then discovered that injecting the interspinous ligaments gave pain similar to injecting muscles of the back, and soon found that it was a much better method. He injected all the ligaments in turn from the fifth cervical to the second sacral, and by so doing he was able to construct an accurate map of the segmental areas of deep pain. (Fig. 14.4) The two papers describing this work appeared under

*J. H. KELLGREN.*

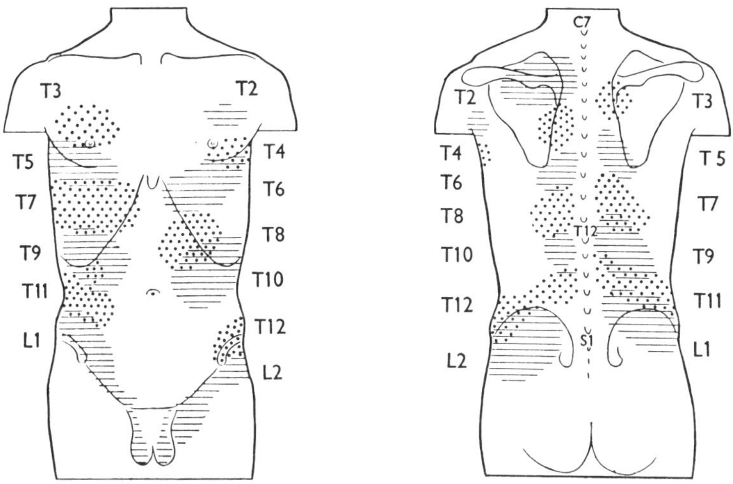


Fig. 1. Shows the distribution of pain arising from the interspinous ligaments T 2 to L 2. Alternate areas have been hatched and stippled.

*Figure 14.4 Segmental areas of referred pain produced by injecting inter-spinous ligaments. (From* Clinical Science *1939;4:35–46.)*

Kellgren's name alone.[93,94] Lewis would not put his name on a paper unless he had actually done the work himself even though, as in this instance, it was part of a larger study which he had initiated and was directing. In this respect he followed the precept of his chief, Sir Victor Horsley.[293] In October 1938 Kellgren was appointed to the 196th Beit Memorial Fellowship for Medical Research of which Lewis had been the first holder from 1910–1912. He was the first person on Lewis' staff to get this prestigious fellowship, though Dr Janet Vaughan obtained it just after leaving his department. Why other of his full time workers did not have it is probably explained by the fact that they had no need of a grant because they had salaries from the MRC. Professor T.R. Elliott who was the 11th holder in 1911–1913 was now secretary of the Trust and three of the assistants on his Medical Unit gained a Beit Fellowship. F. Horace Smirk was awarded one to study the functional pathology and physiology of diuresis from a biochemical standpoint, John McMichael studied the inter-relationships of liver and splenic diseases and Harold P. Himsworth worked on the activation of insulin and the effect of various diets in diabetes. This shows the strength of clinical research in the medical school at that time, remembering also that there were five Fellows of the Royal Society on the staff.

## Relation between somatic and visceral pain

The next step, and it was one in which Lewis was especially interested, was to search for similarities between somatic and visceral pain. It had been well known from Mackenzie's time that visceral disease was associated with muscular rigidity and cutaneous tenderness, and attention was now paid particularly to these features. By injecting the first lumbar ligament they were able to reproduce the retraction of the testis and the rigidity and tenderness of the lower abdominal wall which were known to be features of renal colic. These features were the more remarkable because they cannot be produced by voluntary effort. Then Lewis and Kellgren studied patients who had pain of visceral origin in order to compare their natural pain with that of interspinous injections.[243] Most of their subjects were doctors, who could appreciate the object of the study, and who suffered from angina pectoris. Although the pain from injecting the left eighth cervical ligament was naturally more obvious in the back than the front, it did spread down the left arm and impressed them as otherwise closely resembling their anginal pain. Furthermore it could be accompanied by numbness and tingling of the hand, by a sense of constriction in the chest, and by hyperalgesia of the skin on the inner side of the arm. As an example of a referred symptom which he could not explain, he mentioned a subject who had previously had an attack of neuritis with pain and tingling in the hand and in whom years later these recurred on evacuating a full bladder. That subject was in fact himself.[230] Kellgren then investigated referred pain and tenderness in patients with fibrositis or myalgia, and showed that these symptoms were eliminated by injecting a local anaesthetic, 1% novocaine, into the tender spot from which the pain arose.[92] Some of this work was briefly recounted in a paper entitled 'Suggestions relating to the study of somatic pain' which Lewis published in the *British Medical Journal* thus continuing his life long discipline of presenting his work to the profession as a whole.[211] He explained this approach in a letter to Gerald Horner the editor of the *Journal*.

> Your Journal is the medium I long ago selected as that through which I like best to approach the general practitioner. I try to select from our work at UCH topics that have a bearing on practical work; it is in my view an essential part of a research workers duty.[396]

## Work on renin by Pickering and Prinzmetal

Pickering was appointed as an 'independent lecturer' on cardiovascular disease in the department in October 1936 and Lewis described him as 'a man of very unusual ability and a hard worker, his research is of great interest'.[411] This opinion fully vindicated the comment made in 1930 by Dr John Fulton[(2)] who wrote to Lewis from Oxford saying, 'George Pickering writes me saying he is going to be with you this year. I am very glad to hear the news for he is an attractive and exceedingly able fellow and I am sure you will understand one another'.[365] The research referred to was on hypertension and Pickering had five papers on it in *Clinical Science* that year. One showed the lack of a pressor effect when blood from hypertensive subjects was transfused into patients with anaemia. In the following year, 1937, Dr Myron Prinzmetal[(3)] from Los Angeles came to the department having been attracted to Lewis' work whilst still a medical student when he read *The blood vessels of the human skin and their responses*. Prinzmetal assisted Pickering in his work and they made important observations on renin and notably developed a method for its biological assay in addition to studying hypertension of renal origin in the rat.[280] Several years later Prinzmetal became noted for his experimental work on cardiac arrhythmias and for his discovery of 'variant' angina pectoris which is named after him.

## Lewis' dominant position in clinical research

Lewis served on the Medical Research Council from 1933 to 1937 and became secretary of its Clinical Committee. At its second meeting in November 1933, with Wilfrid Trotter in the chair, it was decided to implement Lewis' proposal that a new unit of clinical research should be established at Guy's Hospital with Ronald T. Grant as its director.[457] Lewis definitely wanted to have more departments like his own, but it was also suggested that he thought Grant's research had become pedestrian and he wanted to move him on. By now Lewis had become the most powerful figure in clinical research in Britain and his opinion was often sought.[22] For example he was twice asked about appointments to Regius chairs in Glasgow by their principal Sir Hector Hetherington. The first was a request about Dr John McNee, a Glasgow graduate who had been at UCH for 17 years firstly on the Medical Unit and who was now a consultant physician. Lewis replied, 'He is a cultured man always well in the swim, knows what everyone is doing and a competent judge of young men who would build up a good show by using his juniors rather than his personal efforts. He has plenty of brains but is inclined to dilettantism.'[406] McNee (later Sir John) became Regius professor of medicine. The second concerned the chair of materia medica and pharmacology. Lewis favoured Wayne who then held a chair at Sheffield, even though he was not an applicant saying, 'He has a highly critical mind, heaps of energy and is much liked by all who work with him'. Smirk, said Lewis, had neither a first class brain nor an easy personality, but McMichael was 'a very keen and capable worker and a very nice fellow but of junior standing for your pos'.[413] Dr Noah Morris was appointed, but Wayne later went to Glasgow to succeed McNee. Lewis' involvement in academic appointments is also shown by a letter he wrote to the Vice-Chancellor of the University of London, Sir Robert Pickard, about the election of professors. He said it was not satisfactory for referees' letters to be read out at the interview and that they would serve their purpose better by being circulated beforehand. But in saying this he overlooked the problem of confidentiality. As secretary of the MRC's Clinical Committee Lewis dealt with grant applications. In 1936 Dr Bruce Perry from Bristol came to see him to obtain a grant in order to follow up many patients of Dr Carey Coombs.[(4)] The suggestion had been made that patients with chorea later got pure mitral stenosis, whilst those with rheumatic fever developed mixed valve lesions. Lewis took him to lunch at the Athenaeum. Indicating a sideboard loaded with food he said 'take what you like, I always have bread and cheese' – which Perry diplomatically had also. But the only discussion on the grant consisted of Lewis saying that one would not be forthcoming 'because you will not be able to diagnose mitral stenosis'.[462] No explanation was offered for this enigmatic remark and the young Perry did not like to challenge it. Not surprisingly his opinion was still being sought about electrocardiography. Sir Robert Robinson, the Government Chemist, wrote in 1936 to ask whether an ink pen recorder developed in his department might be used for this. Lewis replied that several such amplifier driven systems had been developed but they were less accurate than the photographic records and had 'failed to attract'.[410] The episode is of interest because it shows that Lewis was aware of developments in that field and probably knew about the first commercially available direct writing electrocardiograph which had been invented in Geneva in 1932 by Duchosal and Luthi.[25]

## Letters to friends • Helps German Jewish doctors

Other correspondence at this time shows that he was keeping up with friends at home and abroad. In 1936 Lewis sent a letter to Eugene Landis in Pennsylvania to introduce Dr Arthur Wesson who had the Bilton Pollard Travelling Fellowship from UCH.[407] His former student, Dr William A.H. Rushton, wrote to say that he was using the triple response and muscle ischaemia as practical work in his physiology classes at Cambridge, and Lewis' reply ended with the warm comment, 'I hope you are enjoying life again in your old abode'.[416] The growing menace of Hitler had been apparent to Lewis ever since he had warned Paul Rothschild in 1932 of the danger he faced by staying in Germany, and it is clear from his correspondence that he was eager to help other Jewish refugee doctors.[101] For example in 1936 C.J. Rothberger wrote from Vienna to ask his help for Adolph Schott who had arrived in Britain.[464] Schott was well known as the co-author with David Scherf of a book on arrhythmias and he continued with this work in London. Lewis kept in close touch with the German Jewish Aid Committee and helped several others, some of whom went on to the United States. Other letters included one from the renowned neurosurgeon Dr Wilder Penfield of the Montreal Neurological Institute requesting criticism of a paper he had written on the cerebral circulation. Penfield went on to say he had noticed that the pulse disappears during a fit and asks why.[461] Lewis replied that he did not know 'but it *must* be explained'.[415] Dr Chromow wrote from the United States to ask his opinion about the use, in teaching students, of heart sound recordings and was told that they were not of much use, auscultation being best learnt at the bedside.[351] A brief letter to *The Lancet* in 1940 about an article on sympathectomy caused trouble when three words which Lewis added to the proof were not printed because it arrived too late.[209] Lewis said the journal should have waited for the corrected proof but he got a firm reply from Dr Theodore Fox, then assistant editor, who said that 'the sending of a letter for publication gives us authority to publish it in that form'.[429] Lewis had clashed with editors previously, but on this occasion he made no rejoinder.

## Training in clinical research

In February 1937 he wrote to Lord Dawson, president of the Royal College of Physicians of London, in order to point out the problem posed to those entering full time research of the need to pass the Membership examination (MRCP) of the College. He complained that this delayed their start in research by one year at a time when they might be very productive.[412] One wonders why the clinical experience of an extra year in the wards was apparently felt to be of lesser importance. But we know that Lewis wished to establish a university degree in clinical science, probably a Master of Science, and although this never came about he may have visualized it as an alternative to the Membership.

Lewis was keenly aware that the lack of suitable training posts with proper remuneration, was a considerable obstacle for the young men and women who wished to do clinical research. He therefore persuaded the MRC in 1936 to establish and finance such posts.[286] They created six postgraduate fellowships, tenable for one year at a salary of £200. In addition there were four more senior research fellowships at £250 for the first year and renewable at £300 for a second year. A poster was printed to advertise these posts in the medical schools. Dr Alan R. Kelsall, a student from St Bartholomew's Hospital, was appointed to a fellowship at UCH and went for an interview with some apprehension having heard of Lewis' fierce reputation. A.J. Honour remembers that Kelsall was sitting at a table when Lewis entered the room and before any word was spoken he collapsed to the floor in a profound faint. Kelsall later wrote of his time with Lewis as follows:

> He proved to be very kind and agreed to my taking the MRCP exam which delayed for two months my start in his department. He thought it a foolish exam but necessary for a hospital based career in medicine. He said that an ability to read German was essential for anyone going into research and that he would tell the MRC it was study leave if I learnt the language the quickest way by going to Germany for two months. In 1937–8 the first chest leads were being introduced in the USA and to my surprise Lewis was astonishingly sceptical. I must confess I was not impressed with Lewis as a clinician. He never seemed nearly as interested in making a diagnosis as in the mechanism of the symptoms, and in fact not many patients seemed to be referred to his O P clinic. But of course he had a superb research mind being endlessly inquisitive and able to recognise quickly whether a line of investigation would yield results – and ready to drop it if it would not.[519]

## Other work in the department in 1938

In 1938 Pochin did his last joint work with Lewis, and this was on the effects of asphyxia and pressure on sensory nerves. He then undertook by himself a study on the delay in pain perception in patients with tabes dorsalis, which he showed to be due to extinction of the first pain response with preservation of the later second one. He was assisted in this work by A.J. Honour who devised a method of registering the time of the response which greatly facilitated the study, but as was then the custom this useful technical advance was not acknowledged in the paper.[304] Pochin next developed an interest in the ophthalmic features of Graves' disease and Lewis returned the draft of a paper on lid retraction with the comment 'I cannot see the point of giving meticulous attention to a lot of rubbish because it happens to have been published'. It was also in 1938 that Lewis had what was to be his last visiting research worker, who like many before him was from the United States. This was Dr Milton Mendlowitz from New York who studied the mechanism of clubbing of the fingers.[288] At first this seems an unusual topic for Lewis' department, but his work with Pickering on vasodilatation in the limbs and his clinical acquaintance with it in endocarditis, chest disease and congenital heart disease may have led to the choice. He obtained some of the patients from Dr Frederick G. Chandler at the London Chest Hospital, which was the hospital of his own first consultant appointment and where he had been consulting physician since 1913. Mendlowitz used a very sensitive calorimeter made by Honour and showed that the maximal heat elimination of the distal phalanges was increased in all cases of clubbing except the hereditary ones, and concluded that the condition was due to increased blood flow to the fingers. Lewis kept up his contacts with former pupils in the United States and he wrote to Dr Soma Weiss in Boston to introduce Max Rosenheim[(5)] who was going to work there with a Bilton Pollard Travelling Fellowship from UCH, describing him as 'one of our brightest men'. Rosenheim later became the professor of medicine at UCH and the President of the Royal College of Physicians of London.

## The journals *Clinical Science* and the *British Heart Journal*

Policy discussions about the journal *Clinical Science, incorporating Heart* had been going on since 1937. The MRC were responsible for appointing the editor as they had been with *Heart*, but in November 1938 acting on Lewis' recommendation the Medical Research Society took over this obligation. The publisher, Mr H. Morten Bond of Shaw and Sons was able to tell them that the journal was making money, albeit not very much. This was also the year that the *British Heart Journal* was founded by the British Cardiac Society. The Society had been established in 1937 as the Cardiac Society of Great Britain and Ireland, when the Cardiac Club decided to enlarge its activities and its membership. Initially Lewis had advised against a new journal because he thought that enough good material might not be available in Britain but in 1938 he wrote to John Parkinson agreeing with the proposal and saying 'may such doubts as I have had be confounded'.[418] He wrote a spirited foreword for the first issue of the *British Heart Journal* published in January 1939 part of which reads:

> The success of the new journal will depend upon the quality and not primarily upon the quantity of the matter which it publishes. Originality of observation and of view will be the touchstone of quality. The work of editing is uncreative; an editor can publish only what is offered; he will use most of what is offered. The journal's success is governed therefore from the source of the material. The best contributors will submit for publication only sound and original matter and thought. They will edit their own work; will judge their own text impartially and will prune it ruthlessly, thinking of the standard of work accomplished and to be reported and not of personal interest; they will prepare their manuscript in all particulars to save further labour; they will facilitate the reading by every device of conciseness, of simplicity, of clarity, and of accuracy, in composing text, figure explanation, and reference; for every hour so spent by one who writes, will save countless hours by the many who afterwards read. They will remember that the work of editing is a gratuitous and unenviable task, and they will bow loyally to editorial decision.
>
> To express the hope that the new journal will come to possess many contributors of this kind is to give the fullest wishes for the journal's real and lasting success.[214]

By now Lewis had himself been an editor for 30 years and his advice to the authors of papers must have been heartily appreciated by the new editors. Indeed there can hardly be an editor of any current journal in the world who would not say Amen! to his message. Maurice Campbell, who was joint editor with D. Evan Bedford, told Mr Bond of their regret at not being permitted to use the title *Heart* which was owned by his firm.[88] The title must have meant a lot to Lewis and it may well be that he did not wish to remove it from the title page of *Clinical Science incorporating Heart*. One can assume that Mr Bond would have consulted him.

## Film on heart failure • Pickering leaves

Lewis' interests in teaching and in photography came together with his decision in 1938 to produce a cine film on heart failure which he entitled 'The signs of venous congestion'. The decision also reflected his conviction, which he made clear in *Diseases of the Heart*, that the early recognition of congestive heart failure was of paramount importance.[208] Certainly it was the commonest topic for his bedside teaching rounds and one which was often remembered by former students for its excellence. The film started off with fluid filled models which showed how the jugular veins reflect the right atrial pressure and then indicated that by using the sternal angle as the reference point the pressure may be measured with the subject in varying positions. Then followed clinical demonstrations which confirmed these features in normal subjects and in patients with heart failure. Finally there was a section showing the use of the ink writing polygraph. Cine photography was an ideal way of demonstrating the topic, and the film, which is silent, was made in 16 mm black and white by Mr Macdonald the medical school photographer. Fortunately there is one sequence which shows Lewis as he adjusts a pivoted table, but there does not exist a recording of Lewis' voice.[419]

In 1939 Pickering was continuing his work on hypertension by studying prolonged renin infusions in the rabbit. He showed that when the infusion was stopped the blood pressure returned to normal in the same time as that following the removal of an ischaemic kidney. He also wrote papers on high blood pressure in man and on experimental observations in headache.[297] In October he left to take up the post of Professor of Medicine at St Mary's Hospital, London thus ending a decade of work in Lewis' department.[280] He was undoubtedly Lewis' favourite colleague and was addressed as 'My dear George' in letters at a time when surnames only were the rule, and certainly so for juniors. He and his wife went on the Lewis family holidays which no other assistants did, and he later wrote 'Those who gained his friendship and who knew him in his leisure, devoted to his wife and three children, knew a warm hearted man...who was a delightful and witty conversationalist on many topics'.[299] Why did Pickering get on so well with Lewis when others found him difficult to know and understand? Kellgren told me that Pickering's good relations with his chief were due to the fact that he was a very pleasant and friendly man whose company was always enjoyable. To this one can add the important point that Lewis admired the quality of his research, that from the first Pickering was not afraid of him, and as Lady Pickering said 'George was always absolutely devoted to Tom'.[463] He was later the Regius Professor of Medicine in Oxford and was a noted leader in medical education as well as being a world authority on hypertension.

## Professor T.R. Elliott retires

In 1939 T.R. Elliott (Fig. 14.5) retired from the chair of medicine at UCH Medical School which he had held with great distinction for 19 years and Lewis marked the occasion by writing a charming farewell notice in the *UCH Magazine*.[215] He recalled their early friendship and commented in warm tones on Elliott's career which had been so closely linked with his own. They had now been colleagues on

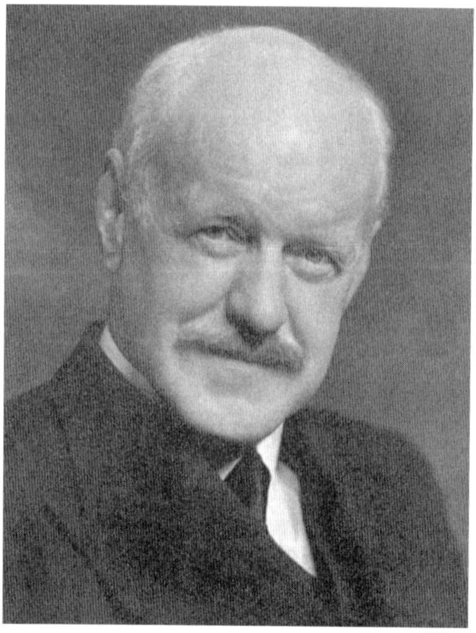

*Figure 14.5 Professor Thomas R Elliott, director of the Medical Unit at UCH and Lewis' close friend and colleague.*

the staff of the hospital and medical school for 26 years and he had helped Lewis to avoid much of the administrative and committee work. It was Elliott who attracted the great Rockefeller Endowment to UCH and with remarkable foresight arranged that the monies provided for the upkeep of beds for the academic units should go to the medical school in the event of the government taking over the hospital service. Elliott's flair for organisation and the soundness of his advice led to him having an especially long period of service on the MRC. It had been entirely his own suggestion that led to Walter M. Fletcher being appointed as its first Secretary.

## Portrait

In 1939 Lewis sat for his portrait which was painted in oils by Evan Walters. (Fig. 14.6) The original hangs in the Welsh National School of Medicine in Cardiff and there is a copy, made by the artist, in University College London. It is a good likeness of Lewis and shows well his penetrating gaze.

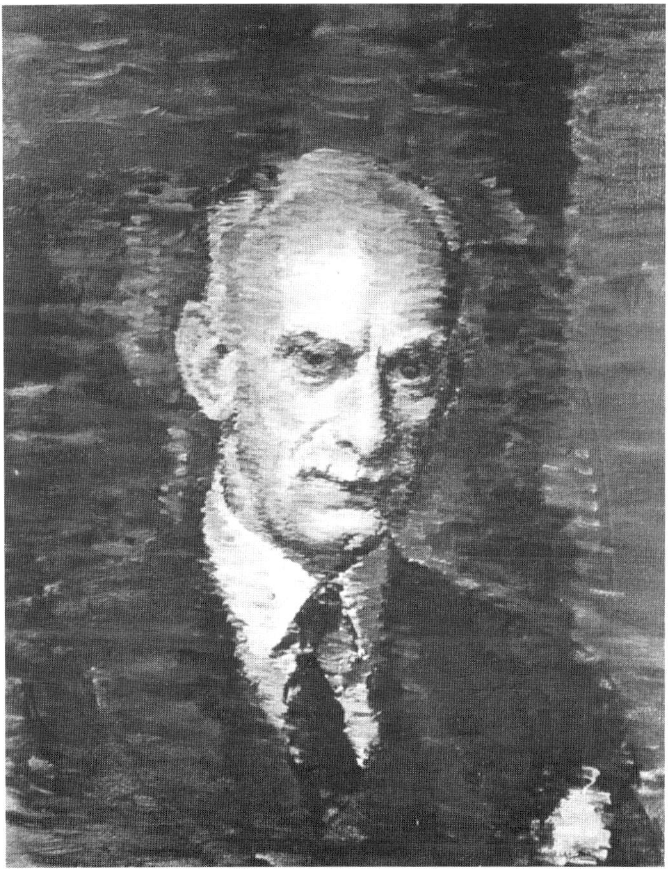

*Figure 14.6 Portrait of Thomas Lewis in oils by Evan Walters, 1939.*

# Notes to Chapter 14

(1) Jonas Henrik Kellgren, 1911–, was always known by his nickname of Yonki. He was interested in surgery and became a Fellow of the Royal College of Surgeons of England whilst still only a casualty officer at UCH. Later he had a distinguished career as Professor of Rheumatology in the University of Manchester.

(2) John Farquhar Fulton, 1899–1960, was an American physiologist who worked under CS Sherrington at Oxford with a Rhodes scholarship. He became professor of physiology at Yale University and was author of a standard textbook *Neurophysiology*. He was also a good medical historian and wrote the biography of Harvey Cushing.

(3) Myron Prinzmetal, 1908–1987, was an American cardiologist who did experimental work on the mechanism of atrial arrhythmias using high speed cine-photography. He is well known for his identification of the electrocardiographic features of angina due to coronary spasm, which is known as Prinzmetal's angina, or variant angina.

(4) Carey Franklin Coombs, 1879–1932, was a Bristol cardiologist with an international reputation who made a 20 year study of rheumatic fever and rheumatic heart disease which he summarized in a fine monograph in 1924. He described the mitral diastolic murmur of acute rheumatic carditis which carries his name. Charles Bruce Perry, 1903–, who is emeritus professor of medicine at Bristol University was his research fellow and later also became a great authority on rheumatic heart disease.

(5) Max Leonard Rosenheim, FRS, (later Lord Rosenheim), 1908–1972, was an outstanding physician who became a world wide ambassador for British medicine. He succeeded HP Himsworth as the professor of medicine at UCH. His great distinction led to him being elected President of the Royal College of Physicians of London.

# *Chapter 15*

# The Cardiographic Department and the Department of Clinical Research • Hospital duties and teaching

THE OUTBREAK of the second world war in September 1939 effectively saw the end of Lewis' department, when the hospital was given over to emergency work and the medical school closed. Elsewhere he undertook clinical work and teaching and did a certain amount of research, but the department was never re-established in his lifetime. This then is an appropriate time to review his work in the medical school and the hospital in the previous thirty years.

## The original department

When Lewis started his electrocardiographic work in 1909 the apparatus was housed in what had been a cleaners' room in the basement of the medical school but soon after the Cardiographic Department was founded in 1910 he was given a larger area, which had been used as a common room for the technical staff. It was there that he continued to do all his early work, both experimental and clinical, and it also had to serve as his office. There was a large main room with a marble fireplace and two inner rooms leading from it, one of which housed the big Cambridge electrocardiograph apparatus. This had to be a dark room because the photographic plates needed to be loaded directly into the camera, and it was lined with galvanised mesh as protection against static electricity. The other small room was also darkened so that electrocardiographic plates could be projected onto the wall for accurate measurement of time intervals. This room was also used in 1928 by Craib for his research on the electrical activity of the tortoise heart. The tortoises themselves were kept in a tank under a radiator. These inner rooms were indifferently ventilated by noisy fans that on occasion sucked in refuse from the street. A corridor of sorts, lined with shelves and cupboards, led to a small workshop located in some cellars under Gower Street. One cellar was used to prepare and anaesthetize dogs prior to an experiment with the electrocardiograph. Various other pieces of equipment were around the main room or fixed to its walls including a large respiratory pump for animal experiments. A carbon microphone enclosed in a sawdust filled box hung from the ceiling which was used to take phonocardiograms. Sometimes it failed to work because the carbon granules stuck together, whereupon the box was tapped with a hammer to shake them up. There was also a device of his own invention which could deliver rhythmic shocks to an animal heart, at rates ranging from 60 to 1000 per minute. It was marketed by C.F. Palmer Ltd as Sir Thomas Lewis' Rotary Contact, price £7.12.6.

Drury worked there from 1920 to 1926 and wrote a vivid description of it:

> The laboratory was an unattractive half basement and low ceilinged room with an inner dark room for the galvanometer and experimental animals. It was dark, crowded with equipment and uninviting. Into it came patients for electrocardiography, dogs for experiments, trays with coffee and buns for lunch. It was hot and dusty in summer and cold in winter. True a large fire burnt brightly in the winter but anyone who found time to warm his backside at it was not beloved by Lewis. It was no good to try and look out of the window for relaxation, for it was glazed with opaque glass. The scientific peaks were our only scenery, and it was our job to try and find the pathways to the top.[49]

Another worker remembered the situation when a dog experiment was being done.[516] The animal was brought in already anaesthetised and the open chest wall seared with a hot iron. The smell of burning from the cautery mingled with that of chloral, ether and tobacco smoke to produce an unsavoury atmosphere which, with an open fire nearby, seemed to pose the hazard of an explosion. But an accident never happened. Certainly it was remarkable that such excellent electrophysiological work, requiring delicate operative technique and the difficult use of a string galvanometer, was done under these circumstances.

Each week there were one or more sessions when outpatients attended for electrocardiograms. This was, after all, the Cardiac Department of University College Hospital even though it was also used intensively for experimental work. For several year patients also came for direct venous pressure measurements when Lewis was developing his method of assessing cardiac failure from the jugular venous pressure. Subjects would be tilted back and forth on a swing couch whilst their forearm venous pressure was measured with a glass manometer. This room, only about 20 feet square at the most, was also used for some of the experiments in the Harvey Film in 1928. It all showed how top class work could be done in a cramped and inadequate environment by dedicated workers.

## Various types of electrocardiographs

In order to take recordings from patients confined to bed, Lewis' two wards had terminals in them which were connected by lead-covered wires back to the medical school about 200 feet away. This method had been used by Einthoven whose laboratory was one mile from the hospital. Once the patient was connected to the terminals, the technician would go down to the department where a three-lead switch on the wall was used to record the electrocardiogram, or sometimes one of the assistants such as Dr Wayne would be in the ward and telephone the department when all was ready. But there was an obvious need for a mobile instrument and in 1920 the Cambridge Company introduced one. It was in effect a massive wooden table on wheels, about five feet long and three feet high, weighing around 330 pounds (150 Kg), and powered by a 12 volt battery. (Fig. 15.1) Until then it had been thought that the quartz or glass fibre, 'the string', in the galvanometer was fragile and sensitive to vibrations, but it was now clear that although only 0.003 mm thick, it was robust and some of them eventually lasted

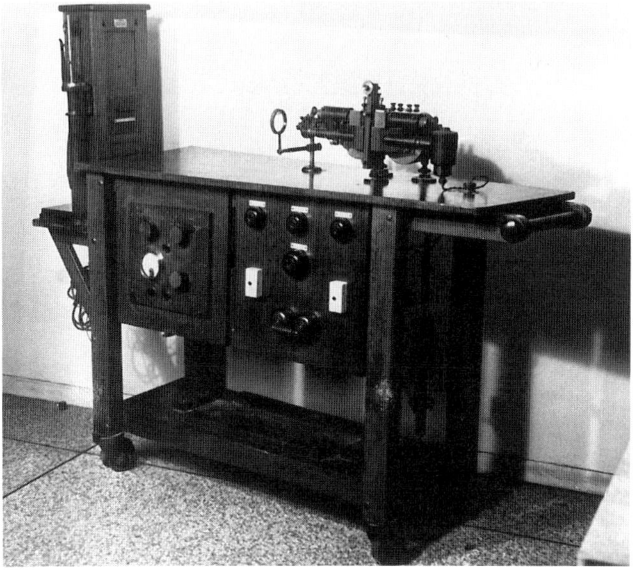

*Figure 15.1 The unwieldy portable electrocardiograph produced by the Cambridge Instrument Company in 1920.*

for 20 years taking many thousands of tracings. When electrocardiographs were taken on the wards it was impractical to use the saline bath electrodes and they were replaced quite satisfactorily in 1920 with a flexible copper mesh strap electrode enclosed in a saline saturated flannel jacket. This, in its turn, was replaced in 1930 by a small plate electrode made of German silver. It was used with an abrasive electrode paste devised by Dr Ashton Graybiel of Boston who worked with Lewis in 1932. The mobile machine was in fact very difficult to move around. At UCH there was a sloping corridor leading to the hospital and it took two men to push the apparatus up it. So the stationary apparatus remained in routine clinical use at UCH, and as late as 1928 Lewis was still using the cumbersome immersion electrodes, even though A.E. Cohn had devised a strap electrode in 1920. Lewis was often reluctant to change an established practice. In 1929 the whole apparatus was radically re-designed, and by using a new type of steel the heavy electromagnet was replaced by a much lighter permanent magnet galvanometer and photographic film was used instead of glass plates. This new model which weighed just 63 pounds (28 Kg) could be carried and it remained the standard ECG machine in Britain for the next 20 years. (Fig. 15.2, *overleaf*) For hospital work it was mounted on wheels and this trolley outfit as it was called was purchased by Lewis in 1932 for £224, certainly an expensive piece of apparatus.[399] A good smaller model had been produced in the United States in 1921 by the Hindle Instrument Company which became the Cambridge Instrument Company of America in 1922. The delay in producing one in Britain was due to the fact that Lewis had no interest in the need for a portable equipment. He thought that a lighter machine would be at the expense of accuracy and the Cambridge Company delayed production until his approval was obtained after extensive prototype tests.[15] It is worth mentioning here that Lewis' original

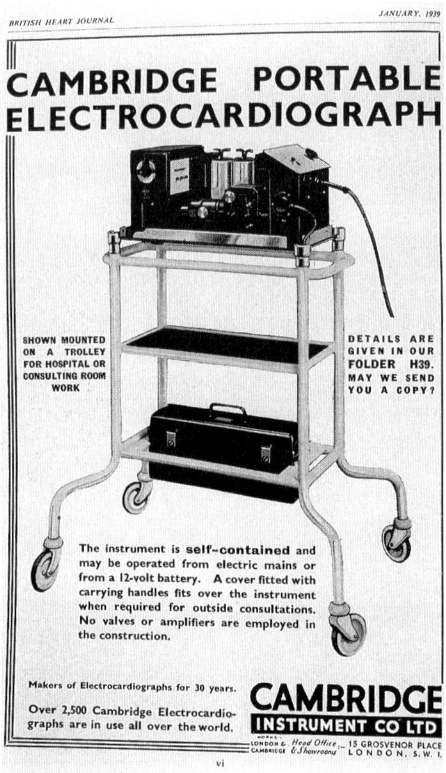


*Figure 15.2 An advertisement for the excellent portable electrocardiograph designed in 1928 which was still in standard use over 20 years later.*

electrocardiograph outfit was loaned to him early in 1909 by the Cambridge Company on the condition of helping to introduce improvements and also that the apparatus might be shown by the company to intending customers. By 1923 that outfit was obsolete and the company gently reminded Lewis of the loan.[14] He was offered the apparatus for £150, half it's value, and he paid for this himself but soon asked the MRC to take it over and recompense him. In that year the total expenditure of his department, excluding salaries, was £1160. The Cambridge Instrument Company took that title in 1924, having been called the Cambridge Scientific and Instrument Company from its foundation in 1881 until 1919 when it became the Cambridge and Paul Instrument Company. Mr S.L. Barron of that company was responsible for collaborating with Lewis, and his accounts of the development of the electrocardiograph are valuable sources of reference and worth quoting from:[14,15]

> The approval of Lewis was sought for any modifications or improvements made in the Cambridge equipment, and he made a thorough and discriminating test on every occasion. Lewis was responsible only for suggestions of improvement: he knew precisely what he wanted, but had no part in the design. At first Lewis had no great leaning towards the necessity for a portable equipment, largely because he had

doubts as to the practicability of retaining the necessary characteristics in a much smaller instrument. He feared that the designers whilst straining for lightness and compactness would, in some degree, forego accuracy, and he would not allow himself to be associated with anything that would be regressive in this sense.

He was not a mathematician, had limited electrical knowledge, and required such explanations involving these subjects as were necessary to be given in a simple manner. The writer clearly remembers, about 1919, spending a considerable time explaining Ohm's law and the method of calculating resistance from current and voltage etc. by the aid of diagrams drawn on the blackboard fixed behind the door of his instrument room. It was some time before he was clear, and, at intervals afterwards he would go to the board and pose himself small calculations of paralleled resistances in order to satisfy himself that he was now competent in that direction. When he had finished he remarked that many erudite scientists had tried to make him understand these simple laws but they never spoke in terms he could readily follow. On occasions, later, at meetings such as the Royal Society Soirees, where research scientists were showing experimental equipment, he would often seek me out to ask me to explain some of the exhibits, always with the remark that he could scarcely ever follow the highly technical descriptions, and that simple straightforward explanations were rarely proffered. He was a most kindly and courteous man, although many, at first introduction, were disconcerted by the straight rather piercing look from his steady eyes, and his slow, deliberate, but very positive manner.

## The department's new location

When the Cardiographic Department was re-established in 1919 and the Department of Clinical Research founded, further space was required. Initially two small rooms nearby were acquired. One served as the secretary's office and remained as such for the next 25 years. The other was a laboratory and in the late 1920's it had a large concrete plethysmograph in the centre whose water bath was heated by a gas ring which occasionally set fire to the parquet floor. In the corner Dr George Brow from Montreal wrestled, largely unsuccessfully, with a Van Slyke blood gas machine which filled the room with a loud clattering noise and perfumed it with caprylic alcohol. The department then acquired a set of rooms on the first floor of the medical school and later had the whole of the floor when the photographic department moved down to their former room in the basement. (Fig. 15.3, *overleaf*) One large room, called 'the long room', which was initially quite bare was later fitted out with benches which were unusual in being placed at a height which allowed one to sit at them in a chair. Also the water supply was arranged so that an arm could be completely immersed in a sitting position. It was here that electrocardiograms were measured with travelling microscopes. It was also used for a variety of clinical experiments and often occupied by Pickering. Further along the corridor Grant had his own fairly large room and this was where the newly arrived assistants had the use of part of a table, and certainly not a desk, for their year or so in the department. There was also a smaller laboratory and then at the end of the floor, over the entrance to the school, Lewis had his own room about 20 feet square. Initially this served both as a laboratory and his office, and there was a big slab of slate in the centre standing on upturned drain pipes, with a dissecting microscope above it. When Lewis came to study Raynaud's disease he often failed to induce an attack in

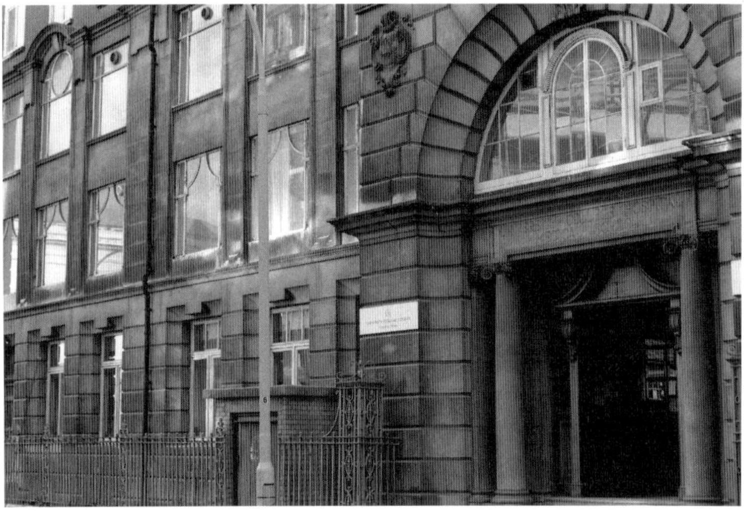

*Figure 15.3 University College Hospital Medical School. Lewis' department was on the first floor with his office over the entrance.*

this room and yet the patient would get the typical white fingers on leaving the building. This exasperated Lewis and so a pane of glass was removed from the window and replaced by a panel with a hole in it through which a finger could be exposed to the outer air. The darkness of the room meant that passers-by were surprised to see just a protruding finger. The panel was later replaced by a small hinged window which is still there.

## Lewis' method of work

The pattern and method of his work has been described by some of his associates and colleagues. 'First came the period of indecision lasting often for weeks during which he considered what to do and how to set about it; he was moody and fretful and nothing was right; he would pace to and fro, appear in a room, stand silent for a few minutes with lowering brow, and pass on. Then, his mind made up, work began and, once begun, nothing was allowed to interrupt its progress...'[299] 'This second phase was one of intense and unremitting activity for the whole laboratory. Sundays and public holidays were grudged as time wasted and which seduced his colleagues from work and he hated any interference that lessened the hum of activity in the laboratory. He spent his days in observation and experiment, being disappointed if he returned home without having learned something new.'[50] 'To see Lewis at his happiest one had to see him at work on his investigations. His experiments were always so clearly planned and the arrangements so complete that there was a total absence of fuss and hurry. He appeared, as he certainly was, to be enjoying himself.'[76] The evening hours were devoted to recording and thinking over the day's work and planning ahead. It is said that he once told his assistants that because they would not be having their Christmas lunch at home until 3 p.m., it would enable them to do a half day's work beforehand – but

Lady Lewis heard of the idea and scotched it. On one occasion the hospital secretary came unexpectedly to the department with the hospital's patron, the Duke of Kent, and asked someone to inform Sir Thomas of their arrival. 'Tell them you haven't been able to find me'. On a typical day Lewis would arrive at 10 a.m. with a list of the experiments to be done that day and an account of the previous day's work. Together with an assistant who might be a research worker, or his laboratory assistant, the experiment would be done with hardly a work spoken. On one occasion, when both he and Grant were the subjects, it consisted of sitting still for over two hours with a weighted strap on their legs. Beforehand Grant asked what they would do during this long period, 'Chat', said Lewis and remained silent for the rest of the morning. While the experiments were still in progress he would start entering them up for publication, so that the final paper was often ready within a week or two of the work being ended.

Lewis took as much trouble with his writing as with his experimental work. Most of his papers were rewritten once or twice before he deemed them finally fit for publication'.[299] He had a very effective method of reading. 'He would read and abstract all articles on the particular subject. Then from memory he would write an essay which later he would check by his abstracts. The abstracts and corrected essays and any relevant reprints were then bound together and from time to time methodically brought up to date. At first sight his method seems laborious, but in the long run its efficiency rendered it economical. He effected economy also by having the strength of mind to relinquish unproductive work.'[76] Lewis received many reprints of articles, and his assistants were encouraged to go into his office to look at them. He sorted them into three piles, labelled 'good work', 'important if true' and 'poor'. Those in the first two categories were retained and bound into volumes. Eventually there were 84 of these and they are now in the Wellcome Institute for the History of Medicine – a useful source of reference, with Lewis' comments written in the margins of some of them. When he was in the wards or outpatients' clinics he would make it his practice to write notes on anything that interested him, always carrying sheets of paper in his pocket for this purpose. On returning to the department these notes would be put in box files under appropriate headings. From time to time he would review these files and maybe get an idea for a new line of investigation. They are now in the library of the National Institute for Medical Research.

When work was being done in the department in which he was not personally engaged, for example Wayne's study of angina, he would discuss the work at least once a week and quickly put his finger on any weak point. But he did not discuss his own work except with the people he was doing it with, and in this respect he was a loner. His human experimental work as we have seen was brilliantly conceived and gave important results, but it tended to be done on only a few subjects with a limited number of observations. This led Arthur E. Boycott, FRS, the professor of pathology, to say, 'The trouble with old Tom is that he doesn't do enough experiments'. This view was supported by Edward S. Stern whom he asked to join him with work on cold and the skin before becoming his house physician in 1929, 'He counted an observation as established if we obtained three consistent positive results. I remember once when things were going well I remarked that the only thing that could upset us now was a single negative observation. He replied, curtly, no. I knew, as he did, that if this happened he might screw the paper with the unwanted observation on it into a ball and throw it into the wastepaper basket. Indeed I have seen him do this'.[535]

## His associates tell of their work with him

Grant worked in the department for 14 years when Lewis was in his prime and his recollections are a valuable source of first hand information:

> He found it easy to see and put things clearly and if you didn't – well you were just a fool and you were pretty well told so. I think part of the discomfort was that you were all the time aware of your own deficiencies when you were with Tom. At times you felt you might as well get out of it but you didn't because you found the man a challenge. You knew that if you sat down under him he would sink you but if you fought back and showed reason he would take it easily. You had to stand up for yourself and your own ideas if you were sure they were right. If they weren't right you got it of course. I once showed him that my method of recording skin temperature was much better than his and he accepted it without any bother.
>
> You felt the place was humming with work, you were really stretched and working hard and we thought it was worthwhile work we were doing. There was a feeling of accomplishment of being able to get it done, and of getting your paper past Tom which was no easy business. There was a zeal for the truth which appealed I think to my Presbyterian upbringing and you felt that this man is really serious about it and you put up with a hell of a lot from a man who was of that quality. He was a wise man, you know.[366]

Wayne said that on the days when Lewis was in a bad mood he had the habit of chewing his moustache and the staff took care to avoid him if they could. On such occasions if an assistant went to him with even quite an important matter he would stare at them with his penetrating eyes, listening in silence and then say 'Well, what of it?' No reply was possible. He could also be abrasive to his staff. On one very hot day Honour came into the laboratory with an open necked shirt. On being asked what he was wearing Honour said it was a tennis shirt. 'You don't come here to play tennis, go out and buy a tie'.[479] But this was probably the only time when he was rude to Honour to whom he was otherwise always courteous and considerate. He was once doing an experiment using the plethysmograph with Grant making the kymograph recording, 'According to him I was doing the thing all wrong, not doing it neatly and properly, and he was needling me all the time. I as near picked up a wet sandbag and threw it at him, but I just didn't thank God. He had that quality of constantly getting under your skin'. It was thought that his often gruff manner was due to the fact that he was inherently a shy person and this is probably true. However he certainly could be deliberately rude. Once two Spanish doctors came to see him but when they apologized for having little English he just walked away without a word. On another occasion his rudeness was a reflection of his own mistaken action. In 1931 he telephoned William Evans, then registrar at the London Hospital to Parkinson who he later succeeded as head of the cardiac department. He invited Evans to apply for the vacant post of assistant physician at UCH. Evans had done good work and was a Welshman too. The local candidate was one of his former assistants, K.E. Harris, of whom Lewis had a poor opinion. Evans recalled that occasion:

> He asked me to meet him to discuss the matter. An appointment was made and I duly attended on a Monday morning at his basement room. When Sir Thomas arrived he took no notice of me, entered his room, sat at his desk and left the door open. Presently I knocked at the door and walked in. I was not invited to take a chair and as I stood before him seated at his desk, he looked up and spoke 'I don't know why you are applying for this post, you have no chance of getting it'. My

monkey was up! I explained that I was doing it at his advice, apologised for interrupting his work, and said that I was especially sorry to be wasting my own time. I turned to walk away and made for the door. Instantly he was out of his chair and invited me to sit down, and we discussed fishing at length.[363]

## The recollections of his personal assistant, John Honour

When John Honour was appointed as a laboratory assistant in January 1926 he was only 15 years old, but within a few years he became Lewis' personal assistant and later was his indispensable right hand man. (Fig. 15.4) In fact, in 1935, Lewis described him in an article as 'my laboratory assistant, Mr A.J. Honour, upon the accuracy of whose observations I have long known I can rely'.[204] It was rare then for a technical assistant to be acknowledged in a paper. In that era when surnames were the regular mode of expression, even between friends, he was of course referred to as Honour. He instructed the newly arrived research workers

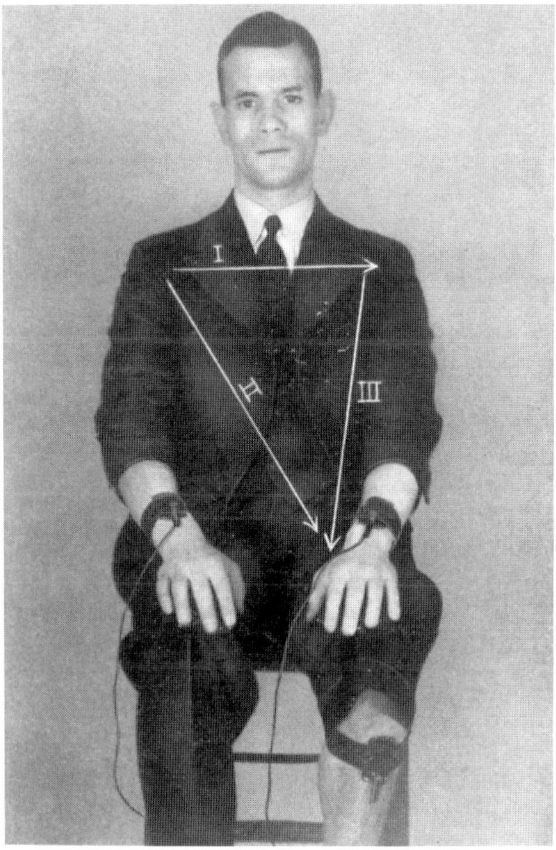


*Figure 15.4 John Honour in 1937 demonstrating the metal skin electrodes and the arrangement of the three electrocardiographic leads. (From* Clinical Electrocardiography, *6th edition.)*

into laboratory methods and several of them, such as Landis and Prinzmetal in the United States, and Wayne and Pickering in Britain, became leaders in medical science. Whenever Lewis did an experiment Honour was there to assist him, and quite often a senior colleague such as Elliott would come into the room to have a discussion. Lewis told Honour that he would not send him out of the room on these occasions, and that he would be trusted never to reveal anything he heard. Honour did hear some outrageous comments being made, but never spoke of them to anybody.

Being Lewis' assistant meant that he was always readily available for experiments on the skin circulation and on pain. Lewis always insisted on having the first experiment done on himself, but after that his research worker and Honour were the next subjects. Honour remembers having his capillary circulation studied. It started with Landis doing a masterly but alarming removal of the cuticle with a razor blade, and then the finger was embedded in a clay block and the arm immobilized with sand bags. In another experiment the head was held secure in a support system whilst the lobe of the ear was studied after blistering with cantharides. These sessions could last for three hours, with Landis and Lewis making observations, and even a small movement or an irrelevant word was frowned upon. Others who learnt about these sessions would try to avoid being enlisted by keeping out of the way but there was a problem in that one of the few lavatories in the school was next to Lewis' room, so it had to be approached with stealth. Sometimes Lewis would go from his room into the big laboratory to consult his clinical notes whilst other work was going on there and his presence was not appreciated. Honour recalled that he was assisting Pickering with blood flow studies which entailed two hours of preliminary work in setting up the plethysmograph. When the patient was comfortable and everything was ready they would hear Lewis' distinctive footsteps in the corridor made by his steel tipped shoes. On entering the laboratory he would try to walk quietly, but the patient's repose was at once disturbed and the resulting vasoconstriction ruined the experiment before it had even started. They came to call him 'The Vasoconstrictor' and learnt to lock the laboratory door whenever his footsteps were heard.

Although Lewis was good with his hands he did not often succeed with operations on the lumbar plexus of cats. Pickering remembered that every Wednesday Lewis went to the animal theatre and afterwards he was would usually sit in Grant's room with his head in his hands because yet again a cat had died on the operating table.[300] Whilst operating, said Honour, sweat dripped off his forehead and his watch chain dropped into the wound which not surprisingly often got infected. In addition to helping with experiments Honour would also record the results, draw up tables of figures and make graphs. When he had been at UCH for only five years he was given, at the age of 20, a testimonial in which Lewis said that he had been much struck by his ability and 'if he chose to do so I think he could obtain a science degree within a few years and have told him so'. In 1935 he thought of leaving but Lewis said it was recognized that he was worth more to the place than he was getting and so his wage would be increased to £4 a week with advances of five shillings a year to a maximum of £5, 'there are very few more highly paid posts as a laboratory attêndant'[516] Honour said that he never had any difficult in working with Lewis who never failed to treat him properly at all times and to whom he was always accessible. He added that Lewis never gave out praise and the only comment he ever received was that, whatever he had done, 'it would do'. However a few months before his death Lewis gave him a signed portrait and thanked him for working so well for him and with him.

## Other memories of Lewis

In 1925 Edward Bridger, then aged 15, became a laboratory attendant and later recalled some aspects of his ten years in the department – after which he became Evan Bedford's first technician at the Middlesex Hospital.[348] He said that Lewis was sometimes charming and at other times 'he could be an absolute blighter'. Soon after joining he was told to get a sphygmomanometer. He had no idea what this was and it was only by looking in an instrument makers catalogue that he could find out. On another occasion he was told to get a ruler. Bridger could see it was in Lewis' breast pocket and said so. 'Go and get the ruler Bridger'. He went away for a while, and on returning with a ruler found Lewis using the first one with no apology or comment. Once he was told to deliver a letter personally but it had only the name on it and he had to find the address from the Medical Directory. One of his tasks was to make prints of electrocardiograms for publication and he did them with a grey background. This was not liked, Lewis wanted black on white. When these were made they were not right, 'I like black on grey'. So the original set was produced, 'These are perfect, why didn't you give them to me in the first place'. But he found that there was also another side to Lewis. During the making of the Harvey film he expected trouble when Lewis' face got covered in blood when an artery was severed, 'but he came out laughing'. During the follow up study a blood pressure cuff was inflated on the thigh of an old soldier who was asked did it hurt. He said, 'You know f...g well it hurts'. Lewis replied, 'Go and get this chap a pint of beer. I've never been sworn at like that before'. Bridger remembered Lewis inflicting severe pain on himself with a faradic current to see if it would produce a change in the electrocardiogram. When he was assisting Craib they could do no work during the day because of Lewis' disapproval and to pass the time Craib converted the electrocardiograph machine into a sort of lie detector. Lewis asked what was going on and agreed to try out the apparatus. After a while Craib, knowing that Lewis disliked Bernard Shaw, said the author's name whereupon the machine reacted briskly. When Lewis was in bed at home with his second infarct Bridger used to take him books from the Royal Society of Medicine and then have tea with him. Drury and Grant gave a useful summary of what he was like to work with:

> Often brusque to the point of rudeness and impeded by deafness in one ear, Lewis was ordinarily no conversationalist; he had a way of countering conversational openings that gave an impression of finality and left the speaker floundering for a new topic. Once the experimental work was finished, and the results being written up, there was a period during which there was much discussion in the laboratory though it was restricted to the problem in hand. This gave him the reputation of being intolerant of general discussion; even light conversation at meals was discouraged: it interrupted the course of his thought. The results written up and the paper in the press, Lewis for a third and short phase was a changed man. He relaxed, talked on all subjects, gave unstinted help and advice from his experience to any one who sincerely asked for it. He moved around the laboratory cheerfully, whistling in the characteristic manner that his co-workers knew so well. But he was soon again restless and seeking a new problem'.[50]

An organ grinder often played in University Street just outside the department and during this period of relaxation Lewis would send him a few coins for encouragement. But at other times Honour was told to instruct the medical school beadle to have the man sent away. Lewis used to go to the refectory for lunch, joining other consultant colleagues, but by all accounts the lunch table was not as agreeable to him as it was to them. Wilfred Trotter, famous as a philosopher as well as a surgeon,[303] had a sharp tongue as well as a brilliant mind and liked to tease Lewis with provocative remarks. (Fig. 15.5) Trotter inclined to the left in politics whilst Lewis was certainly conservative in his views. On one occasion Trotter said that the trouble with Britain was that Marxism had not been introduced here, which led to Lewis exploding in dissent. On another Trotter remarked that people tended to behave at home in an irrational way. Lewis denied this, but was unwise enough to mention that if he spilt beer at table he would throw a drop over his left shoulder, 'I can always rely on you Lewis to supply me with a perfect example of my own contentions'.[515] After Trotter operated on King George V for empyema he declined to accept a baronetcy even though he had saved the King's life. One day at lunch Elliott took him to task for refusing saying that it would have brought distinction to the medical school. Looking towards Lewis, who had a knighthood, Trotter replied that he did not believe in these baubles. However there is no doubt from the evidence of their colleagues that the two men had a good tempered relationship.[53] This conclusion is supported by a letter from Trotter written after Lewis had delivered the Victor Horsley Memorial Lecture in July 1929:

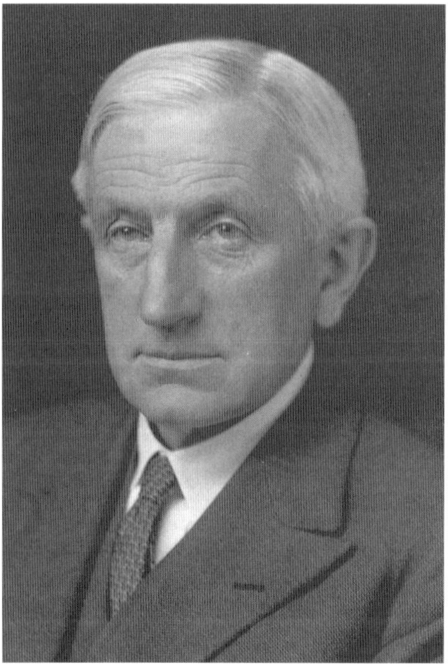

*Figure 15.5 Wilfred Trotter, a fine surgeon and teacher, who is best remembered as the author of* Instincts of the Herd in Peace and War, *and for his essays on the philosophy of medicine.*

Dear Lewis,

I must give myself the treat of writing you a few words to express the intense pleasure it was to hear your lecture yesterday. You can combine the direct exposition of fact with an easy power of thought in a way I hope you won't think me sentimental to call very beautiful. I enjoyed it enormously and was proud it should be given where it was and on such an occasion.

Sincerely yours,
Wilfred Trotter[473]

This compliment clearly meant a lot to Lewis because he kept this letter in his personal files at home. There is no record that the lecture was published, nor what its content was. Pickering recalled, 'when deep in thought at the lunch table or corridor, it was a lesson soon learned that to try to make conversation was to court a look and a few cutting words that soon closed the incident'.[299] Himsworth added, 'He avoided controversial discussion on nonmedical matters, and, if attempts were made to involve him, he would terminate the conversation by dogmatic statements of unexceptionable orthodoxy. To accept such as his considered opinions would be misleading. Many he never considered, apart from deciding that any discussion of them would necessarily be inconclusive and therefore futile'.[76]

Miss Lena Searle had a most important, though unobtrusive role in the smooth running of the department and Lewis acknowledged his indebtedness to her in the preface to *Diseases of the Heart*, 'My grateful thanks are due to my secretary, Miss L.M. Searle, upon whom the arduous task of making accurate copies in type has mainly fallen, and who has given me other and considerable help'. If someone in the department wished to see the chief then they went through her, except for Honour who had direct access, and it was she who typed all their papers. But Lewis made sure that it was only the final and always much altered draft that they were allowed to have typed; all the intermediate ones had to be hand written. Miss Searle entered up his appointments, for example a council meeting of the Royal Society, in his personal diary. On one occasion a tall, distinguished looking man came to her office and requested to see Sir Thomas. He did not give his name and although Miss Searle was well aware that Lewis disliked having his work interrupted she nevertheless thought the visitor might be important and asked Lewis to see him. He was Sir Walter Morley Fletcher and afterwards Lewis expressed his pleasure at her initiative.

## Clinical duties in the ward and the outpatient department

Lewis was meticulous in attending to his duties in the wards and the outpatient department, and even an intensive period of laboratory work was not allowed to interfere with them. His clinical 'firm'[(1)] comprised himself and his house physician together with five or so junior students, known as clerks, and the two or three full time assistants from his department. The house physician, who was chosen after an examination, was given a list of duties.[423] They were told to write a preliminary summary of the physical findings and to make sure that the students did not do this, nor write any progress notes, except under supervision or dictation. This ensured the accuracy of the findings, which Lewis would check and amend himself on his visit to the ward after which the house physician had to enter the diagnosis and record any chief points of interest. The notes contained a detailed account of how to complete the case sheet forms. No operative treatment, for example lumbar puncture, was to be undertaken except 'with the sanction of the physician', and any death should be reported at the earliest opportunity.

It should be mentioned here that when Lewis became a full physician, UCH was one of only three teaching hospitals in London to take women students. Prior to the war only the Royal Free Hospital took women, but during the war others had to do so to meet the shortage of doctors. Afterwards, however, only Kings College Hospital and UCH retained this policy, as well of course as the Royal Free. But even at UCH, which had been founded on the liberal traditions of UCL, there was opposition to the idea. The men students voted against it, Elliott thought it lowered the standard and other consultants were hostile. However in 1918 six women were admitted and Lewis' first house physician in 1920 was one of them, Ruth Dingley. During his career Lewis had 48 house physicians and 11 of them were women.

Lewis held an outpatient clinic once a week and this was run on different lines from the other physicians, being arranged chiefly with a view to student teaching. On other firms the old patients were seen by the houseman, but at his own clinic they were looked after by the assistants. It was the job of the house physician to see all the new patients before the clinic began and select two or three for Lewis to teach on. For a newly qualified doctor this was quite a responsibility and of them said she found it terrifying. However the patients' interests were not neglected and a former student remembered an episode in 1940 when there was a middle aged man with precordial pain, which Lewis thought was of functional aetiology. He took the patient into a side room away from the students and after 20 minutes or so he came out and explained to the class some of the environmental anxieties and so on which had contributed to the man's symptoms. 'This was at a time when it was by no means the custom for a consultant to take the time and trouble for this kind of personal talk and it is my main reason for describing Sir Thomas as a humane and understanding doctor'.[537] The inpatients were in two 28-bed wards, one male and one female, which he shared with Elliott's Medical Unit. (Fig. 15.6) From time to time he would complain that he had too many beds to look after, whereupon Elliott would look after the others. This meant that the assistants then came under Elliott who gave them their training. Lewis wanted a maximum of six beds in each ward and seemed to regard a total of six as even better, designating this number as one which would be desirable for his successor.[479] The main ward round was on a Monday morning and the houseman was expected to admit the patients over the weekend and to personally do tests such as blood counts. Lewis and his assistants came over in silence from his department and took the lift to the third floor where the houseman and students would be waiting. On the ward round the house physician read out the case history which was expected to be full and accurate and which he accepted without any questions. Then he examined the patient thoroughly, pointing out anything that the house physician had missed, and then gave his opinion and the reasons for it. Once the diagnosis had been established he usually left details of the treatment to the house physician, though he always looked at the treatment sheet – usually without comment – but occasionally he said with a smile, 'You're a believer in such and such a drug are you?' However Lewis' assistants such as Pickering and Wayne were always around and they helped the houseman with the treatment

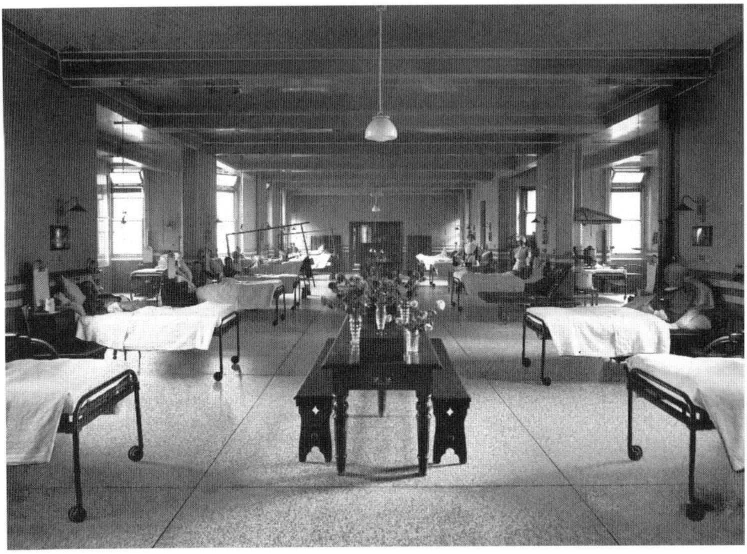

*Figure 15.6 A typical ward at UCH in Lewis' time. The wards were spacious and had plenty of natural light and fresh air.*

and general management of the patients. Lewis had an especial interest in cardiac pathology and if a patient of his died he and all his staff would attend the post-mortem examination. If a patient without heart disease was admitted to one of his beds he did not concern himself with them, leaving their management to an assistant. But he did have an interest in general medicine and a good knowledge of it. Once he was taken by mistake to the bed of a patient with multiple sclerosis but instead of accepting the houseman's apology and moving on he stayed and gave a fine talk on the signs and the nature of that condition.

## Clinical teaching for the students

His rounds were more concerned with teaching than patient management and the second round of the week was used especially for teaching his students. Unlike other physicians such as Dr Batty Shaw who went from bed to bed on the round, he selected just two or three patients to teach on, going into the problem very thoroughly. Lewis usually stood silent whilst his clerk read out the history, chin on chest and with an outstretched arm resting on the head of the bed. Then came abrupt questions which got to the heart of the matter and next a student was asked to examine the patient. This was usually one of his own clerks because quite a few students found it was something of an ordeal to be picked on 'to take a case' on his rounds and this was one reason why so few students outside his firm came on his rounds. Another reason was that he did not teach with a view to getting the students through their examinations, and often a student would say later that they regretted he did not do this. The student had first to inspect the patient and tell what he or she saw. If the answer was that they could see nothing, the reply could be 'Well it's a man isn't it?' or something like that. Inspection could even take some minutes before one was invited to start the examination. It had been known for a student who started off with auscultation to have his stethoscope taken and thrown away. The physical examination was checked minutely and then came the discussion with its insistence on a logical interpretation of the facts. Priority was given to interpreting the mechanism of the symptoms and signs, rather than in reaching a diagnosis. Although he usually taught on a cardiac case he had a special interest too in the genesis of physical signs in the lungs – for example in pneumonia or tuberculosis. Throughout the ward round which usually went on for nearly two hours he stood at the bedside and the students of course had to stand too. One ward sister, who was tall, found she could kneel on a chair without this being noticed – or at any rate commented on. At times his beds were largely filled by patients who were the subject of his current research and so one condition such as Raynaud's disease might be taught at every ward visit. Carola Seward, who married George Pickering, was one of his

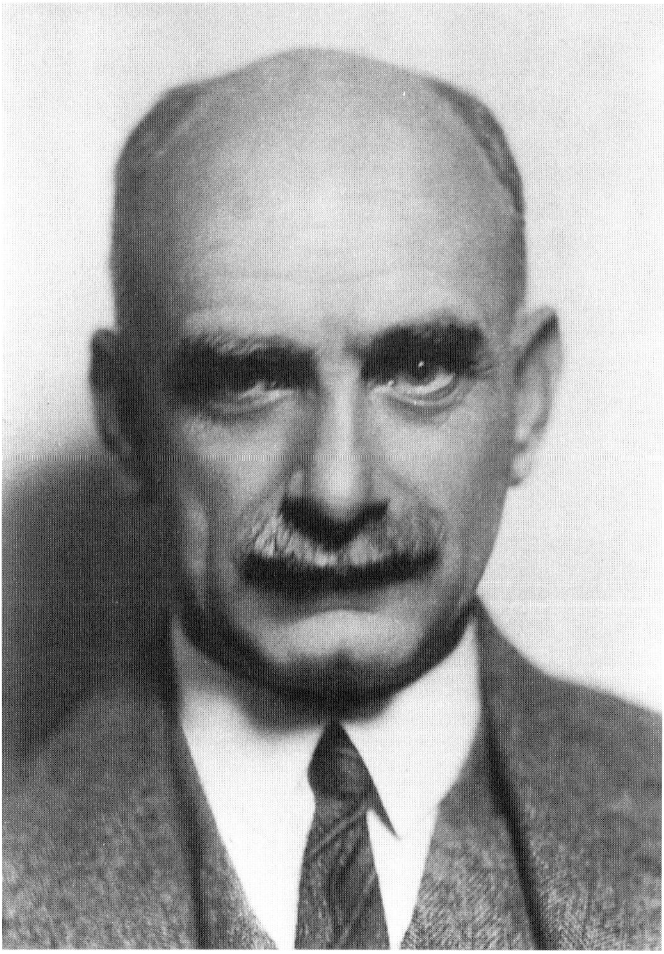

*Figure 15.7 Lewis' penetrating gaze which some students found intimidating.*

clerks. She said that she found his rounds pretty forbidding because the piercing blue eyes were on you all the time and would not relent until you had answered the question. (Fig. 15.7) You might give a silly answer and he would let you know it was silly, usually because one had not correctly observed something. Following on his usual question, 'Have you noticed...?', you felt anything you were going to say was foolish and she found him frightening because he could reduce you to an absolute jelly.[463] Another former clerk confirmed that he had the reputation of being rather a fierce teacher (Fig. 15.8) but said that he had a true humility as shown by an occasion when he spent several minutes checking that a cardiac murmur which an unskilled student claimed to have heard was indeed absent.

He was a very keen observer and had a sharp eye for petechiae which in his patients often meant endocarditis. On one occasion there was surprise when having only observed the patient he said that he would give her digitalis. This went against the accepted teaching that you never prescribed a medicine without examining the patient completely. But he pointed out that the patient was breath-

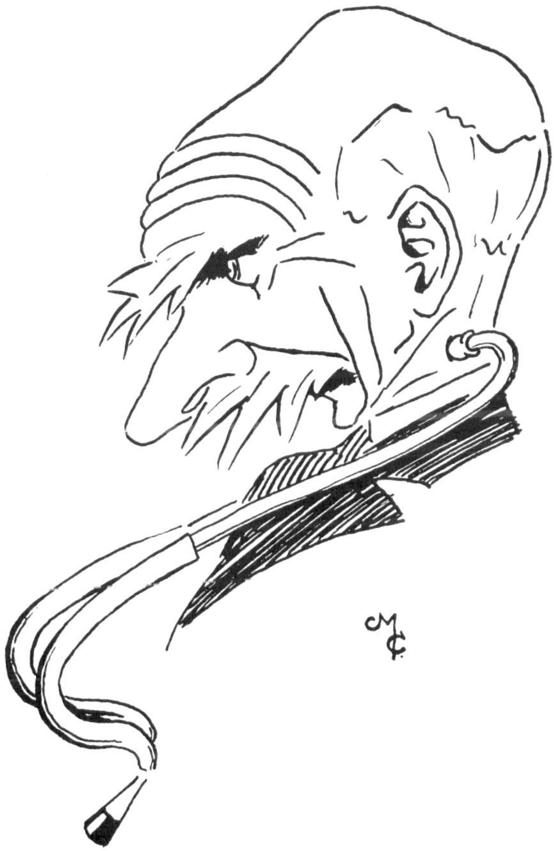

"TOM."

*Figure 15.8 A cartoon of Lewis in the* UCH Magazine, *showing him as a 'rather fierce teacher'.*

less, had a raised venous pressure and rapid atrial fibrillation, so whatever else was found by examination it would not alter that decision. On another occasion he stopped at the entrance to the ward and indicating a patient a few beds away he said that the man had aortic regurgitation – he had seen the capillary pulsation in the face and forehead. But he was not a showman and he never tried to appear clever in any way. He was remarkably lucid as a teacher and the excellence of his teaching was acknowledged and admired by staff and students alike. One colleague said, 'Tom ought to be made to spend his entire time teaching'. His teaching had two aims, namely the inculcation of technique and the displaying of principles, but he was no airy theorist and believed that technique was the least understood thing in science. One of his ward sisters said to a new houseman, 'Sir Thomas teaches you not just for today, but what will be taught in 20 years time'. The hallmark of his bedside teaching was its simplicity. He had the gift of making the complex appear simple, clear and interesting. Everything was put so simply that a student fresh from his second MB could understand every word and concept and yet it was so advanced that a consultant could learn something new. The clarity of his teaching in cardiology made an especially deep impression on the new student because his questioning and experimental approach showed so well how their preclinical training could be applied in treating patients. Together with the student he took each symptom and sign and worked out its significance, and demonstrated the case as a natural sequence of ideas and not just as a series of disconnected facts. He stressed the importance of thinking logically, of taking nothing for granted without evidence, and of examining the validity of that evidence. He disliked terminology which implied an understanding of the mechanism of a phenomenon, having a particular antipathy to the phrase 'cardiac decompensation'. You should say what you found and not what was possibly behind it. A student who was on his firm in 1933 later wrote, 'To a student he seemed to have a tremendous driving force, but was always friendly and approachable. I never remember him being sarcastic. He taught us hard and no slipshod thinking got past him. He made cardiology seem an exciting, logical and rapidly expanding area of medical knowledge, and we felt it was a great privilege to have been trained by him'.[534] The comment about not being sarcastic was echoed in my own experience when as a junior clerk I was invited to 'take the pulse if you will' on a patient who was later found to have the so called 'Pulseless disease'. I could not feel a radial pulse and naturally felt bad about such an elementary fault. Lewis then quietly said I should try the brachial at the elbow. But I felt for it in the upper arm and when he asked why was I trying there I blurted out, being now pretty anxious and a bit sweaty, that I had been taught that as a pressure point in first aid. A sarcastic teacher – and there were some at UCH – would have made this an occasion for a sharp comment, but Lewis just led me on to find that even the carotid pulses could not be felt. He then gave a masterly exposition of the effect of ischaemia on the forearm muscles and the eyes, the unfortunate young woman having arm pain when using a broom and transient blindness on exertion. She also had continuous murmurs on both sides of the neck. He later wrote up this case in his only paper in the *British Heart Journal*, under the title 'A curious syndrome, with signs suggesting cervical arteriovenous fistula and the pulses of the neck and arms lost'.[253] The patient died after he did, so he never knew that she had aortic arch arteritis, Takayasu's syndrome, and that he had misinterpreted the murmurs which were in fact due to severe carotid stenoses. He was obviously unaware that arterial narrowing could produce a continuous murmur especially when there is hypertension which he knew she had, having measured the blood pressure in her legs.

He missed another diagnosis too, in a young woman called Eileen Carney who had long standing ascites which successive housemen on the Medical Unit had learnt how to tap. When Smirk was on the Unit he noticed that she had a high jugular venous pressure and asked Lewis for his opinion, reminding him of his statement that a high venous pressure meant heart failure. Lewis agreed with the finding but said he could not explain it, there was no evidence of heart disease. A year or so later in 1935, a UCH registrar, Dr L.P.E. Laurent, heard Dr Paul White give the St Cyres lecture on constrictive pericarditis and at once realized this was Eileen's diagnosis. Lewis then saw her again and said, 'Why haven't I been shown this patient before?' A young doctor was brave enough to tell him that he had. In 1936 she became the first patient in Britain to have a pericardial resection, which was done by Trotter's assistant, Mr Robin S. Pilcher, later professor of surgery at UCH.

A student in 1933, Dr Mary Savory wrote 'In caring for patients I remember him as having a personal, friendly and quite classless approach which put most people completely at ease, and made them trust him absolutely. (Fig. 15.9, *overleaf*) He was closely concerned with the details of their lives and the exact history of their illness. His advice was detailed, practical, put into simple language and given as kindly as possible. I do not think of him as becoming particularly emotionally involved, but this is something he might well have concealed'.[534] A house physician said that although he did not have an especially good 'bedside manner' his patients realized that they were being looked after by someone special and felt fortunate to be under his care. He was very friendly with his old patients and used his influence with them to ensure that those in heart failure conformed with his requirement for proper rest whilst in hospital, and he would make sure from the ward sister that they were getting adequate hours of sleep. However, long before rehabilitation became part of the medical scene, he not merely prescribed but arranged for his patients to have work that was suited to their capabilities. Another student was impressed that before the class was taken to see a man with a leaking aortic aneurysm they were told to be very careful not to say or ask anything which might upset the dangerously ill patient.[512] Dr Sheila Howarth says, 'Criticism has been expressed by some in recent years of the way Lewis treated his patients. Of this all I can say is that on his firm in 1942 I saw nothing but a kindly doctor–patient relationship'.[517] However it is fair to add that not everyone viewed it that way. Dr Alan Fowler, a student in 1943, writes, 'I was impressed with the contrast between Tommy Lewis, the dedicated technocrat indifferent to bedside manner and Kenneth Harris the suave and polished consulting physician. Lewis did not seem to communicate with his patients, he just regarded them as interesting material for the clinical science he was demonstrating'.[514]

## His course of formal lectures

In addition to bedside and outpatient teaching he also gave a series of lectures which took place, not in the medical school, but in a small clinical lecture theatre on the top floor of the hospital. It was semicircular with steeply raked seats and well suited to his purpose of demonstrating patients as a part of most lectures. In particular he might show a patient connected with his current line of research. For

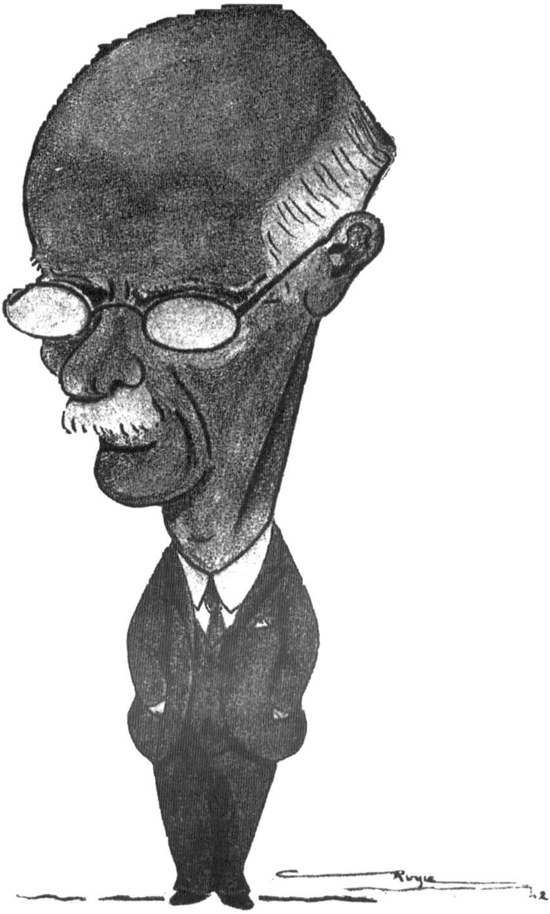


*Figure 15.9 A cartoon of Lewis in the* UCH Magazine, *which shows Lewis in a contemplative mood.*

example a patient with cold haemoglobinuria would have a limb immersed in cold water and the resulting red urine demonstrated. Cardiac patients were naturally often shown and students never forgot his masterly demonstration of the signs of cardiac failure, and the different types of jugular venous pulse. Outpatients came up too and were paid for their effort. One of them was a man of 21 with cyanotic congenital heart disease, who 'will come at any time for two shillings and sixpence'.

Lewis' own lecture notes, covering 56 lectures and bound in a loose leaf volume, have been preserved. Each lecture was on one topic, for example angina or digitalis, and the notes are carefully set out under main and subsidiary headings, and running to two or three pages. His lecture slides, numbering over a thousand, were all numbered and contact prints of them were mounted in a separate book. Their place in each lecture together with their numbers were noted in red type, and often there was a description of what they showed. These detailed notes reveal a man who made sure that his lectures would always contain everything that he thought should be in them, leaving nothing to chance, and certainly taking his teaching duties very seriously. The 30 lectures on the heart refer to most of the main conditions such as endocarditis and hypertension, but as one might expect they are not the usual systematic account. For instance there are individual lectures on sudden death, heart strain, syncope, shock and hypertrophy. A complete lecture was devoted to digitalis and another to quinidine. The other lectures dealt with circulatory disorders, the effort syndrome and with pain and of course covered his own work in these areas. But the most remarkable feature were the four lectures which dealt with the history and philosophy of medicine.[78] This was certainly a most unusual topic for any course of lectures in a medical school and it disposes of any suggestion that Lewis was just a narrow minded technocrat. The first lecture was on the nature of disease when the contributions of Sydenham, Brown, Broussais, Cohnheim and Bernard were all quoted. The next two were on the identification of disease covering its purpose and use in research and using Pinel's classification as an illustration. He spoke of the need to study the history of medicine and showed his good knowledge of it by, for example, referring in detail to the controversy over typhoid fever between Broussais, Louis and Bretonneau. Finally he dealt with treatment and cautioned the students that the human weaknesses of credulity, irrationality and superstition still had strength even in the face of modern scientific therapeutics. Instances of fallacious remedies included Abram's box and Baine's dielectric oil – both of them strongly supported by doctors of repute – and Perkin's metallic tractors which sold at five guineas a box leading Oliver Wendell Holmes, he said, to comment 'A man who pays £5 for a whistle is likely to blow all the harder on it'. Rather surprisingly there was no lecture on clinical science.

## The opinions of his students

Lewis gave the impression to many students of being austere and intimidating, but others found that this was not always the case. Dr William Phillips was a student in 1927 and later wrote, 'I knew about him from childhood because my family lived near his, and although Tom was supposed to have no soft side to his nature in fact he did have one which he kept pretty securely hidden for he was always more than averagely civil to me'.[531] Dr Richard Philps who became a noted bird photographer said that in 1936 when he was a student, 'I don't really remember how he discovered that photographing birds was a mutual interest; certainly I was far too much in awe of him to broach the subject directly but somehow he got to know of it. Having passed this hurdle he was most happy to show off his pictures to me in his room at lunchtime'.[532] Jeremy N. Morris, later a cardiovascular epidemiologist, was his house physician in 1934, and remembered that Lewis was always accessible for advice. Lewis, he said, was a great man and it was an extraordinary opportunity to work under him. 'Life was truly marvellous at UCH, we were very privileged and we knew it'.[530] On one occasion Lewis had somehow come to learn that Morris had been seen one evening at a coffee bar in a nearby street. He was clearly concerned to protect Morris from undesirable characters, and took him on one side after a ward round and said in a fatherly like way that 'Nice people don't frequent Southampton Row'. Morris remembered this with gratitude as evidence of Lewis' concern for his staff, especially because, he said, Lewis clearly found it something that was very difficult to do. He thought Lewis had a shy and inhibited personality. Indeed Morris's opinion echoed that of Jonathan Meakins 20 years previously when he commented on Lewis' shyness and reticence.[281] It was well known that Lewis was very fond of the company of good looking, intelligent, women, and although the female students were treated equally with the men on his teaching rounds he was happy to be with them and his female house physicians on social occasions. When Eleanor Woodford-Williams became a student in 1934 she started attending his clinics and after one of them he said he had heard that she came from Cardiff, and that he would like her to meet his family. 'Two weeks later I received an invitation from Sir Thomas and Lady Lewis to spend a weekend with them and during my undergraduate years I spent a number of very pleasant Saturdays and Sundays with them at Loudwater; to me it was just like home.' In 1937 another woman, Joan Rooke (now Dr Joan Stokes) became his house physician, and he used to enjoy having lunch with her at the nearby Maple's restaurant and also taking her to the cinema on some afternoons.[471] Lewis did not have much to do with the medical students in respect of their societies, sporting activities or social events with one exception. I well remember the Saturday night dances, 'hops' as they were called, in the medical school. Lewis would bring his daughter Pat to this and she was looked after by the houseman who was obviously expected to turn up. He would then dance with any female student who took his eye, leaving her partner little choice in the matter.

The students had their own society within the medical school which published a good journal called the *University College Hospital Magazine*. It had a regular feature 'Sayings of the Great' for which the students assiduously collected comments they heard made by the consultants. Some of them were often good for an amusing quote, such as the neurologist Sir Francis Walshe whose entertaining ward rounds were crowded with students. But Lewis featured only twice. On one occasion he emphasized the need for concentration when trying to hear a cardiac murmur by saying, 'You don't go into the woods with a girl if you want to listen to the nightingale singing'. On the other he said 'At 45 a change takes place in the cerebral vessels. They become more rigid and perhaps as a consequence our ideas become fixed. You will find it very difficult to get a man over 45 to listen to a new idea. That is why the writers of textbooks are always behind the time'.[171] That remark was made when he was 43 years of age, and seven years later he wrote his own textbook *Diseases of the Heart*.

## Note to Chapter 15

(1) The term 'firm' is one which is still applied to the basic clinical unit in a British teaching hospital which comprises a consultant in charge of beds, together with junior doctors and a group of students. Up to 1939 the only junior doctor was the house physician and the students would be on a firm for three months. It was therefore a close knit and fairly long attachment when they would get to know the consultant and the house physician very well. It was usual for students to work on two medical and then on two surgical firms. The origin of the term 'firm' is not known. Perhaps it was originally used as a joke, in relation to retail firms such as grocers and tailors with a proprietor and employees.

# Chapter 16

## Marriage • Family life • Holidays • Hobbies

It was in 1914, soon after his 33rd birthday that Lewis first met his future wife, Alice Lorna Treharne James. She was born in 1889 in the small mining town of Merthyr Tydfil, 20 miles north of Cardiff, being one of four children. Her father, Frank Treharne James, was a solicitor and one time Mayor. He was the son of Frank James, also a solicitor. Her mother was Agnes Mary Powell. The family belonged to the Unitarian Church and this led to her attending the famous boarding school at Roedean which had been founded by Unitarians and at which her aunt had been a founder pupil. It obviously suited her well and she became the head girl of her house. On returning home she became a keen volunteer nurse, taking part in public demonstrations of first aid in Wales. (Fig. 16.1) At the outbreak of war she became a member of the Voluntary Aid Detachment of nurses and served in France at a convent hospital in Saumur.

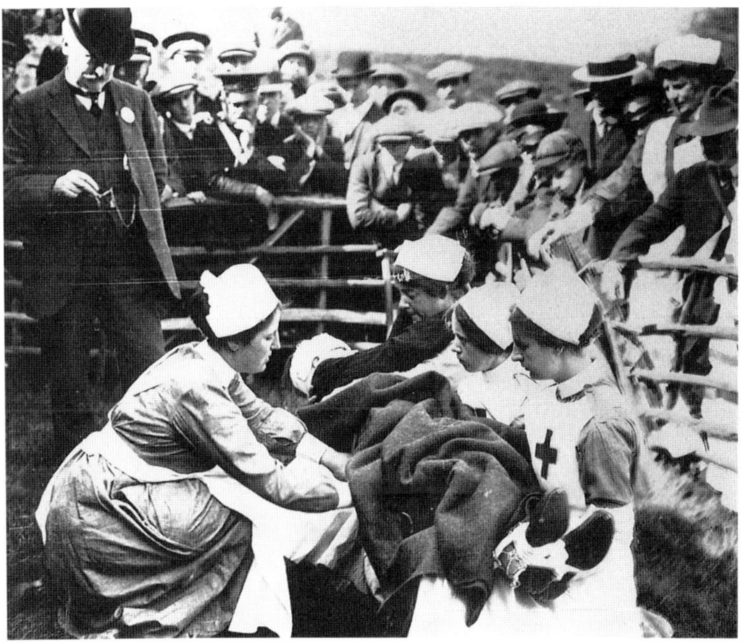

*Figure 16.1 Miss Lorna James in charge of a first aid demonstration in Wales in about 1910.*

Mr James belonged to the same Cardiff club as did Mr Lewis and their wives became friends. On Boxing Day 1914 Lorna was reminded by her mother of a promise to go to Cardiff and see Mr Lewis who had been ill, and as she later recalled, 'When I arrived Tom happened to be there'. This was the start of their courtship and 'after only about four meetings I decided I would like to marry Tom'.[377]

## Engagement and marriage

They became engaged in August 1915. (Fig. 16.2) His pocket diaries for 1915–1916 are available and they give us a few glimpses into their day-to-day life.[526] On August 28 they went house hunting for the first time. An October entry, 'smoking reduced', may have reflected Lorna's disapproval, but if so it had little effect because he was to remain a heavy smoker for the next ten years. In November they had a busy twelve days in London which included having Sir James and Lady Mackenzie to tea one day and lunching with them on another. They had four evenings at the theatre, one at the cinema, dinners at the Savoy, Frascati's and Berners Hotel and a visit to see Sir William Osler at the Canadian Army's Duchess

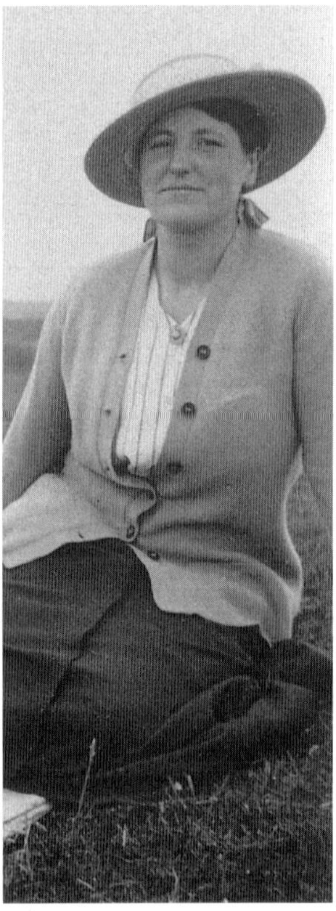

*Figure 16.2 Lorna aged 26 at the time of her engagement.*

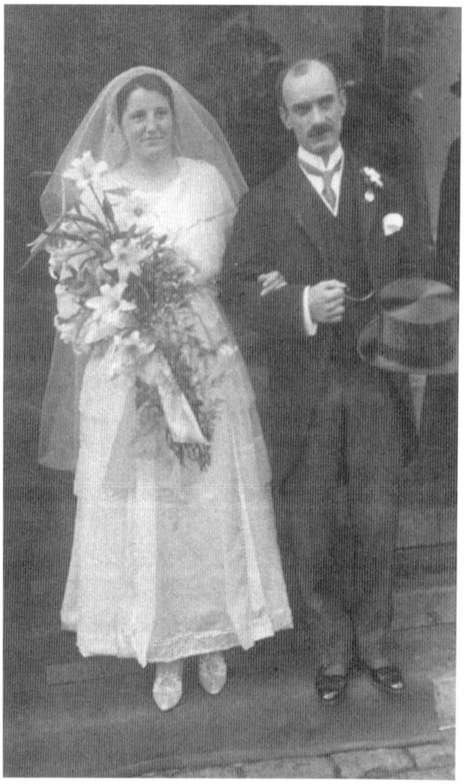

*Figure 16.3 The newly married Dr and Mrs Lewis.*

of Connaught Hospital at Taplow. On February 1st 1916 they rented a house at No. 1, Reddington Road, Hampstead, which was to be the first of their three homes and which also housed his secretary, Mr H. Vernon Jones. They were married at St Marylebone Church on March 30, London being a more convenient war time venue than Wales for many of the guests. It was a traditional white wedding and the bride was a handsome lady of 27, taller than her husband and his junior by seven years. (Fig. 16.3) His consulting room, now at 27, Queen Anne Street, was used for the last time to shake off the confetti and change for the honeymoon. This was spent in the west country, some of it at Bude where he had laryngitis for a week and 'sat on the verandah in a big coat with an astrakhan collar looking very gloomy'.[377]

## Bird watching

But once this was over they were able to enjoy themselves with his boyhood hobby of bird watching. Probably his scientific life had been so full up to now that it had given him little time for this, but now he not only had the leisure but also an enthusiastic companion to share it with. However it would be a mistake to equate hobby with relaxation because he worked at ornithology with the same intensity as his research. Each day the diary recorded their findings, such as 'Dunster, long tailed tit building', 'Coombe Woods, buzzard's nest empty now', 'Slapton Sands, ring plover, curlew on estuary'. They arrived home after three weeks and were then out every weekend at nearby places such as Burnham Beeches, Cookham and Radlett with the emphasis, in April and May, very clearly on bird nesting. Their meticulous notes state if birds are building a nest, whether eggs are fresh, slightly or very much incubated, or hatching, and if there are fledglings present. The species with eggs included sparrow-hawk, jackdaw, chaffinch, jay, bullfinch, whitethroat, blackbird and mistlethrush. An excursion further afield to Aldeburgh in Suffolk yielded eggs of swallow, lark, pheasant, greenfinch, willow wren, brown linnet, wren and nightjar. They used a mirror on a long stick to search out nests in hedgerows. Eventually they had a very large collection of eggs in a cabinet, numbering over 200 and all carefully labelled. This collection is now housed in the British Museum at Tring in Hertfordshire. As a reference book he used *A History of British Birds* by William Yarrell published in four volumes in 1884.

## Photographing birds

Bird photography was a natural extension to bird watching and Lewis had a top quality camera for this work, a quarter plate Dallmeyer with an f 4.5 lens. (Fig. 16.4, *overleaf*) It was he who usually took the photographs but they shared the tasks of developing the negatives, printing and enlarging. It was not an easy matter then to take bird photographs, especially as he did to take good ones. Focusing had to be done on a ground glass screen, exposure times might be too slow to record movement crisply, and furthermore the shutter was operated pneumatically by squeezing a rubber bulb. Lewis got over the problem of photographing the moving wings of a bird by combining two features. Firstly he carefully

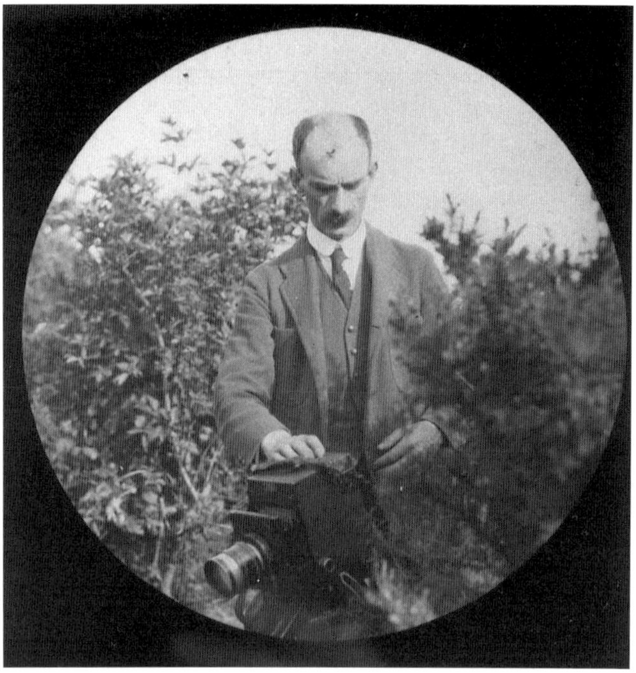

*Figure 16.4 Taking a photograph with his Dallmeyer camera.*

observed when the wings of a particular bird would be at the point of least motion. Secondly he knew the time delay from squeezing the bulb to the shutter actually opening. (Fig. 16.5) He took the photographs from a portable hide which had his name on the back, or sometimes he would use a more easily carried small

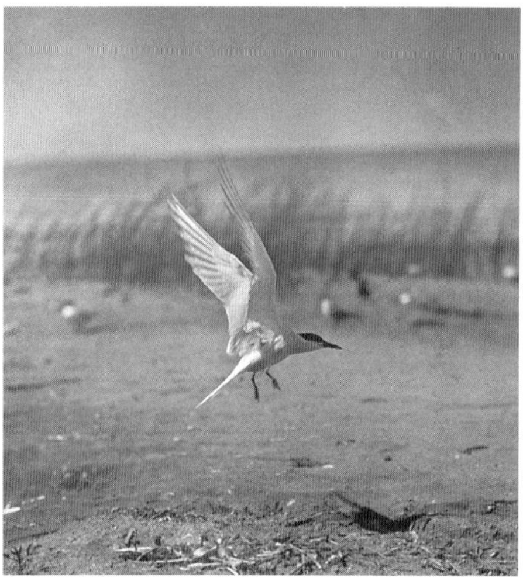

*Figure 16.5 A fine action photograph of a little tern leaving its nest.*

'gypsy' tent. (Fig. 16.6 and 16.7) On one occasion he noticed that cuckoos were in the habit of perching on wheat stooks so he made his hide inside one and got good pictures the next day, and as he told a friend 'I said to myself, cuckoos yesterday, cuckoos today, why not cuckoos tomorrow'. He had very keen eyesight and could spot a small bird many yards away. His bird watching activities were recorded in great detail on large index cards which eventually numbered over 120. They were arranged according to individual species. For example, dippers were seen on a stream at Taff Vechan on July 17 1917 and again at Merthyr in April 1918 and then at Bude in May 1919. A typical entry reads, 'They fish up stream as a rule wading sometimes in fast running water up to their wings. Old

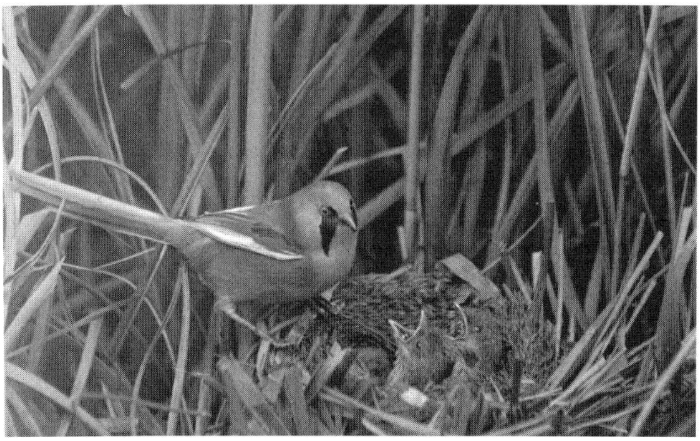

*Figure 16.6 A bearded tit and its young.*

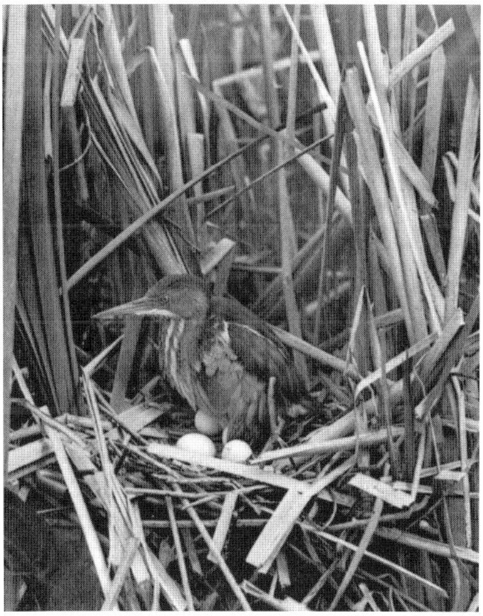

*Figure 16.7 The bittern is a very shy bird and difficult to photograph.*

birds fed young at nest with small fish, etc hovering while feeding, not still an instant'. The notes reveal his capacity for long and continuous observation as in the case of a lesser tern's nest in June 13 1920. Starting at 10.47 there are 29 entries up to 4.15 with details of the birds' movements and the exposure times.

After the Heart Hospital moved to Colchester there was gradually less work to do and also more opportunity for ornithology. In May 1918 he found a sparrowhawk's nest built against the trunk of an oak tree thirty feet from the ground. To avoid disturbing the birds he waited three weeks for the eggs to hatch and then with his American colleague Frank Wilson he constructed a platform up in the tree covered by a green tent, from which an excellent view of the nest could be obtained. They observed the nest for a whole month and would spend up to four hours at a time in the hide in order to analyse what the three young hawks were fed on. The total for the period was 46 thrushes and 66 smaller birds. He wrote a 20 000 word article on this study and of the many photographs taken 43 were selected as illustrations. It was never published but the manuscript has been kept.[385]

The text reveals his close sympathy with nature and displays the usually well concealed emotional side of his personality. For example, 'The hen bird usually assumed a proud posture, a fine bird with an outline of comely proportions moving with dignity, her mien was bold almost to defiance. On the contrary the male came furtively, his attitude skulking'. And writing of a blue tit's visit to the tree, 'the plucky little fellow actually perched on the nest, a courageous but thoughtless little bird, the click of my shutter drove him to safety'.

His wife used to join him at Colchester at the weekends and they would take his colleagues from the hospital with them on their bird watching expeditions. He once made a photographic portrait of everyone who worked in his unit and produced copies for each of them. But when the prints were laid out to dry they were chewed up by his wife's highland terrier 'Stodger' who was jealous of him. She also had a pet rat, 'Juggins', which she carried about with her, even when they went to a restaurant. At about this time they bought their first vehicle which was a 3 HP Sunbeam motor cycle and sidecar. It carried the heavy photographic equipment and they used it for their visits to Wales. Early in their married life his wife got accustomed to seeing her husband waiting rather impatiently for her with a raincoat over his arm and this, she said, was when she learned the art of punctuality.

Another intensive bout of bird watching took place in June 1920 at Horsey Gap on the Essex coast and he published the observations in the journal *British Birds* under the title 'Notes on the breeding habits of the lesser tern'.[152] It is illustrated with splendid action photographs, (Fig. 16.8) and his index cards record that they were taken at 1/1000 second with an f 11 aperture – his camera could be fitted with a focal plane shutter when necessary for such a fast exposure.[(1)] The only other bird article appeared in *Country Life* also in 1920 and was signed 'ALTL and TL'. It is a charming account of how two woodpeckers had their previous year's nest hole in an old ash tree taken over by a pair of starlings, forcing them to create a new one higher up. 'Strange neighbours these; the tenants of the upper flat a shy dignified and aristocratic pair; the tenants of the lower flat a pair of cheeky and incessant chatterboxes'.[109] Again the photographs were excellent.

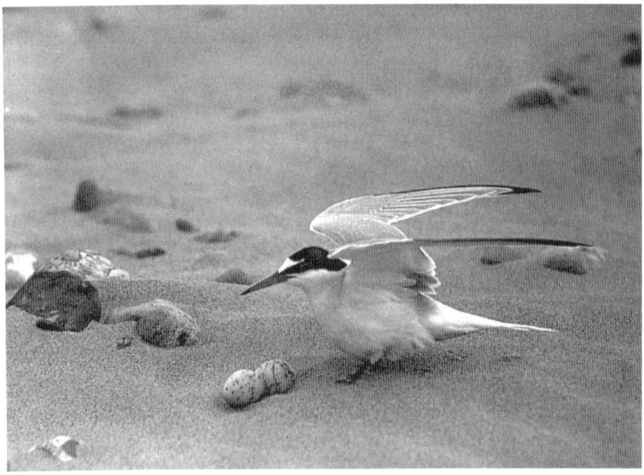

*Figure 16.8 A little tern with two eggs. (From reference 152.)*

## Fishing was his other great hobby

Apart from photography his other great passion was fishing, another hobby which continued from boyhood throughout his life. As one might anticipate from this intense and energetic man, it was fishing with a fly or a spinner that held his attention. Watching a float would not have been his idea of relaxation. His pocket diaries are only sparsely annotated and most of the entries are records of the fish he caught. These were mostly trout, but there is one note of a 15lb salmon and others of pike and greyling. His reference work was *A History of British Fishes* by William Yarrell, a book published in 1836 and which he had been given as a child. Occasionally he annotated it, for example by recording a sapphirine gurnard which he caught at Abersoch in August 1929. Lewis was impressed by the keen observation of country folk and he liked to recount one instance of this which happened when he was fishing, as he liked to do, on the River Tyfi near Tregaron in mid Wales. One hot summer's day he and his ghillie, Dai Evans, approached his favourite pool and found that cows were cooling themselves in it. He was annoyed but Dai said, 'Oh, it's alright sir' and directed his fly near a cow's tail where it was immediately taken by a nice trout. Dai explained that on a hot day there were many flies on a cow's tail and that an occasional one would be knocked onto the water where the expectant trout was waiting for his meal. Lewis was very impressed.[363] He was also keen on sea fishing and enjoyed the challenge of fishing off the rocks which required a good deal of expertise. But he preferred to avoid any activity which he could not master and this was illustrated when he watched James Mackenzie play golf near his home at Northwood. After the round Mackenzie said 'Well now Lewis, why don't you take up golf', and was displeased to have the reply, 'I gave it up because I could not play any better than that'.[377]

## Leisure reading

In his professional life Lewis spent a good deal of time in reading the literature and also in assessing articles submitted for his journals, but in his leisure time he

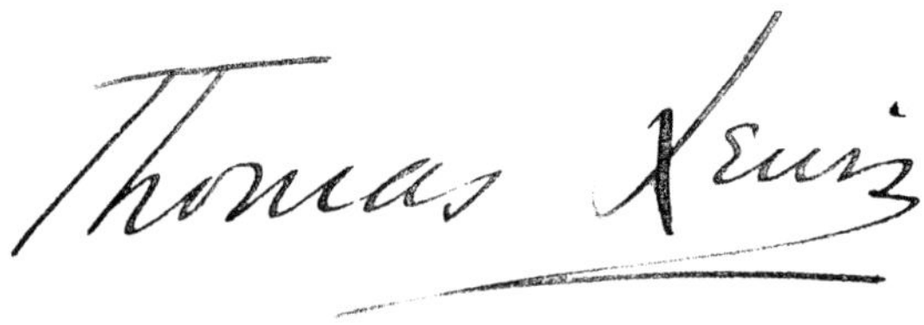

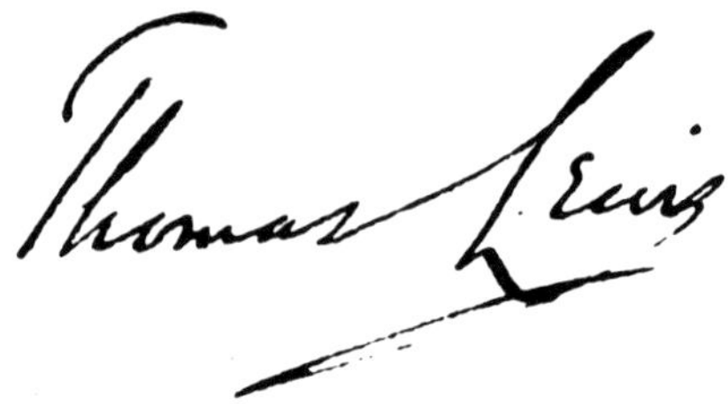

*Figure 16.9 Lewis' signatures at age 19 and at age 26.*

also, perhaps surprisingly, did a lot of reading. But as far as one can judge he seems to have taken this up after the age of 55. Maybe the pace of his medical life was slowing down and with less photographic work there would have been more time to relax with books, which he got from the Times Book Club. But relax is perhaps not the right description because he wrote a detailed summary of each of nearly 100 books on cards which have been kept in his personal papers. They were all indexed under the following headings: Critical, Memoirs, Modern History, Biographical, Science, and Novels. The books were mostly nonfiction, and biographies were clearly a favourite. They reveal a considerable range of interest and include ones on Torquemada, Oscar Wilde, Count Zeppelin, Cecil Rhodes, Elizabeth Fry, John Wesley, Voltaire and Mussolini. Among the few novels there are *The Moon is Down* by John Steinbeck, described in his note as 'Quite a little classic', and *Anne Vickers* by Sinclair Lewis. He was a good letter writer and wrote fairly legibly in a small sloping script. (Fig. 16.9) Two of his former house physicians kept a dozen or more letters which he wrote to each of them,[525] whilst Hugh Sinclair and George Pickering were others he corresponded with. Pickering said '(he) made few friends until his later years when he formed warm attachments with the younger people working in his field; and they had reason to know how affectionate and considerate a friend he could be'.[299]

## The young family

Their first child, Patricia Treharne, 'Pat', was born on December 1st 1918 and, in a letter to Einthoven, Lewis wrote 'only last week a little girl came to our great joy'. A year or so later they purchased a large four storey house in Hampstead, at 10, Chesterford Gardens, where they stayed for the next 14 years. (Fig. 16.10) A childrens' trained nurse was engaged as a nanny and Pat remembers her, Miss Marjorie Weekley, as a good looking young woman of 21 who stayed with them

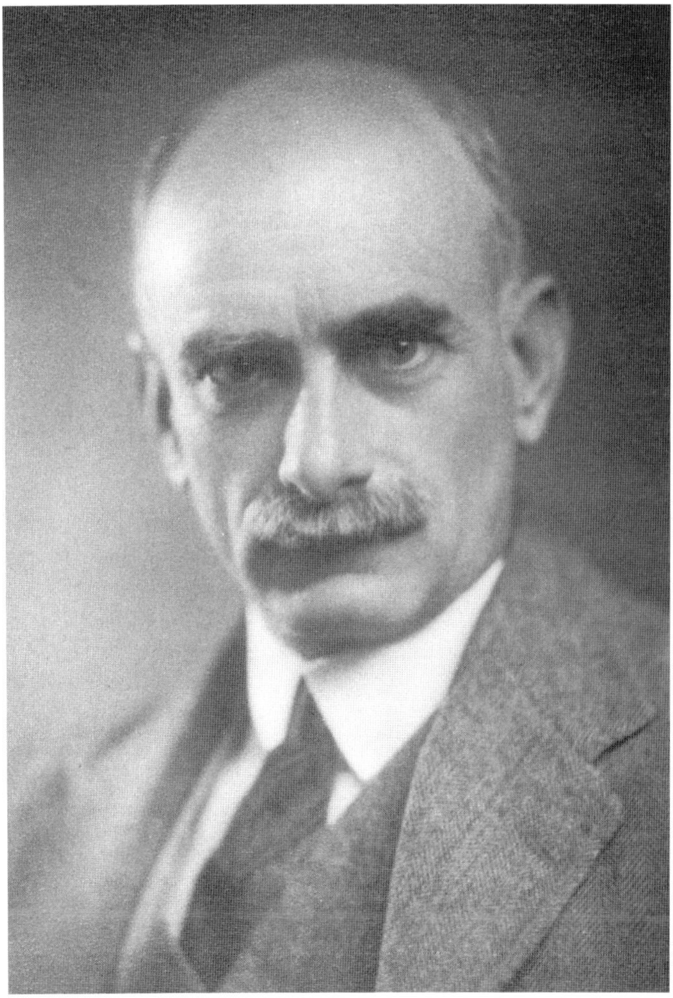

*Figure 16.10 Lady Lewis' favourite photograph of her husband.*

for 15 years. They also had a nurserymaid, a house parlourmaid and a cook all of whom lived in a large bedroom at the top of the house. Their second child, Thomas Henry Christopher, 'Chris', was born there on July 17 1923 and their family was completed with the birth of Katherine Phillipa, 'Pip', on January 5 1929. During the week the children would see their father only for a short while before supper after which their nanny would take them up to the nursery, where their mother would read to them before they went to sleep. Lewis would usually spend every weekday evening working at his papers. Although he had his own study he chose to be in the lounge with his wife who nevertheless had to be quiet. She passed the time reading or knitting, but above all she was able to listen in silence to the radio with an early crystal wireless set and headphones, which she said retained her sanity. When Pat was older she too had to be in the room and was encouraged to read *The Times* though if the pages rustled too much she got a severe look from her father over his glasses. Occasionally he would read with irritation from an author's manuscript and ask, without expecting an answer, 'What *is* this fellow talking about?' and then throw the paper over to his wife.

Now that they had a family the motor cycle and sidecar had to replaced with a car and they bought a four cylinder Austin 12 with a collapsible hood and draughty mica windows. Lady Lewis had been the first woman in Wales to hold a driving licence and she had taught her husband how to drive on the broad hard surface of the Pendine Sands. At the weekends their parents devoted all their time to introducing the children to the natural world and to broadening their education. There would be trips in the car to the countryside and these often involved bringing back small fish, tadpoles, newts and snails to place in a large aquarium which had been made out of old glass battery tanks. This was a constant source of interest and delight. In the same room he had a primitive laboratory where he would demonstrate simple experiments such as mixing clear chemicals to produce a coloured fluid, or show how to melt lead and make castings of it. Sometimes they went to Epping Forest to collect fungi which then had their spore patterns examined back home. If it was wet they would spend the day in the London museums. The London Zoo was another popular place to visit. Their garden shed had a nesting box built into its side which could be opened from the back so that the nest with the young birds could be inspected from the darkness of the interior. Chris said, 'My father was a mine of information on natural history. Life in his company was always a learning experience as his encyclopaedic mind encompassed most flora and fauna'.[262] The one attempt that failed was when a tutor was engaged to teach the piano and German to Pat and Chris, neither of whom could master these disciplines. Their parents did not have a lot of interest in music and did not go to concerts, though they did listen at home to a mechanical pianola. Sometimes at the end of the week the children would be taken to the local cinema, at first in their small Austin but later in a Riley, a quite expensive car that had something of a sporting image. On the way there Lewis would drive slowly in spite of urging by the children to get there in good time 'Please go faster Daddy'. However on the return trip he would not allow any other car to remain ahead of him, whilst delivering a strong criticism of the films they had seen. He is remembered as a rather aggressive motorist.

## Their home in the countryside

The Lewises' third and last home was in a small and secluded housing estate called Loudwater located in a wooded valley in the Hertfordshire countryside 20 miles west of London. He was essentially a countryman and he disliked London, and his wife too loved the country. Also, following his heart attack he had realized, or at any rate had been told of, the need for more leisure. But their move was in fact made more or less by chance when they happened to call on Welsh friends during a drive through Hertfordshire and found their house was for sale, and they moved to it in 1933. He was able to get to work quite easily by taking the Metropolitan railway from nearby Rickmansworth to Euston Square station, a few minutes from the hospital. The house, 'Clearburn' (Fig. 16.11) was on three stories and not particularly well designed having rather dark living rooms. His study had several framed engravings of famous physicians and scientists. One

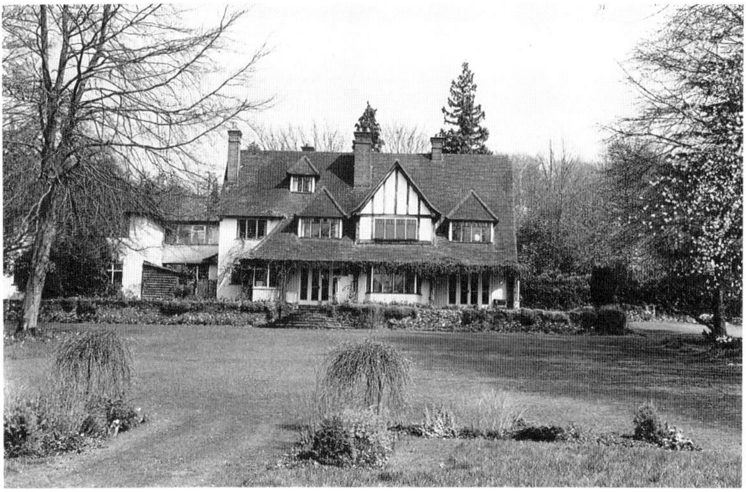

*Figure 16.11 Their house and garden,* Clearburn *at Loudwater.*

naturally was of his hero William Harvey and the others were of Thomas Willis, John Locke, Richard Boyle, and Samuel Garth. The lounge had a narrow sideboard in it which had previously been used to mount his first electrocardiograph machine. The attraction of the property lay in the large sloping garden of nearly three acres with a trout stream, the River Chess, (Fig. 16.12) at the bottom, and another one and a half acres on the other side of it. The acquisition of this property made a considerable change as to the way in which the family spent its leisure time. Lewis and his wife both liked gardening, and they often went to local nurseries to make a careful selection of plants. She spent a lot of time on the several flower beds, rose beds and a large rockery, whilst he had an especial interest in trees and shrubs. The children enjoyed helping him plant these, and he

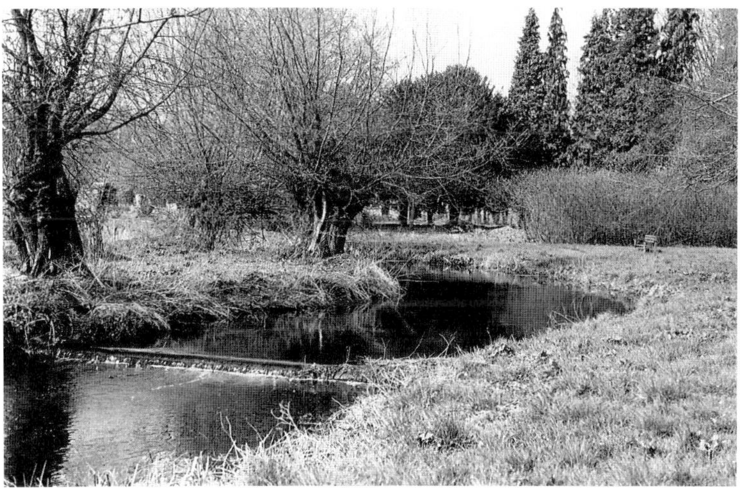

*Figure 16.12 The River Chess at the bottom of the garden.*

used to insist on digging a large hole, 'to give them plenty of room', although quite often they would later be moved to a new location when their progress in the difficult chalky soil, full of flints, seemed unsatisfactory. There was plenty of room for a full size tennis court and the whole family used to play on it wearing the regulation white clothes for the game. A swimming pool was made early on and Lewis planned its design and located it by the side of the stream, which provided the water. He and the two older children worked on it though a lot of the digging and mixing of concrete was done during the week by Lady Lewis and the full time gardener.

But of all the domestic activities it was fishing that took first place, and Lewis would go down to the stream for an hour or so when he got home from work. The children were taught fly fishing on the stream, and they also used to practise casting on the lawn trying to pick up a handkerchief or some other light weight object. He would show them how he painstakingly tied his own flies for fishing and they spent a lot of time watching him do this. He deduced that fish did not see the colour of flies but appreciated only the dimpling pattern of the hackles and so he developed his own dry fly without bright colours. It was dark brown and had white hackles added so that it could be seen by the fisherman as it floated through turbulent water. The numerous willow trees on the river bank used to entangle the lines and they had to be pollarded every spring with Lewis wielding the axe himself. He also taught the children how to climb trees safely by placing pieces of wood on the trunk as footholds if the branches were not low enough. This was often with the objective of finding a bird's nest, and then they would be shown how to blow out a bird's egg and to carefully label and store it. Every year the stream had to be weeded so that the trout could be caught without being entangled in the Water-crowfoot plants. One year when Chris was helping him Lewis noticed that their hands became swollen after working in the cold water for some hours and this initiated a new line of research into the mechanism of oedema produced by cold. Chris is mentioned in the introduction to the paper.[225] The stream certainly kept them busy because in addition to fishing it, they had to restock it with trout every year and at the same time get rid of the pike and perch which had migrated into it.

## Social life

The Lewises' social life was on a modest scale, because he preferred to spend his evenings during the week working at home. Only occasionally did they go to the theatre or concerts, and he avoided official dinners if he could. But they did entertain at home to a certain extent and they gave dinner parties for medical visitors and for colleagues. Einthoven stayed with them in 1921 and they gave a supper party so that he could meet some of the younger men. After it he wrote to say, 'I enjoyed my visit to England and my stay in your hospitable house extremely; I appreciate all the kindness shown to me very much. How are you and Mrs Lewis and little Pat?'[317] Certainly his research workers from abroad greatly appreciated the hospitality and kindness that was extended to them. For example Harold Marvin wrote, 'I wish there were some way in which I could reveal to you how often and how pleasantly you and Lady Lewis are present in my thoughts',[454] and in a later letter he said, 'In that happy time in London you and

Lady Lewis created bonds that have not grown weaker with the passing of the years'.[455] William Kerr wrote, 'Mrs Kerr and I appreciate all that you and Lady Lewis did to make our stay in London enjoyable'.[371] However for some of his own staff an invitation to dinner might be a preliminary to an evening in his study and these occasions were not always appreciated. Wayne recollected going to dinner with his wife, Drury and Grant. Afterwards when they were talking Lewis said, 'I think Grant we would be more profitably employed in going through your paper'. It was, said Wayne, a rude thing to do. Drury, perhaps jokingly, once said that before going to dinner with Lewis he always had a large whisky and two aspirins.

At Clearburn they often had guests at the weekend. His students, house physicians and younger members of his staff were glad to be invited and some of them even chose to walk the two miles or so from the station. They were very useful in helping to construct the swimming pool, and with heavy tasks in the garden such as planting trees, and then joined the family for a traditional lunch of roast beef, with a bottle of beer. Lewis and his wife drank very little alcohol. At weekends they might have sherry and beer at lunchtime and in the evening. Lewis always made a point of never drinking at lunchtime if he was working in the afternoon. During World War II when sherry was unobtainable he would bring alcohol from the hospital pharmacy and mix it with orange juice. The Lewises had been regular tennis players for some years and now that they had their own court they became quite proficient. (Fig. 16.13) They were joined for tennis by their old friends the Dales with whom they had played for years. Sir Henry was Chris' godfather. Other

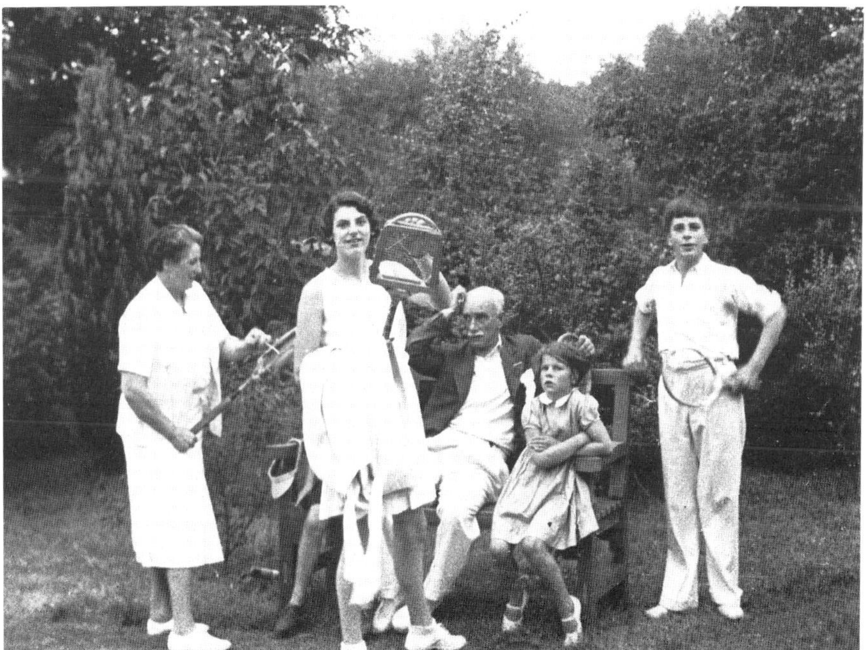

*Figure 16.13 A family tennis group. The children from left to right are Pat, Pip and Chris. This photograph was taken by the late Dr Charles Fletcher, son of Sir Walter, in 1939. It is the only picture of the Lewis family together.*

guests would often include the Pickerings and the Cottons and sometimes there would be old colleagues and friends from abroad such as Paul and Ina White and Samuel Levine from Boston, and Charles Best from Toronto. Lewis' bachelor brother Clifford often stayed with them as did a variety of cousins of the childrens' ages, and sometimes a favourite lady house physician would be invited for the weekend. All their visitors found Lady Lewis to be an excellent hostess, but Lewis himself was not a naturally good host. Although he was good at talking to individuals his shy and inhibited character was not well suited to social conversation. As a result, and also because he could on occasion be a difficult person, he would get irritated to the point of rudeness on some social occasions at their home. One visitor recalled an episode when the conversation lapsed and after a while someone tried to start it again with a trivial comment. Lewis glared at the person and said, 'I cannot understand what caused you to make that remark', whereupon of course there was an even longer silence. But if he did get into a bad mood like this his wife would say, 'Well if you're feeling like that Tom you had better go out for a long walk'. But he was a different person when he was with a friend, and Pickering wrote that 'those who gained his friendship and who knew him in his leisure, devoted to his wife and children, knew a warm hearted man, whose support once gained was unstinted, and who was a delightful and witty conversationalist on many topics'.[299]

## Lady Lewis

Lady Lewis had great charm and she devoted her considerable energies to supporting her husband in his work and hobbies, and to their children and their home. (Fig. 16.14) For several years she worked every week in the Child Welfare Department at UCH, and then on leaving London she became active in local affairs at Chorleywood near their new home. She was elected as a Councillor and eventually served for 50 years, being chairman of the council on two occasions, and was appointed a Member of the Order of the British Empire (MBE) for these services. She had a special interest in creating public housing for the poor and the pensioners, and surprised her colleagues on one occasion by climbing into suggested types of baths to try them out. She knew many of the tenants personally and would call in on them to see how things were going. Her scheme became a model for other small communities. She was a wonderful organizer who led by her enthusiastic participation. During the war she became head of the Womens Voluntary Services in her area and arranged the meals on wheels service for the disabled. At home she milked the goats, making butter and cheese and supplying goats milk to local children who were allergic to cows' milk. She too had a strong personality and indeed Sir Thomas was referred to in the neighbourhood as Lady Lewis' husband.

## Family holidays

Holidays were an important aspect of Lewis family life. In the early 1920's there were holidays with a good deal of bird photography in the Scilly Isles and in Norfolk but when the children were older this was not a good occupation for

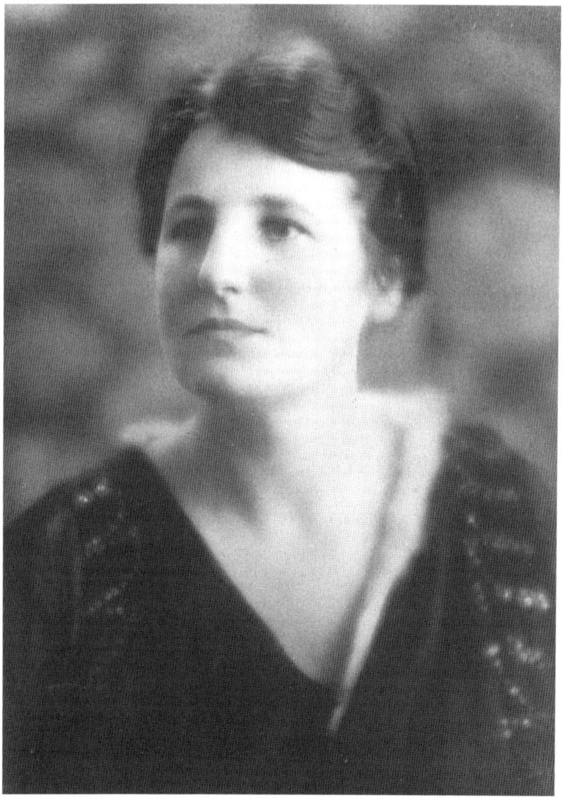

*Figure 16.14 Lady Lewis aged 35.*

them and it was then largely given up. At Easter and Christmas they would often go to Merthyr Tydfil and stay with the James family, whilst a long summer holiday was usually spent at the seaside. Pat remembers that 'Mum and Dad spent a lot of time with us on the beaches. He made us beautiful castles in the sand with very expert turrets'. Abersoch in North Wales was a favourite venue where, when Pat and Chris were old enough, they were shown how to fish off the rocks. Lewis did not like to sit down on the beach for very long and he would soon be looking for shells. When they were at Newquay in Cornwall he and Chris took up crabbing. This involved swimming around the rocks, and with the initial guidance of a local fisherman, pulling the large edible crabs out of their holes with a crab hook. A holiday in Ireland was spent fishing in Loch Foyle when they were accompanied by the Pickerings and their first child. Lady Pickering recollected that each day was carefully planned by Lewis and his wife who, she said, worked very well together.[463] Their nanny, Miss Weekley, always came on holiday with them. Lewis' assistant secretary Miss Truebody also came a few times and Lady Lewis described her as a good looking and capable young woman who almost became one of the family, adding that 'Tom seemed to be quite attracted by her'. Butterfly hunting was another holiday pastime, and this too was taken seriously with the insects being killed in a cyanide jar and then carefully

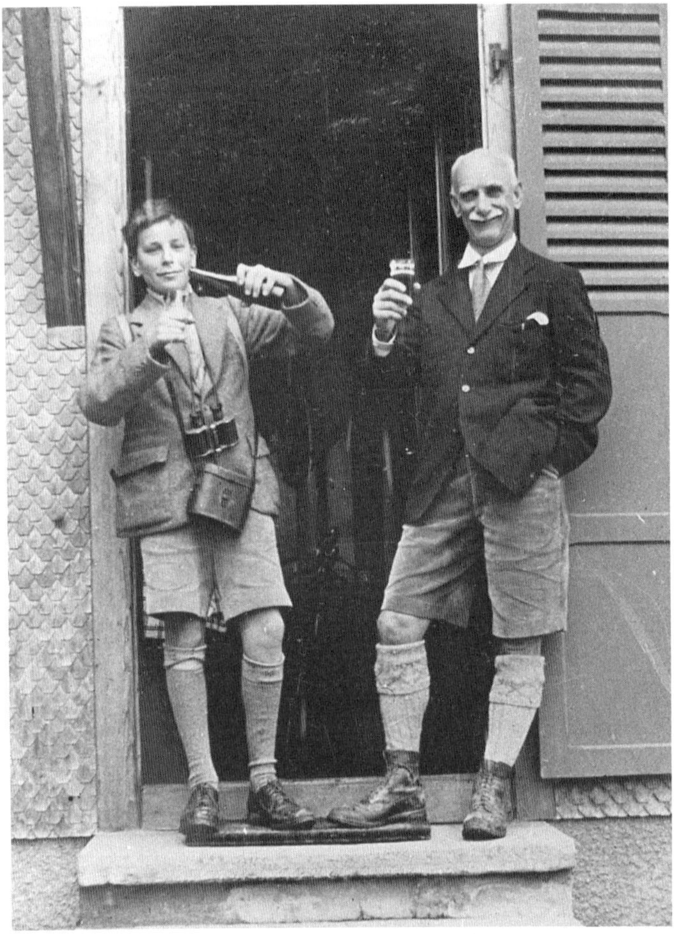

*Figure 16.15 Chris with his father walking at Wengen, Switzerland in 1934.*

mounted. This was a painstaking operation using fine pins on a special mounting board after which they were labelled and placed in special boxes. In addition to natural history there were also frequent visits to castles and ancient churches. Lewis did not take work with him on holiday and in the evenings he would read detective stories and other books or play cards with the family. He was an expert at Lexicon, a word game with cards, and could sometimes put down an entire hand at once. One of their best holidays was to Switzerland in 1934 which was planned as a walking tour to see the alpine flowers. (Fig. 16.15) The snow was late that year and this enabled them all to do some ski-ing. Lewis had been ski-ing with his parents over 20 years previously, and on this occasion he was soon ski-ing with the more advanced groups. Afterwards they went to Paris where 'Dad seemed well versed in French history and the paintings'. For several years Chris and his father used to go fishing together in Wales every spring, either to Talybont, or on the Usk near Crickhowel. Chris remembers with affection how they sat on the river bank together at lunchtime comparing notes and observing the bird life around them, and the quiet evenings when 'Dad usually read a book whilst I spent hours sketching the other guests in the hotel'.[262]

## The children growing up

The two eldest children both went away from home to boarding school. Pat went to her mother's old school, Roedean, for five years whilst Chris was at Stowe. When the war started in 1939, Pat joined the Land Army and worked single handed on a farm for the whole four years. Pip was then only nine years old, and Lewis was uncertain whether Britain could resist a German invasion. So he arranged with Paul and Ina White for her to stay with them in Boston. This was not unusual. Quite a few British families who could afford it, and had friends or relatives in North America, sent their younger children to Canada or the United States. Dr and Mrs White were delighted to help, and had in fact had the same idea themselves, but even so the initiative was his and Lady Lewis felt rather hard done by and would have preferred to have kept her daughter at home. Many years later Pip, now Mrs Phillipa Althaus, recollected her childhood:

> My best recollections would begin around 1936–7 when I began school at the age of five. My father was a wonderful story teller. I had a wooden hobby horse which lived behind my bedroom door and he wound many of these stories around Hobby as he was called. Hobby would engage in all kinds of activities after I had gone to bed, such as going down the valley to meet some real horses which used to be in a field there, returning to his place in my room by morning. I can still visualise a picture he drew of Hobby behind that door. I even remember one letter he wrote to me while I was in the States which was illustrated with drawings of Hobby swimming across the Atlantic to visit me. Dad was a wonderful teacher and he instilled a love of nature in me which I have tried to pass on to my own children.

Chris went from Stowe to read medicine at Oxford. He had often been a subject for his father's research on the skin and on pain, and had been to the laboratory and occasionally on ward rounds, and several times had gone to soirees at the Royal Society. He found all this fascinating and always assumed that he would have a medical career. But like his father he was a good artist and he had a considerable interest in that too. Whilst at Stowe he was not doing well in biology and was forbidden to do any more art until he had passed his first MB examination. He never regretted the decision to do medicine but found the comparisons with his father were inhibiting, with phrases such as, 'We expect great things of you' or, 'This is Sir Thomas Lewis' son'. Lewis got in touch with his former pupil Hugh Sinclair, by now a Fellow of Magdalene College and asked him to be Chris' tutor. Sinclair said that Lewis once stayed in Oxford to encourage his son in an examination and that the outcome was predictable. After Chris had failed Sinclair had the task of suggesting to Sir Thomas that it would be better if he stayed away at the next attempt. In Sinclair's opinion Chris loved and respected his father, but was also rather intimidated by him.[470]

Lewis gave constant guidance to his son, much as his own father had given him, and his letters are worth quoting from because they give a good insight into Lewis' character[262] They start when Chris was at Stowe at the age of 15:

> To acquire good habits of work and to come to like work at your age is to lay the foundation of a successful and happy life.

A year or so later when Chris was promoted to a higher class he got more detailed advice:

> I expect you will find the work a bit stiff at first. Don't go too fast or try to, getting through the days work and understanding it. The last is the most important thing and you will find yourself on top of it all in time. Don't mind, for the moment, where you are in the form. Good luck to you in the exams. Don't forget to leave a little time for reading through what you have written to make sure there are no obvious slips.

Whilst still at school at the age of 18 the war had started and he was exempt from military service because he was studying medicine, but the exemption depended on passing the necessary examinations:

> I am a bit disturbed to know you are doing dramatic stuff this term. If this is anything but a very small part you are ill advised to be doing it. Everything must give way to your exam.

He did pass the first exam for a medical degree, the 1st MB, and then went to the University of Oxford:

> Don't forget to keep a bright eye open for good friends at Oxford. Go slow in making them, but once you are sure cultivate them. Your country is in great peril. Many of your contemporaries are or will be dying in the services. Being exempt from fighting places a very big obligation on you to give your very best to your country now, and in the future, in other ways. Think this over dear boy and, whatever you do, don't cultivate the idea that you are just lucky and can proceed on the path of enjoying play (that is of course beyond reasonable recreation) whilst less fortunate young men are risking or giving their lives.

When Chris was starting his second year at Oxford his father wrote him a long letter in November 1942 on methods of work, of which the following are extracts:

> This will be the time of the most important development of your mind. It is hard not to believe that the chief acquisition at this stage is information; there seems so much to gather in. But there are two other things of more importance. 1) *is getting to know how to learn*, so that for the future you will require no teacher, but books and objects of study. It is important to get a habit of selecting for study things which matter most, from the best books etc. Of course your teachers will guide you, but my point is that you should try and form your own judgement as well. 2) *is forming proper habits of thought*, and the most important things here are (i) a complete understanding of the things you do tackle. I mean not taking things for granted or using rule of thumb methods; every good method has reason behind it, and the reason of it must be seen if you are ready to be served by the method. (ii) a critical sense and understanding of evidence; so that a conclusion is not accepted without knowing why it is formulated. I think the laws of evidence are more soundly learned by examining examples, than by studying them in the abstract. Think these things over from time to time in your work from now on, and be persuaded that they are the very essence of your present training if you can master them. It is very important because at this stage your teachers are men who recognized these matters; whereas when you come to the clinical stage, most of your teachers will not.[262]

Lewis consulted his colleague Harold P Himsworth, the professor of medicine, as to which medical school Chris should go to and got the reply, 'Send him to the best one', meaning UCH. He went there in 1945, shortly after his father had died, and did his house jobs there. Later he went to Canada where he met his wife, Helga Ritter and after marriage in 1958 they settled in Vancouver where he practised as a physician. The artistic bent which he got from his father found further expression when he became a first class sculptor.

When Pat was age 33 she married Sinclair Watson, whom she had known as a near neighbour since the age of 14 and who had been at Stowe with Christopher. Together they managed a small farm which had been created after Lewis' death with the purchase of adjoining land. Phillipa married Peter Althaus, a German citizen, later a naturalized American, whom she met in Australia, in 1959 and they live in California. Altogether there are eight grandchildren, and Chris' daughter Dr Andrea Lewis is in the medical profession.

Lady Lewis survived her husband by 44 years and continued to live at Clearburn, with Pat and Sinclair until her death in 1989 a few months short of her hundredth birthday. She was buried by his side in the grave at Llangasty Churchyard, Breconshire.

## Note to Chapter 16

(1) It is surprising to find that in 1920 there was a photographic emulsion which was sensitive enough to permit of an exposure as short as 1/1000 of a second, at an aperture of f 11. However this fact is well documented in a book, which Lewis could well have read, entitled *Photography for Bird Lovers* by Bentley Beetham, published in 1911 by Witherby and Co London. It contains detailed information as to what shutter speed should be used to photograph birds in various modes of flight. It states that 1/1200 of a second is the highest speed at which a focal plane shutter will work and adds that it is not often that the light will permit one to use such a brief exposure.

# Chapter 17

## The war years • Effort syndrome • Llandough Hospital • Monograph on Pain • Views on digitalis • Copley Medal • Final illness and death

The probability of a war with Germany and the likelihood of large scale air raids on British cities had led to the Emergency Medical Service (EMS) being set up. It was planned to use the central London hospitals chiefly as casualty clearing stations and to transfer most of their staff and patients to locations outside the metropolis. UCH was in sector IV which covered north west London and the surrounding districts, and practically all the clinical staff enrolled either as full time or part time members of the Service. Beds for UCH patients were allocated at Stanborough's Hydro near Watford and at Leavesden Asylum nearby. On the declaration of war on September 3 1939 UCH was emptied of patients, and all the medical staff reported to their allotted posts in the EMS except for those who were to remain at UCH to man the casualty clearing station.[289] On September 4, Lewis wrote from home to Mellanby saying 'I have been posted to a hospital at Leavesden. Simultaneously I am running the Casualty Services for West Hertfordshire. I will do any work the MRC considers more suitable for me'. He wrote again to say 'Honour, the head lab man, is little employed but he is much too valuable to release as I shall want him for any work I engage in and wherever it is'.[503] Lewis now had his patients at the Leavesden hospital, 20 miles north of London, where he also made regular teaching rounds. But his work with the first aid casualty services in his home district of Chorleywood was less satisfactory because of a dispute as to who directed them. Lewis had been commandant since 1938 and had written a 32 page document covering every aspect of their organisation. Naturally he considered that he was in charge, but the local Medical Officer of Health (MOH) also claimed that position. Lewis threatened to resign and he sought the support of Professor Francis R. Fraser, a leading clinical research worker, who had been seconded from the Post Graduate Medical School at Hammersmith to be director of the EMS. Fraser would no doubt have liked to help, but he had to uphold the general rule that the MOH was in control and that exceptions could not be made, 'There is only one Sir Thomas Lewis' he sympathetically added. So Lewis continued in post with the comment 'These long standing medical officers are more encased in protective mechanism even than the Ministry itself'.[421]

# Effort syndrome and other problems in the war

However the war presented a much more important problem to Lewis than this parochial matter. It was the problem of recruits and soldiers with 'supposed affections of the heart' which he had investigated so thoroughly in the First World War, and he quickly produced a second edition of *The Soldier's Heart and the Effort Syndrome* saying in the preface, dated April 1940, 'I had hoped never to be called upon to re-edit it. But a new war has come upon us, and in these first few months of it I have become increasingly aware that we are wrestling with the same old problems'.[216] The book was revised, and a new chapter added on 'Definition of effort syndrome' in which he said that symptoms such as breathlessness, giddiness, fatigue and 'in cases of extreme effort pain over the precordial region' which occur after exercise in healthy people occur also, though after much less effort, in 'a large class of patients in ill health' who were therefore said to suffer from the 'effort syndrome'. The comment about chest pain was made to forestall criticism, such as Levine had made in 1918, that it did not in fact occur in normal subjects. He made it clear that the effort syndrome was a 'very mixed group'. Some patients had unrecognized infections or were convalescing from an acute illness, others were played out by the 'constant strain and jar to body and nervous system which work in the front line brings'. With eloquent prose he told how the enforced training and the unnatural conditions of war submit men to a most drastic test:

> Who then can affect surprise if many men fail when so tested? The test in its entirety selects, it selects the weaklings in the general sense and marks them down. It grasps those who lack physical strength or nervous stability; it grasps those seemingly in full health and yet the subjects of incipient disease. Many it breaks at once, some it breaks only in the end. Healthy men break when the trial is too long continued; there is a limit to the endurance of each and all.[216]

However his views were challenged by Dr Paul H. Wood[(1)] who undertook a precise analysis of 200 cases from 1940–1941. He disputed that the symptoms were similar to those found after exercise pointing out for example that normal people did not especially sweat on cold palms or in the axillae, not did they usually get inframammary pain. Wood considered that Da Costa's syndrome, as he preferred to call it, was nearly always associated with psychoneurosis with the features closely resembling those of emotion, and especially of fear. Wood claimed that after the war 'the recognition of this syndrome, as such, will die'.[335] But Lewis and indeed Mackenzie had pointed out that it was often present prior to entry into the Army, was not peculiarly a soldier's malady, and was frequent among civilians both women and men. There were letters in the *British Medical Journal* following Wood's article but not from Lewis.

Lewis' concern about Britain's chance of defeating Hitler and of his hope that the United States would join in the war was expressed in a letter to his former research associate Dr Duckett Jones in Boston in September 1940. 'We are sometimes fearful that we shall not suffice however good a show we put up; the forces against us are terrific', and saying that the entry of the United States would ensure success. He added, 'But our chins are well up and there is not a sign of faltering anywhere, in fact quite the contrary'.[427] His anxiety about the war was reflected in his recommendation to his wife that their youngest child Pip, then aged nine, should go to the United States and she went there in June 1940. Lewis thought up two ideas to help with the war. He designed a metal plate which fitted into the back of the gas mask haversack on the chest and which he predicted, from careful calculations, would protect the heart from 31% of bullets coming from any direction.[426] This idea, which was quite a good one though not taken up, may have come from his study of the soldier with a bullet embedded in his heart, and it was well known that soldiers' lives had been saved by the metal cigarette case in their breast pocket. Another idea was to suggest that delayed action bombs could be rendered ineffective by freezing them with liquid carbon dioxide.[428] His work with the casualty services made him acquainted with the type of tourniquet being issued for the first aid treatment of limb haemorrhage. This was the Samway type which required considerable force to stretch the thick rubber tubing and place it in a metal anchor. Lewis was appalled by it and tried without success to get the Ministry of Health and the Home Office to withdraw it, saying he would make his views public if they failed to act. He was after all a world authority on the limb circulation and after giving them their chance he wrote first to the *British Medical Journal* about 'this instrument of torture'[218] and then to *The Times* newspaper in May 1940. His solution was to use a stout rubber strap three inches wide and three feet long and he obtained a large amount of this for trial from the Dunlop Rubber Company.[422]

When the air raids failed to materialize UCH gradually resumed its role as a general hospital. Although Lewis remained at Leavesden, work started again in his department where Pochin was joined by John Squire,[(2)] as the only two remaining members of staff. Kellgren, to his dismay, had had his Beit Fellowship abruptly terminated by Elliott but he managed on the strength of his FRCS to get a job as a surgeon in the EMS even though his surgical experience was minimal. Whilst still a student Squire had worked in Lewis' department whilst still a student, and he became his house physician in August 1939. He had a distinguished later career. Pochin and Squire's work was done in relation to the programme of the Committee on Traumatic Shock of the MRC and they developed a simplified method of estimating blood volume with Evans' Blue dye. It was later used to measure blood volume in air raid casualties.

## A monograph on pain

The onset of war put an end to his plans to continue with research on pain. In particular he had wanted to investigate further the phenomena of visceral pain and tenderness which presented an unsolved challenge to him. So he used his enforced leisure to signal the end of that era of work by writing a monograph on it, as he had done before with his other two main periods of research, on the electrocardiogram and on the blood vessels of the skin. The book was entitled simply *Pain*, (Fig. 17.1) and in the preface he wrote 'Reflection tells me that I am so far from being able satisfactorily to define pain, that the attempt would serve no useful purpose. Pain, like similar subjective things, is known to us by experience and described by illustration'.[230] The chief purpose of the book was to review modern ideas on the mechanism of pain whilst recounting the work done in his own laboratory during the previous ten years. It contains excellent chapters on referred pain and the pain of visceral disease and the difficulty of these topics did not blunt the clarity of his writing. He was clearly impressed by evidence about pain from abdominal structures produced by surgeons when operating under

PAIN

BY

THOMAS LEWIS, M.D., F.R.S.

PHYSICIAN IN CHARGE OF DEPARTMENT OF CLINICAL RESEARCH, UNIVERSITY COLLEGE HOSPITAL, LONDON; FELLOW OF UNIVERSITY COLLEGE, LONDON

THE MACMILLAN COMPANY

NEW YORK

*Figure 17.1 His last monograph, published in New York because of the war, in 1942.*

local anaesthesia and the work of Mr John Morley, a surgeon in Manchester, and James Mackenzie is often mentioned. Mackenzie's work as a general practitioner had included major surgery and it is clear that he and Lewis had discussed pain because one reference is a personal communication from him. The final chapter is entitled 'Principles in the clinical use of pain' and in it he was concerned with improving the diagnostic value of pain by enhancing the accuracy of its description. He said that trying to remember what a previously experienced pain was like could be difficult – it should be described when it occurred and the description revised if it recurred. Another source of inaccuracy arose when the pain was described by terms such as tearing, boring, stabbing and crushing which the subject 'imagined to be capable of causing it' but which were in fact outside their own experience. He emphasized the value of what he called the time- intensity curve of pain, a feature which in his view had been given too little attention. This was illustrated with a diagram comparing the pulsating pain of toothache with the longer phases of intestinal colic and the unfluctuating pain of angina or burnt skin. (Fig. 17.2, *overleaf*) It is an impressive work which must have been difficult to write

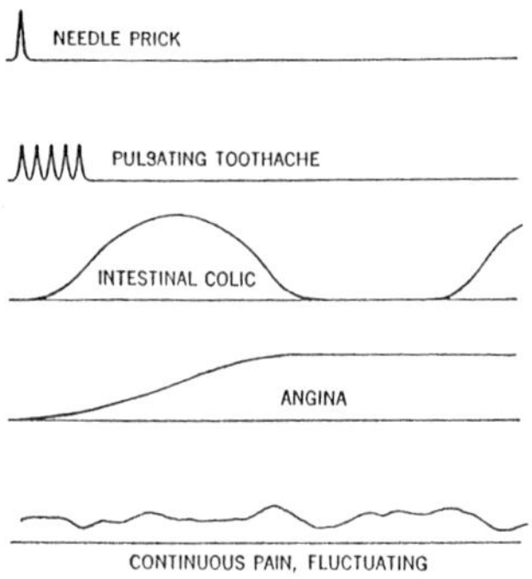


Fig. 26. A diagram illustrating time-intensity curves of various well-known pains, namely, needle prick, pulsating toothache, intestinal colic, angina, and continuous fluctuating pain.

*Figure 17.2 A figure from* Pain *to show different varieties of pain.*

and yet he seems to have completed it in only a few months, a testimony to his continuing capacity at the age of 58 for incisive thought and hard continuous work. By April 1940 it was finished and he decided to get it published by Macmillans in New York, who had produced the American edition of *Diseases of the Heart*. His unease about Britain's wartime capability showed up in May when he told Macmillan to proceed with publication if Britain was invaded and to have the royalties held by Paul White, Harold M. Marvin or William St Lawrence. He had already discussed the question of royalties with Mr Daniel Macmillan in London saying that whilst the British house of the firm gave him 15%, the American one gave only 10%. Lewis seems always to have had a close concern about financial matters.[495] In 1940 he corresponded with two American doctors. Somehow he had found out that Dr Alfred Blalock, professor of surgery at Johns Hopkins, had stated in his book *Principles of Surgical Care*, that Lewis had said that the H substance was a single substance. Lewis replied that he had never said it, and that the error came from Krogh.[424] Blalock agreed and offered to correct the error in the next edition.[346] The other letter was to Dr F. Boys in the United States who had asked for the names of clinical scientists in that country. Lewis replied that there were very few now that Cushing was dead: he did not name any.[425]

## Karel Wenckebach dies in 1940

The death of Professor Karel Wenckebach in 1940 at the age of 76 broke an important link with Lewis' early career, and he wrote an affectionate obituary notice in the *British Medical Journal*. Whilst still a young man he had made a special point whilst in Holland, on his way to meet Einthoven, of going to see Wenckebach whose book *Die Arrhythmie*, published a few years previously, he described as a brilliant achievement and the foundation of much that followed. 'Venkie', as he liked to be called, was a great friend of Mackenzie and came to be a good friend of Lewis too, who now spoke of him as 'a genial, good hearted fellow, full of enthusiasm for work, inspiring to others and a great teacher of

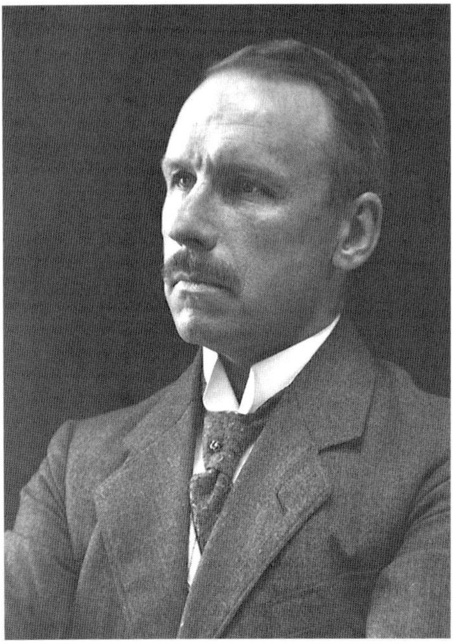

*Figure 17.3 Professor Karel Wenckebach, one of his first friends in cardiology.*

students'. (Fig. 17.3) This great Dutchman, he said, would be remembered in Britain with affection and admiration.[221]

## Teaching and working at Llandough Hospital in Wales

The teaching of medical students had naturally been disrupted by the outbreak of war. In 1939 and early 1940 they were taught first at Cardiff in Wales, and then back in London and also at Leavesden, but the onset of heavy and persistent air raids on London in September 1940 made it necessary to move all the teaching out of UCH. The October entry of clinical students were sent to Cardiff. Lewis took charge of this group and he went to live nearby at Llwyn Crwn Farm, Llanishen. He was accompanied by his devoted personal assistant John Honour who, as always, was a great support to him. Dr John Squire came too and acted as medical tutor. The clinical work was based at Llandough Hospital where Dr David A Williams was one of the consultant physicians. He was charged with making sure, at a preliminary visit, that Lewis did accept the position and aided this by offering, to Lewis' surprise, any number of his own 68 beds. At the end of the visit Williams said he hoped that Sir Thomas would not be afraid to come back to Wales to work with the wild Welsh. 'He turned, stared with his typical piercing stare, and then laughed'.[536]

The success of that clinical year was ensured by having Lewis in charge. He loved teaching and it proved to be a very happy time for him. The students felt they belonged to a closely knit group and knew they were privileged to have Lewis as their chief. They also got excellent teaching and guidance from Squire. Otto Wolff, later a professor of paediatrics, was one of the class and he remembers that Sir Thomas became almost a father figure, often inviting a few of them to join him on a Sunday walk. But they were expected to know, as Lewis did, the name of every flower or bird they saw, and this he says could be a bit frightening.[537] It is said that his very attractive girl friend made Wolff always welcome on these walks. Dr Williams remembered several episodes at Llandough, and one of them became a familiar situation:

> Sir Thomas was always in the lounge at coffee time, with a newspaper. If a person came in whom he did not like he put the paper up firmly, apparently reading it, but with someone he did like he put the paper down and had a chat. But even when the paper was up he was listening to the conversation and if he heard any loose statement the newspaper would go down and the person was told quite forcibly that he should be precise. But having expressed himself strongly he would later on be having lunch quite amicably with a senior doctor he had previously shaken too brusquely.[536]

One day Lewis sought medical advice for himself. He had twice experienced severe pain in the calves on walking 25 yards that morning and was obviously quite concerned about himself believing he might have arterial disease. But Williams found nothing wrong and diagnosed cramp due to Lewis having walked a long distance on the previous day. The diagnosis was accepted and Lewis took a train to London. 'I asked him to see one of his colleagues there, but he just laughed'. Lewis was never one to leave anything to chance and this is well illustrated by another of Dr Williams' recollections:

> Sir Thomas told me that he would be asked to see patients in the vicinity of Cardiff, and if that person had in any way helped the hospital he would see them, but not otherwise. So from time to time in the doctors' lounge I would listen to Sir Thomas being asked by a small group of senior people to see someone. I would be standing nearby facing Sir Thomas and waiting for him to look in my direction, and then I would either nod or shake my head.[536]

Research at Llandough was at a low level, though Squire did a study with Williams of asthmatic patients sensitive to foreign proteins, and with Lewis he investigated the protein content of exudates and transudates. He also studied the effect on patients with the nephrotic syndrome of transfusions of blood plasma, but none of this work was published.[287] Williams said that although Lewis held Squire in high regard he gave him little encouragement to do research. Certainly the year in Wales was an unusually quiet one for Lewis. Although he was able to do important research with the simplest of apparatus, he in fact did little. No issue of *Clinical Science* was produced and he wrote only one paper. But he was certainly more active on the wards than at UCH, and Williams was impressed by the very conscientious care that he gave to his patients. Furthermore the students had plenty of teaching. One can only assume that the closure of his department, Pickering's departure, the new environment, the need to leave his home and the uncertain future of Britain all conspired to neutralize his investigative drive. However the abrasive side of his character had not diminished as was shown by yet another encounter with the editor of a medical journal. He had written a letter to *The Lancet* about an article on visceral pain and it had been slightly changed.[219] He wrote to the editor, Dr Egbert Morland, saying, 'Your office boy or another has altered a sentence…I say office boy because the grammar as it now stands would disgrace a junior schoolboy. I protest against your slack editorial method'.[429] This letter shows how deliberately rude Lewis could be when he chose. But he did write one paper in 1940 on 'Caleb Hillier Parry MD FRS (1755–1822). A great Welsh physician and scientist' which arose from an address he gave to the Cardiff Medical Society. It was published in their proceedings which explains why this good account is so little known. It is headed with a quotation from Parry which reads, 'The most dangerous state incidental to the human mind is a calm acquiescence in the accuracy and extent of its own attainments'. In the article he emphasizes that Parry's book on angina pectoris in 1799 contains the first recognition of myocardial ischaemia in relation to effort or emotion. He also underlines Parry's other priorities in describing hyperthyroidism well before Robert Graves, and in demonstrating that bradycardia occurs with carotid pressure prior to Karl E. Hering and Augustus Waller. The article concludes with the words, 'His was a truly great, a noble, career; the man remains for us a shining example and inspiration, to whom I invite the enduring attention and reverence of his countrymen'.[224]

Lewis' desire to help in the fight against Germany was put to the test in May 1941 when the British Council asked him to undertake a 3–5 month tour of South America, especially Argentina where a senior physician was keen to have a visit from him. The visit was designed to enhance British prestige in this neutral country. The route, they explained, would be by plane to Lisbon and then onwards by boat. For a man of 59 this was quite an undertaking in war time, but in his reply Lewis clearly recognized his duty to assist the war effort.[430] However when T.R. Elliott was asked for his opinion he pointed out that a medical tour would not help very much and also that after two coronary attacks it would be unwise to go. Furthermore, 'You are needed to nurse the growth of clinical science'.

Air raids were now infrequent and the summer term of 1941 was the last at Cardiff. He was appointed Honorary Consultant Physician at Llandough Hospital and he wrote that 'the appointment will give me a feeling of lasting association with the hospital at which I have worked so happily during the last 12 months'. Although he was away from home this certainly had been a very agreeable time for him. The lack of research work meant that he spent much more time in the wards both in clinical work and teaching than he was accustomed to do at UCH. He may even have realized that his previous intensive laboratory work had divorced him to some extent from a closer involvement with bedside medicine which he was now enjoying. In addition he was back in the Welsh countryside which he had loved and known so well in his boyhood.

## Research on shipwreck, chilblains and frostbite

His faithful secretary Miss Lena Searle wrote to say 'It will be good to see you back' and by the autumn of 1941 he was at the UCH Sector Hospital which was housed in the former Stanborough's Hydro near Leavesden. This had been made into a 70 bed hospital with a library and lecture rooms. His laboratory was in the gardener's potting shed which the ever resourceful Honour had converted by installing some equipment and benches from UCH. Squire remained with him and continued his work on protein sensitivity which had started at Llandough. He joined the Royal Army Medical Corps in May 1942 and Lewis ensured that he could continue research whilst in the Army.[22] Pochin had remained at UCH working on thyroid problems and on shock, and he now went to the MRC Physiological Laboratory at the Armoured Fighting Vehicle Training School,

Lulworth, Dorset. This was in line with the policy of the MRC in relation to war service, minuted by the Council in 1939 and re-affirmed in 1940.[287] This stated that previous research work should be continued as far as possible, though attention should also be given to new subjects of research which were directly related to the war. This policy fitted in well with the research on the effects of cold on the limbs which Lewis had commenced a few years previously, and now took up again, because there were important war time applications, especially in relation to shipwreck. His interest in the topic had first been aroused, like other of his research projects, by a personal experience, which has already been referred to. Whilst weeding his trout stream, with a water temperature of 12°C, he had found that his hands became swollen with pitting oedema. But if one hand was used it was only that hand which became swollen even though the other one was always wet, showing simply but conclusively that the swelling was due to cold and not to the hand being wet. His present experiments were designed to throw light on the phenomena and treatment of 'immersion foot', a condition of extensive damage and swelling of the limbs which was occurring in shipwrecked crews who had been exposed to cold water in the North Atlantic. Honour devised a sensitive method of measuring the volume of the hands and feet, which were kept dry with gloves. Lewis showed that the swelling of an extremity in cold water was due to a direct injury of the skin and subcutaneous tissues by cold, producing oedema which was judged to be inflammatory because of its high protein content, and resulting presumably from liberation of H substance. Sailors in swamped boats might lose substantial amounts of protein and fluid into their limbs.[225] He served on the MRC committee on the Care of Shipwrecked Personnel. Cold was the subject of three Holme Lectures which he gave in the medical school that autumn and which were published in December in the *British Medical Journal.* The first was on the reactions to cold and injury of normal skin, the second on chilblains and the third on frost bite. He found that chilblains were not easy to explain and did a lot of experimental work on subjects who were prone to them. He showed that prolonged or repeated cooling was an important causative factor, and that chilblain subjects seemed to owe their predisposition to the malady from the readiness with which the temperature of their fingers fell to that of the surroundings and to the long delay in warming after general vasodilatation had set in. He pointed out that limbs which had become cold from disuse, such as in poliomyelitis or syringomyelia, were limbs in which chilblains were common. But his conclusions were limited by the difficulty of producing chilblains experimentally. In discussing frostbite he showed that skin could be cooled to minus 15°C for ten minutes, or minus 25°C for ten seconds, and yet remain unfrozen, from a protective mechanism against freezing called supercooling. The capacity to supercool was connected he thought with the relative dryness of the horny layers of the skin because it was diminished by washing, and he commented that Arctic explorers left their skin unwashed. The acute reactions to supercooling had to be distinguished from frostbite. His experimental studies on freezing the skin enabled him to give detailed recommendations on the treatment of frostbite.[222] His interest in cold continued with a question to Professor John B.S. Haldane, a member of the staff at UCL, who recounted how he had immersed himself in cold water to the limit of his tolerance to which Lewis replied with 'thanks for the account of your heroic bathing'.[433] He also wrote a paper on Trousseau's phenomenon, a condition where spasm of the hand muscles occurs when the arm circulation is arrested in a patient with tetany due to a low blood calcium level.

This sign had been known for over a century but the mechanism had always been disputed. His study of the sign was a classical Lewis type investigation, simple and conclusive. By placing two blood pressure cuffs on the upper arm, and inflating them alternately, he proved that the tetany was due to a loss of the blood supply to the nerve underneath the cuff, and not to any direct effect on the muscles.[226] However the change from Llandough was not all to his liking as is shown in a letter to Eugene Landis, 'I am working at a makeshift place outside London but chiefly at teaching, and at routine which as you probably guess I hate'.[431]

## The Copley Medal of the Royal Society

In November 1941 he had the great honour of being awarded the Copley Medal of the Royal Society of London. (Fig. 17.4) This is the premier award of the Society and its distinction lies in the fact that it may be awarded to a Fellow of the Society, anywhere in the world, for eminence in sustained work done in any branch of natural science. He received it for his clinical and experimental investigations upon the mammalian heart. Only once in over 100 years had it previously been awarded to a clinician, namely Lord Lister, also a former student at UCH and who like Lewis had also gained the Royal Medal.[54] Lord Lister was awarded it in 1902 and the clinician before him was Sir Benjamin Brodie in 1811. The other medical scientists who received it during that period read like a roll call of the

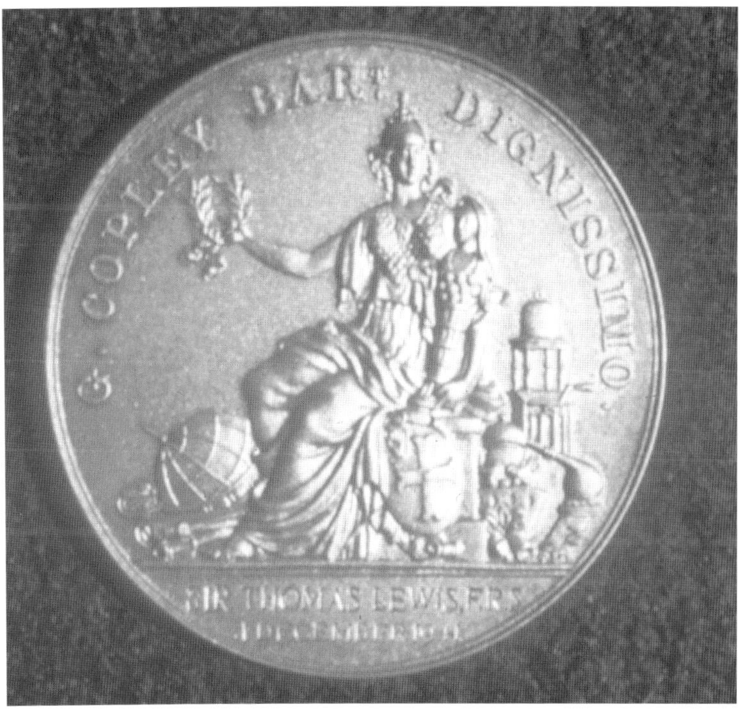


*Figure 17.4 The Copley Medal of the Royal Society of London.*

famous, with names such as Louis Pasteur, Claude Bernard, Carl Ludwig, Rudolph Virchow, Ivan Pavlov, Charles Sherrington and Henry Dale. He received several warm letters of congratulation. The one from A V Hill was addressed 'My dear Tom'.[368] Hill was the only person outside his family to use his Christian name. T.R. Elliott wrote, 'My dear T.L. At least you never dreamed of that when you were in Mornington Crescent' – where they had shared rooms.[360] The letter from Edgar D. Adrian read, 'My dear Lewis, You have never chosen to rest on your laurels…it has been a fine example to us all and I think this is the sort of occasion when one can say thank you'.[341] C.S. Sherrington wrote, 'I have so long admired your work and so greatly…I remember with gratitude your great encouragement to me e.g. in the scratch reflex'.[469] Sir Charles Sherrington had received the Nobel Prize for his work on the physiology of the nervous system, and the scratch reflex was a life long interest of his. These letters must have meant a lot to him because he kept them and yet when he wrote to Landis at that time he did not mention the medal, illustrating, as Drury and Grant wrote, that 'he was a humble man without conceit'.[50] His correspondence with Landis, to whom he addressed a question about capillaries, extended into 1942. It included a more optimistic view of the war than he previously had, 'Now that we are no longer standing alone in the big conflict' – a reference to the Soviet Union. With a further comment made after America became an ally, 'We are all very hopeful that you will soon get busy with the Japs'. The soft side to Lewis' nature, not often exposed, is shown in his reply when Landis announced the birth of their daughter Barbara. 'I think Barbara is a very pretty name and for me it has the advantage of no past association having never known a Barbara. I think one always tends to associate a name with people one knows of that name'.[434]

## The 3rd edition of *Diseases of the Heart*, and a fierce argument with F.M.R. Walshe

During this winter he was preparing the third edition of *Diseases of the Heart* which came out in March 1942. The brief preface states that 'all recent and relevant advances in our knowledge, which it is judged will be of value to practitioners, have been incorporated'. As the book reviewer in *Nature* had said in 1938 in regard to the second edition:

> Sir Thomas Lewis has not spoiled his book by yielding to the ordinary temptation to add to it every new theory or observation irrespective of whether they have been fully tested and proved to be of value to the medical man. The bane of most of the modern text-books of medicine is their incomprehensible comprehensiveness. Every rare event…is mentioned…every remedy that has been tried is listed…and all the modern as well as many of the older theories of causation are cited…Lewis has deliberately avoided all these faults.[12]

But Lewis did once deviate from this precept by recommending sulphapyridine in bacterial endocarditis, because although this treatment did offer hope for a lethal illness, it was in fact useless. Other changes from the second edition were slight, but there was a cautious acceptance of left ventricular failure 'The idea has value if recognized as still hypothetical'. However he still emphasized that 'failure of the heart as a whole, is the heart's usual method of failing'.[229]

# Lewis has an argument with Walshe

Lewis clearly took some pride in the fact that the arrangement of the subject matter in his book did not follow the conventional pattern. Instead of starting off with anatomy, physical signs and so on he went straight into an account of cardiac failure. When his colleague F.M.R. Walshe produced his book *Diseases of the Nervous System* Lewis thought that Walshe had attempted to model it on his own book and wrote to complain about the lack of acknowledgment. His letter was the first in a remarkable and acrimonious correspondence between the two of them in June 1942 which also contained a second and more important complaint from Lewis.[436] This concerned a 64 page article which Walshe had published in *Brain* – of which he was the editor – on 'The anatomy and physiology of cutaneous sensibility: a critical review'. In it he criticized the concept of the nocifensor system with its lack of evidence of the appropriate nerves, saying Lewis was 'ready to call into existence, as it were, anatomical structures to meet the apparent requirements of physiological observation'.[324] In his letter Lewis said he regarded the article in *Brain* as an ex cathedra attack on himself which misrepresented his views at a time when he was easily accessible to discuss them, and which upset him because of his friendliness towards Walshe with whom he had been on nothing but good terms for years. 'I am not questioning your right to express your own views; I am bringing certain cold facts to your notice; it is to your manner that I take exception'. Walshe sent a long and well considered reply which started by saying he was distressed by his attitude being taken amiss and having his friendship put into question and ending by saying he did not want to quarrel about the matter, 'Life isn't long enough to fight with persons...' Regarding the book he said that many friends had made valuable suggestions and that he had followed the usual tradition by thanking them in general and not by name in the preface, though he did not specifically reply to the comment on the book's layout. On the nocifensor system he said that a year beforehand he had written out a precis of Lewis' views and had got it approved with trivial amendments by Lewis himself.[475] However this moderately worded reply did not satisfy Lewis. In his second letter he accused Walshe of launching a criticism upon him '*your colleague and friend, without discussion and without disclosing to me your intention*', and accused him of an act of discourtesy.[437] This brought another long reply from Walshe saying that although Lewis had forced a quarrel on him 'paradoxically enough in the name of friendship' he refused to get angry about it. But he was obviously upset by apparently being accused of dishonest conduct and said 'you have no right to use language like this to me even in anger'.[476] Lewis' final letter was a brief one to terminate the exchange, to which Walshe replied, 'For you to close the matter at this stage is not perhaps the dignified thing you imagine'.[477] Not surprisingly this entertaining correspondence closed without agreement, but it has to be said that Walshe's letters contain level headed and apparently convincing refutations of Lewis' complaints. Happily their friendship was later restored, for a year later Walshe asked his opinion on the draft of a paper he had written on reform in medical education to which Lewis replied 'I welcome your admirable article'.[441] Furthermore he supported Walshe's election to the Royal Society and accepted his invitation to join the Research Advisory Committee at the National Hospital for Nervous Diseases.

*Diseases of the Heart* continued to be a very popular text and this third edition sold about 7000 copies, bringing the total sales in Britain to over 17 000. The first two American editions, and there was not a third one, sold just over 15 000. Lewis was a good business man and he negotiated very favourable royalties. For an edition he got 15% on the first 2000 copies, and 20% after that in Britain, though only after 3000 copies in the States. His total royalties up to 1943 were £2,156 in Britain where the book sold for fifteen shillings, and $9,574 in the United States where the price was $ 3.50. These were considerable sums of money at that time.

In November 1942 he wrote a review in *Nature* of James B Herrick's book *A Short History of Cardiology.*[228] Herrick, who was well known for his pioneer descriptions in the United States of coronary thrombosis, responded with an appreciative letter saying:

> It pleases me immensely to note that you have really read the book and not simply copied the blurb and that you have not hesitated to point out sins of omission and commission. It is by all odds the best *real* critique of the book I have seen. I agree with you 100% as to the ugliness of the word 'cardiology'. I wish I had used my first impulse which was to use 'heart disease' instead.[367]

## Cardiac catheterization pioneered in Britain; Lewis hesitant to support it

The remarkably bold and new technique of inserting a catheter into the human heart was invented in 1929 by a young German surgeon, Dr Werner Forsmann, who did the procedures on himself. His objective was to give drugs through the catheter, and to study the heart in some way, but his colleagues prevented him from developing his work. However his method was eagerly adopted at the Bellevue Hospital in New York where Dr André Cournand and Dr Dickinson Richards had been studying cardiopulmonary function since 1932.[39] By sampling mixed venous blood from the right atrium it was now possible in the human subject to use the Fick principle to measure the cardiac output, and this unique opportunity was soon appreciated by Dr John McMichael at Hammersmith Hospital.(278) He had been using the difficult acetylene method for some years and was now, with Dr E.P. Sharpey-Schafer,[(3)] using it to study cardiac output after blood loss following venesection. Their first right heart catheterization was done in the autumn of 1942 and a year later they reported three studies using this method at a meeting of the Physiological Society held at UCH on November 27 1943. Two of their papers showed the alteration of cardiac output with changes in posture and venous pressure, and with atropine and adrenaline. The third was on the fainting reaction after haemorrhage, a one litre venesection in a volunteer, when it was shown for the first time that the fall in blood pressure was due to vasodilatation in muscle. The response to their papers was later recounted by McMichael

> Sir Thomas Lewis was in the chair. He described our opening paper as 'startling' and at the lunch table he shook his head hinting that we should abandon the procedure. Sir Henry Dale, also at the table, however, took a different view and said that the total record of experience which we had assembled[394] cases seemed to establish the practicability and safety of the technique and that it was too valuable to be dropped. His powerful and influential support was indeed a great encouragement.[275]

McMichael was very disappointed with Lewis' attitude at that meeting and it is fair to say that he never really forgave Lewis for it. However it is now quite clear from Lewis' correspondence that this was far from being the first time that he had known about the work at Hammersmith Hospital. He had already known about it for several months because Sharpey-Schafer, who had been his house physician and for whom he had a high regard, had written to him about the findings. Of the letters which have been kept the first is dated March 31 1943, and in it Sharpey-Schafer thanks Lewis for a previous letter which gave him advice about the results in cases of anaemia, and goes on to say:

> I hope you are not right about the catheter. It has of course been used by others many thousand times without so far as I know anything happening. Our experience (about 30 cases) does not indicate risks greater than any intravenous injection – indeed perhaps less than some, at least it doesn't give you catarrhal jaundice![467]

That last comment referred to hepatitis being transmitted by syringes contaminated with blood. What Lewis said about the catheter is unknown but from the context it is obvious that he was unhappy about the technique. Whenever Lewis did an investigation on a patient he always without exception had it done on himself first. He may have known that the Hammersmith team had not had it done on themselves. Incidentally Sharpey-Schafer should have written 'a few hundred', not 'many thousand'. The 394 cases referred to by McMichael was the world total at that time. But the correspondence continued and one just wonders whether McMichael knew anything about it. Sharpey-Schafer wrote a long letter about the effects of venesection in November prior to the UCH meeting, which seems to indicate that Lewis had a continuing interest in the studies.[440,468] The last one which has been preserved is from Lewis on August 3 1944. In it he says that the results with digoxin are 'certainly very interesting' and there is no hint in this letter that he disapproves of the continuing use of cardiac catheterization.[444] It was in fact to the contrary, because he was clearly displeased that a paper on the cardiac output with digoxin in man had been sent to the *Quarterly Journal of Medicine*:[279]

> I am very insistent that all your best work in Clinical Science should be published in the journal of that name. It is the journal of our Society, the full-time workers, and it should be fully supported. The Q.J.M. should not be for us. The new movement depends for its success on our holding together. I do not think that Fraser has a proper appreciation of this.[444]

McMichael had experienced an earlier set back with Lewis when he was working in Edinburgh on the cardiac output using the acetylene method. He submitted a paper about it, which was rejected with the comment from Lewis that the readers of *Clinical Science* were not interested in the cardiac output.[456] McMichael used to quote this episode against Lewis but the paper, which got published elsewhere, was a long and technical account out of keeping with the journal, and Lewis' reply should have been better worded to that effect.[274] However McMichael was fascinated by the development of cardiology in the 20th century and gave the Harveian Oration of 1975 to the Royal College of Physicians of London on 'A transition in cardiology: the Mackenzie Lewis era'.[276]

## The controversy about the place of digitalis in heart failure

This is an appropriate place to discuss Lewis' views on the use of digitalis in the treatment of heart failure. He had always maintained that digitalis was usually of significant benefit only when there was atrial fibrillation, but others disagreed with him and a short review of the subject may be useful. The fine investigative work of James Mackenzie had shown that digitalis was of especial benefit in heart failure in that group of patients who had complete irregularity of the pulse, and this led to the identification of that arrhythmia, which was shown to be atrial (auricular) fibrillation when electrocardiography became available. In his textbook *Diseases of the Heart* Mackenzie said that all his patients with extreme heart failure who had obtained great benefit from digitalis had auricular fibrillation. He added, 'In searching the records in literature for the evidence of the good effects of digitalis, I feel fairly certain that it is in patients with auricular fibrillation...that the extraordinarily good results have been obtained'.[266] Lewis held Mackenzie, who was then a much more experienced clinician, in high esteem and it may have been his influence that led Lewis to write, in 1919, 'The principle of digitalis therapy is that, administered to suitable cases, the heart, by means of it, obtains rest. Those who regard digitalis as a cardiac stimulant mistake its character; its chief action is to rest the heart. To the heart foxglove is not tonic, but powerfully hypnotic'.[151] However Mackenzie did use digitalis also in heart failure with normal rhythm as is shown by his comment in 1911 when he wrote, 'Cases of auricular fibrillation are more readily and more markedly affected than cases with normal rhythm'.[268] By 1925, in the 4th edition of his book, he went further and wrote, 'Without knowing why or wherefore, drugs of the digitalis group have occasionally a good effect, so these should be tried in every case'.[270] Looking ahead a few years to 1933, when Lewis was a mature clinician, we find a slight change of emphasis in the first edition of his *Diseases of the Heart*, 'Occasionally, however, cases of congestion that present regular heart action, and that have been treated with the usual measures without success, seem to respond to full doses of digitalis. The remedy usually comes to be tried when others have failed'. But dissent from Lewis' statement of 1919 had already come in that same year from the United States when Henry A Christian wrote a paper entitled, 'Digitalis effects in chronic cardiac cases with regular rhythm in contrast to auricular fibrillation'.[32] This theme was taken up by other American authors.[408] In 1927 H.M. Marvin, who was a good clinical investigator, showed the benefit of digitalis in heart failure with regular rhythm.[273] Paul White, of Boston, in his important textbook *Heart Disease* wrote in 1931, 'Digitalis is often, though as a rule far less dramatically, effective when there is heart failure with normal rhythm. To be sure, digitalis therapy in the presence of normal cardiac rhythm is not always effective and its success averages far below that when auricular fibrillation is present; nevertheless it is often strikingly beneficial and sometimes it is life saving'.[332] These two authors had both been pupils of Lewis. Then British investigators turned their attention to the subject. Clarence J. Gavey and John Parkinson studied the effect of digitalis over a two week period and found moderate or great benefit in 31% with normal rhythm, and in 44% with atrial fibrillation.[66] A year later in 1940 Paul Wood found, as judged by the circulation time, that digitalis improved left ventricular failure in three out of five cases, and right ventricular failure, as judged by fall in venous pressure, in 18 out of 20 cases. His study period averaged one week. Wood denied the previous authors' claim that benefit was more likely with rheumatic heart disease, because most of his patients had hypertension.[336] Then came the cardiac catheterization work, already referred to, by McMichael and Sharpey-Schafer. One of their studies concerned the effect of intravenous digoxin in right heart failure with regular rhythm.[279] They showed that digoxin lowered the right atrial pressure and increased the cardiac output. Prior to publication Sharpey-Schafer wrote to his former chief about this work. In his reply on August 3 1944 Lewis said:

> Personally I am unable to convince myself that very many cases of failure with normal rhythm are benefited by digitalis. I cannot agree that Parkinson has shown this. It fails nearly always when I try it. It is a question of the reaction over days, not hours. You should beware the conclusion that with increasing cardiac output there *must* be improvement.[444]

This last comment was a shrewd one because since then it has become common to make the error of extrapolating from the acute to the chronic situation. In fact of all the studies referred to above, none were long term, though Gavey and Parkinson did mention that it was in those patients with atrial fibrillation that digitalis best prevented recurrence of the failure. In view of his long continued interest in this controversy it is odd that Lewis did not mount his own controlled clinical study. The study of digoxin in his department by E.J. Wayne in 1933 was concerned only with rate control in atrial fibrillation.[326] However as his letter to Sharpey-Schafer indicates he did make observations on individual patients and these were recalled by D.A. Williams at Llandough Hospital:

> Sir Thomas was especially interested in the effect of digitalis on cardiac failure with regular rhythm. He watched every case very carefully and made certain the patient had the correct dose by watching him take it. He told me, laughingly, that he did not get the luck in such cases that some of his colleagues were claiming.[536]

Lewis' last comment on the subject came in the 4th edition of *Diseases of the Heart* published in 1946. Writing about the treatment of heart failure he says:

> The most emphatic action of digitalis and its allies is in the case of auricular fibrillation. Clear evidence that digitalis is useful in failure with congestion presenting normal rhythm has been slower in coming, because success in such cases is less obvious and less frequent. Nevertheless it is now generally recognized that digitalis is valuable in these cases and sometimes succeeds in lowering venous pressure and in bringing relief where other remedies have failed.[237]

One wonders why he decided, towards the end of his career, to give more emphasis than he previously had done to the benefit with regular rhythm. It has been suggested that a personal experience was responsible for the change. In his final illness he developed left ventricular failure, with sinus rhythm, and there is good evidence that he improved when Sir John Parkinson treated him with digitalis.[363]

But even now, in 1996, the discussion continues. Regarding the point about acute versus chronic improvement, a leading British textbook states, 'The place of digoxin in the management of chronic heart failure is a matter for debate', and says that many clinicians are convinced of its short and medium term effects in the specific situation of a dilated, poorly contracting ventricle in patients with sinus rhythm.[47] An American text states that digitalis can give sustained improvement in chronic congestive heart failure with sinus rhythm and that it is of potential value in many such patients. However it adds that 'the clinical response is critically dependent on patient selection' and says that those with impaired systolic function respond well whilst those with reduced ventricular compliance and preserved systolic function are not helped.[314] In general digitalis therapy with regular rhythm is accepted more in North America than in Great Britain, but even in the United States a leading authority on heart failure, writing in 1995, does not use it in failure with normal rhythm.[329] So it looks as if Lewis was correct to be cautious about recommending its use in normal rhythm.

As a final point it was worth mentioning that even in 1946 Lewis was still usually prescribing digitalis as the tincture, that is to say an alcoholic extract of the leaf. This was in spite of the fact that the more convenient tablets of the dried leaf had been in use for some decades. For example White wrote in 1931 that he had used the tablets for years, and knew them to be effective.[332] No doubt Lewis would have said that the tincture was a method he had learnt to rely on, but it does seem to provide evidence that he had a natural reluctance to change his mind on an established position, well shown with the subject of bundle branch block, and with his late acceptance of metal skin electrodes for electrocardiography. However he states that business men find it convenient to carry tablets of digoxin, and he gives conversion rates of tincture to tablets of the leaf. But he was not the only one to be slow in changing. Ten years later in 1956 one of the world's leading cardiologists, Dr Paul Wood, writing in his book *Diseases of the Heart and Circulation*, was still recommending the dried leaf, which had to be biologically standardized, rather than the pure glycoside digoxin, which soon completely replaced it. Wood, like Lewis, had grown accustomed to using a particular preparation.

## Continued interest in arrhythmias

By the summer of 1943 the lack of air raids made it possible for UCH to function more or less normally again in London and in October a new intake of clinical students entered the medical school having done their preclinical work at Leatherhead in Surrey. Lewis again had his own firm of students and was fully engaged in clinical work and teaching but his department had only himself and Honour in it and little research work was done. (Fig. 17.5) However it did offer the opportunity to make a careful examination of the heart of a man with the Wolff–Parkinson–White syndrome who had been a patient at Stanborough's. Lewis had become interested in the syndrome, which was the only important arrhythmia he had left undescribed in 1925, and had tried without success to change the ECG pattern with atropine. Honour cut hundreds of sections but the accessory pathway was not found. Certainly his interest in arrhythmias had not diminished and another patient caused him to write to Paul White asking him if he had come across any patients with almost continuous paroxysms of tachycardia 'breaking back to normal for one to two beats and restarting again at once. I had one case years ago and another one now'. He sent the ECG's and suggested a joint paper, but nothing came of it.[438] In another instance his help was sought by a chest surgeon, Mr Gordon Hesling, who was able with Lewis' assistance to devise

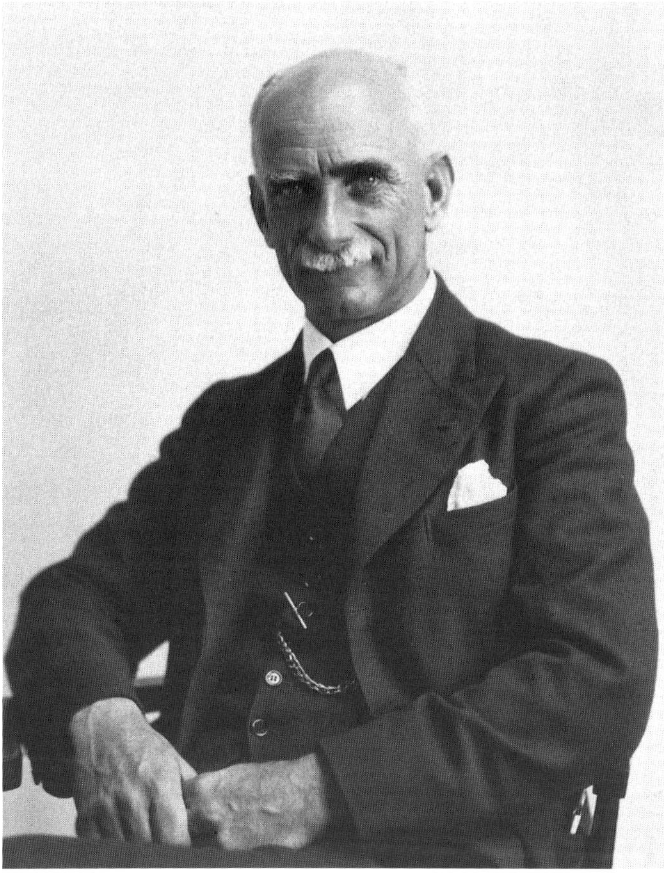

*Figure 17.5 A photograph of Lewis in 1943.*

a rhythmic stimulator to get a stopped heart going again at a thoracic operation.[439]

## New ideas on medical education

Inactivity was never a feature of Lewis' life and he now directed his efforts towards medical education by submitting a memorandum to the Inter-Departmental Committee on Medical Schools chaired by Sir William Goodenough. In it he emphasized the extent of ignorance about the true nature of disease, with the achievement of a diagnostic label being often regarded as more important than an understanding of the disease process. Whilst it was necessary, he said, for the student to have a sound factual knowledge of diseases it was more important, indeed fundamental, for him to acquire sound habits of learning. These would give him independence of thought and judgement and a fondness for understanding which 'is the basis of progress and the vital flame in education'.[233] To achieve reform along these lines Lewis proposed that teaching should be of two types, vocational and theoretical. Vocational teaching would be done by the visiting consultant staff and it needed to be more organized with less factual information, because it 'seems chiefly intent on imposing a colossal burden on memory'. Theoretical teaching would be in the hands of the full time professorial staff whose particular task would be 'to simplify and bring order to the mass of knowledge by establishing general rules and principles'. But he regarded these two systems as complementary and emphasized '*that while all may enjoy the twofold opportunity different minds may make different and appropriate choices*'. Theoretical education, he hoped, would create a strong body of leaders of the profession who were trained to discriminate in what they taught and advised. But the teaching done at present by the professorial units was in his view unsatisfactory and he recommended six ways to improve this. In particular he believed that professors had far too many patients to look after and too much administrative work. Lewis believed that the British full time system had not been a great success, due chiefly to the fact that the universities expected the whole time professorate to be engaged first of all in teaching the practice of medicine. He felt very strongly that this approach was wrong, and that the emphasis should be on the study of disease in man.

## Teaching clinical physiology to medical students

His memorandum was called 'Reflections upon reform in medical education' and it was published in *The Lancet* in January 1944.[233] It was followed by a book, (Fig. 17.6) the last new one he wrote, entitled *Exercises in Human Physiology (preparatory to clinical work)*.[235] The stimulus for this book came from his long held conviction that the most difficult period of a medical students life was the change from preclinical to clinical work. The change was 'from the deliberate and scientific ways of academic study to those of hospital life...where opportunism reigns with the voice of authority (and) where memory is more extolled than reason'.[236] He had spoken on this problem in 1920 during his address at the British Association on the relation of physiology to medicine when he advocated that physiological teaching should be centred on human rather than on animal physiology.[153] This book was his contribution to that aim and it contained a long series of observations and experiments to be done by the students on themselves in the physiology class room, and was based largely on his own work.

He could not satisfactorily cover the whole field but even so the range was considerable and a few examples can be given. There were exercises on the skin noting capillary pulsation, the triple response, vasodilatation with cold, erythralgia and reactive hyperaemia. Cutaneous sensation was examined and the differences shown between superficial and deep pain. There were clear instructions as to how the students could give saline injections into muscle and interspinous ligaments to study referred pain and there were several pharmacological experiments with pilocarpine, atropine and other drugs. The venous and arterial pulses could be recorded with the polygraph, and electrocardiograms could be taken too. It was intended that the teachers should select those exercises which were the most appropriate for themselves to use and supervise, and probably some of the invasive ones would have been little used. The book was a good and certainly

EXERCISES IN
HUMAN PHYSIOLOGY
(PREPARATORY TO CLINICAL WORK)

BY

SIR THOMAS LEWIS
C.B.E., F.R.S., M.D., D.S.C., LL.D., F.R.C.P.
PHYSICIAN IN CHARGE OF DEPARTMENT OF CLINICAL RESEARCH, UNIVERSITY COLLEGE HOSPITAL, LONDON; HONORARY CONSULTING PHYSICIAN TO THE MINISTRY OF PENSIONS; CONSULTING PHYSICIAN, CITY OF LONDON HOSPITAL; FELLOW OF UNIVERSITY COLLEGE, LONDON

MACMILLAN AND CO., LIMITED
ST. MARTIN'S STREET, LONDON
1945

*Figure 17.6 An imaginative book for teaching pre-clinical students. (From reference 235.)*

unusual contribution to a difficult feature in education and it was typical of Lewis to produce a practical solution rather than just write about the problem. 'It has weighed upon my mind' he wrote 'that I may not remain in the position of giving lip service to an idea, and not attempt to contribute something substantial to its working.'

## Resigns as editor of *Clinical Science*

In the summer of 1944 Lewis resigned as editor of *Clinical Science* and was succeeded at his request by George Pickering. He had now been the editor, continuously for 35 years, of *Heart* and then of *Clinical Science* . He explained his decision in a letter to T.R. Elliott, on July 20 1944:

> You may have heard that I have given up the editorship of *Clinical Science*. The editing is getting a bit beyond me, owing to its present scope it has become very dull and hard work. After several struggles with contributors I took the decision, the last straw being the long paper of your successor. You will like to hear that I remain on cordial terms with him and he has since told me (too late) that I was right, with his very unusual and generous frankness.[443]

The person he referred to was Professor H.P. Himsworth, who had succeeded Elliott as director of the Medical Unit. In his reply Elliott said:

> You have carried the journal for a period as long as that of Langley with the J of Physiology, and with the same high ideals of editorship: and now you may watch what the next generation do with the inheritance.[361]

In fact Professor John Newport Langley edited the *Journal of Physiology* for 31 years, four years less than Lewis, and for nearly half of that time he was a co-editor. As fate would have it, Lewis now had only eight months to live and one wonders whether his resignation may not have been an early sign of his impending fatal illness which started just a few months later.

In the spring of 1944 an Allied invasion of Europe seemed to be close and there was a need to prepare for the treatment of battle casualties in British hospitals. The MRC, in association with the Emergency Medical Service, set up a subcommittee on Vascular Injuries with Lewis as its chairman, and MRC War Memorandum No. 13 on 'Arterial injuries: early diagnosis and treatment 'was soon in print. The invasion took place on June 6 and a few days later London was attacked with the pilotless 'flying bomb' which was to kill 6000 civilians in the next eight months. But the hospital and the medical school did not move again, and luckily they were not hit.

## More honours for his work

Lewis' fine achievements continued to receive recognition. In 1943 he was made an Honorary Fellow of the Royal Society of Medicine. In April 1944 the newly founded Institute of Cardiology in Mexico was opened and the entrance hall had two large murals, each of 24 square metres, by the well known painter Diego Rivera with portraits of the most illustrious men in the history of the heart and circulation. Lewis was one of them (Fig. 17.7) and Professor Ignacio Chavez sent him the commemorative medal, together with a book containing detailed colour reproductions of the paintings.[350] In 1945 Lewis was awarded the Conway–Evans Prize. This prize, which was founded in 1925, is jointly in the gift of the presidents of the Royal Society of London and the Royal College of Physicians of London, and is awarded only when an occasion arises to honour a person who has made a valuable contribution to science, especially medical science. On this occasion it consisted of the very large sum of five hundred guineas. The only three previous recipients had been C.S. Sherrington in 1927, J.S. Haldane in 1933 and Gowland Hopkins in 1938. In late 1944, a few months prior to the actual award in 1945, the two presidents sent warmly worded letters to Lewis. Lord Moran wrote to say, 'I have long wanted, in the name of the College, to pay some small tribute to your work. The Conway–Evans Prize at last gives me this opportunity'.[459] Sir Henry Dale of the Royal Society said, 'I regard it as putting you and your work in a succession of which any man might be proud, I think, to join. I am confident that the whole world of medicine and medical research will applaud and rejoice'.[355] In his reply on November 29 to Dale's letter Lewis said:

> I need hardly tell you that I am proud to the point of embarrassment to be placed in line with Sherrington, Hopkins, and Haldane, whose works had set them on

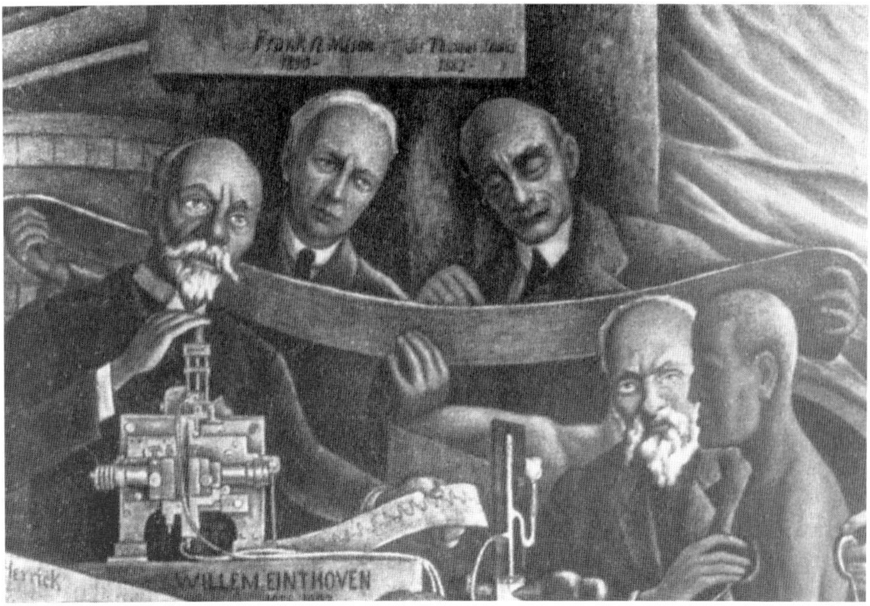


*Figure 17.7 A portion of the mural in the Institute of Cardiology Mexico, showing a group of famous electrocardiographers, left to right, W. Einthoven, F.N. Wilson, T. Lewis and A.D. Waller.*

> pinnacles even in the days when I was a student. There come occasions when it is impossible not to look back and pass in review the results of what cannot be too far from a full life's work; and when one is apt to see, as the worker himself can see, and perhaps to dwell on unduly, the deficiencies. At such times the considered and favourable judgment of one's contemporaries upon whom one has to come to rely, as in your case in unusual measure, is a source not only of comfort but of deep satisfaction. I have valued the friendship and advice you have given me so freely and for many years. They have been and remain among my most valued possessions.[442]

This letter amply confirms the judgement of Drury and Grant[50] that although, as they said, he was suspected of vanity and self seeking, 'He was a humble man, without conceit, courageous and entirely honest; he was loyal to his colleagues'.

## His final illness begins

In the late autumn of 1944 Lewis began to experience attacks of cardiac asthma and was admitted to the Private Patients Wing of UCH with George Pickering as his physician. John Honour remembers taking his electrocardiogram and trying to dissuade him from his request to see it after it had been developed. But he did inspect it, saying nothing, and characteristically pulling thoughtfully on his moustache. (Fig. 17.8, *overleaf*) It is appropriate to recount the words, written at this time in his letter to Sir Henry Dale, 'the results of what cannot be too far from a full life's work'. Pickering suggested that Dr (later Sir John) Parkinson

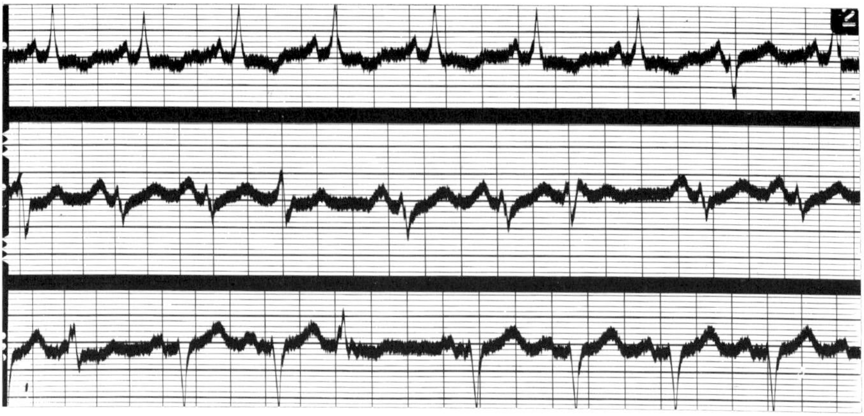

*Figure 17.8 Lewis' electrocardiogram (standard leads) taken ten weeks before his death. Like the one taken nine years previously (Figure 13.9) it shows little evidence of myocardial infarction.*

should be consulted but Lewis would not hear of it saying one could predict his advice – several weeks in bed – so why waste his time. But later on Parkinson did see him and beneficially treated the heart failure with digitalis, even though there was sinus rhythm. So, as a patient, Lewis experienced at first hand that two of his beliefs were at any rate sometimes wrong. Lone left ventricular failure did exist, and digitalis could work with regular rhythm. A pulmonary embolus early in January 1945 prolonged his illness. Pickering said, 'The meaning of these changes was as clear to him as was his conclusion that a life of inactivity and invalidism was unacceptable. Very soon he was out of doors and striving for recovery'.[299]

## New editions of his books

It is likely that Lewis had employed himself with literary work during this long illness because two new editions of his books were published after his death. One of them entitled *Electrocardiography and clinical disorders of the heart beat* (Fig. 17.9) was really a new book because it was a fusion, with revision, of his two small teaching books *Clinical electrocardiography* and *Clinical disorders of the heart beat*. Both of them had first been written over 30 years previously and had gone through six and seven editions respectively, indicating their popularity with students and doctors. He pointed out in the preface that the greatly increased use of the electrocardiogram was a good reason to combine them. Chest leads were included for the first time though they were mentioned and illustrated, with lead CR4, only with cardiac infarction. The publisher's note from Shaw and Sons Ltd, who had published his first book 34 years previously, contains a nice appreciation which reads 'As in his earlier works Sir Thomas prepared the manuscript of this book with great care and precision. Few authors have paid so much attention to the use of words and the construction of sentences'. This was high praise from a firm whose main activity was with legal publishing. The other new edition was the fourth edition of *Diseases of the Heart*, published in 1946 and reprinted two years

ELECTROCARDIOGRAPHY
AND
CLINICAL DISORDERS
OF THE
HEART BEAT

A HANDBOOK FOR
PRACTITIONERS AND STUDENTS

By the Late SIR THOMAS LEWIS
C.B.E., F.R.S., M.D., D.Sc., LL.D., F.R.C.P.
PHYSICIAN IN CHARGE OF DEPARTMENT OF CLINICAL RESEARCH, UNIVERSITY COLLEGE HOSPITAL; HONORARY CONSULTING PHYSICIAN TO THE MINISTRY OF PENSIONS; CONSULTING PHYSICIAN, CITY OF LONDON HOSPITAL; LATELY PHYSICIAN OF THE STAFF OF THE MEDICAL RESEARCH COUNCIL; FELLOW OF UNIVERSITY COLLEGE, LONDON

Publishers:
SHAW & SONS LTD., 7, 8 & 9, FETTER LANE,
FLEET STREET, LONDON, E.C.4, ENGLAND
1949

*Figure 17.9 A new book which fused his previous two teaching books. Published four years after his death.*

later.[237] The main revision in it concerned the classification of heart failure. Lewis had been reluctant to accept that the right or left ventricle might fail alone, and in the 1933 edition this idea was not even mentioned. By 1942, in the third edition, he agreed that the idea had value, but only if it was recognized to be still hypothetical, and he emphasized that failure of the heart as a whole was the heart's usual manner of failing. The chapter headings now were of bilateral failure, predominance of left failure, and predominance of right failure. He also mentioned pure right-sided failure, and his description of one case shows that he knew about the condition which is now called primary pulmonary hypertension.

## Death in March 1945

After leaving hospital he convalesced at home where Honour visited him and was shocked to see how, quite suddenly, he had become old and drawn. Chris recollects that he was, 'really a cardiac cripple, wasted and enfeebled and latterly rarely going far from the house and if it was warm enough sitting on the verandah and enjoying the beauty of their garden paradise from afar'.[262] But in the early hours of Saturday March 17 1945 he had a third attack of myocardial infarction and died at home a few hours later at the age of 63. After the second attack in 1935 he

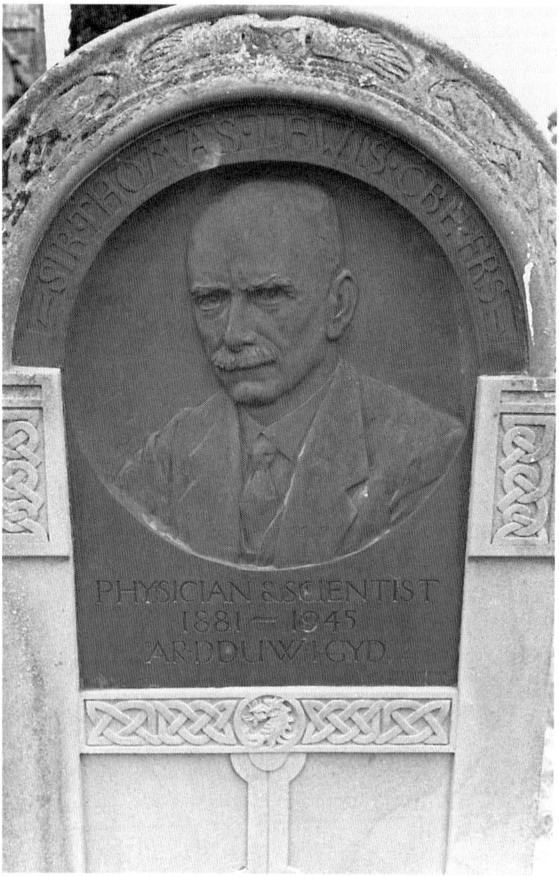
SIR THOMAS LEWIS CBE FRS
PHYSICIAN & SCIENTIST
1881 — 1945
AR DDUW I GYD

*Figure 17.10 The fine headstone to his grave in Llangasty churchyard, Brecon, Wales.*

had said to Henry Dale, 'Another arrow from the same quiver my friend, but there are plenty more to come and one of them will get me in the end'.[46]

There was a Memorial Service in St Pancras Church at which Sir Henry Dale, his friend for forty years, gave a fine and touching address before a packed congregation. At his wish he was buried in Llangasty churchyard which overlooks Llangorse Lake in Breconshire. This is a beautiful part of Wales which from boyhood had been one of his favourite places to fish and study nature. The burial service was a simple one and the only mourners present, apart from the members of his family were Mr Law, Lord Buckland's ghillie, and Mr Davies the boatman on Llangorse Lake, both of them old friends and mutually respected. The headstone of the grave is fine. (Fig. 17.10) Set into it there is a large circular bronze plaque of his head, taken from a photograph, which is surrounded by a carving in stone of birds and animals. The plain inscription records his name and dates together with the family motto Ar Dduw I Gyd, which is best translated as 'All to God'. (Fig. 17.11)

After Lewis' death Dr Samuel Levine of Boston wished to commemorate his teacher and friend, who had given him so much inspiration.[17] He did this by

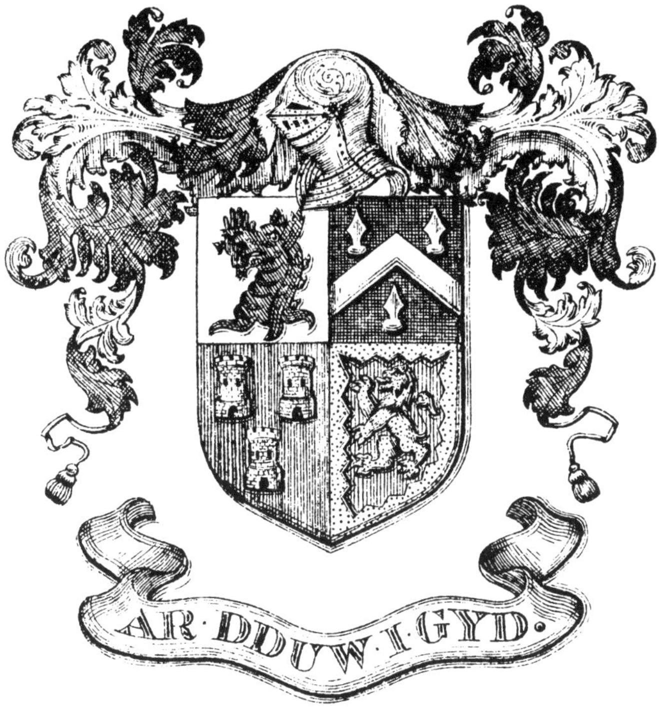


*Figure 17.11 Lewis' bookplate with his family's motto.*

endowing the Thomas Lewis Lecture of the British Cardiac Society. The first lecture was given in 1963 by Sir George Pickering and it has been given bienially ever since. The centenary of Lewis' birth, in 1981, was marked by the issue of a postage stamp. (Fig. 17.12) An attempt to get this done in Britain failed but fortunately the distinguished Prime Minister of Mauritius, Dr Sir Seewoosagur

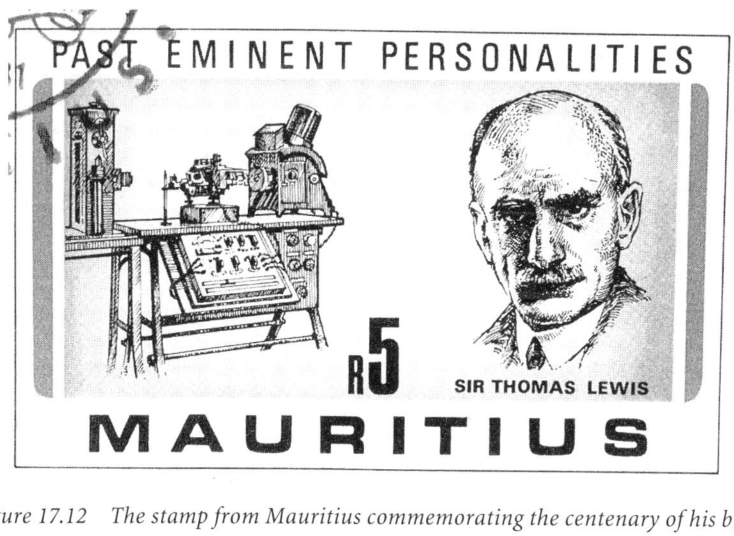


*Figure 17.12 The stamp from Mauritius commemorating the centenary of his birth.*

Ramgoolam, had been a pupil of Lewis at UCH in 1935. He was delighted to be approached with the idea and he instructed the Mauritius Post Office to create a Thomas Lewis stamp as part of their series on Former Distinguished Persons then under preparation. The others in the series are all Mauritians. This elegant 10 rupee stamp shows a portrait of Lewis and his first Cambridge electrocardiograph. Of all the physicians and surgeons who have contributed to the study and practice of heart disease in the last 400 years only 16 have had a stamp issued for them.

## Notes to Chapter 17

(1) Paul Hamilton Wood, 1907–1962, was an Australian born physician, working in London, who became one of the most famous cardiologists in the world. Before the second war he was on the staff at the British Postgraduate Medical School at Hammersmith Hospital and after it he was a consultant at the Brompton Hospital and the National Heart Hospital. He was the first director of the Institute of Cardiology. Among his many gifts was an outstanding ability to elicit and interpret physical signs in the heart . He had a deep understanding of mitral stenosis and of congenital heart disease. Wood had a brilliant mind and in 1950 his textbook *Diseases of the Heart and Circulation* inaugurated a new era in cardiology.

(2) John Rupert Squire, 1915–1966, had an outstanding career in experimental pathology, in which he held a chair at the University of Birmingham. His ability was recognized by Lewis when he was still a student and he became Lewis' house physician and last research associate. His fine academic work and great talent for organisation made him the obvious choice as director designate of the new Clinical Research Centre at Northwick Park. He had done much of the planning for the Centre before his untimely death from coronary heart disease at the age of 51.

(3) Edward Peter Sharpey-Schafer, 1908–1963, had an important career in clinical research. He was a lecturer at the British Postgraduate Medical School from 1935 to 1952 where he collaborated with John McMichael in a pioneer study of cardiac catheterisation. He then became Professor of Medicine at St Thomas' Hospital London where his further work was on the peripheral circulation.

# Appendices

## Appendix 1: Sources of material

A. The Contemporary Medical Archives Centre at The Wellcome Institute for the History of Medicine, London.

a) The Centre has a collection of over one thousand papers relating to Lewis which are designated PP/LEW. There is a 42-page catalogue giving details of the classification and contents of this collection.

b) Sound Archive Collection. The Centre also holds tape recordings of 24 oral history interviews which Dr A Hollman conducted between 1974 and 1990 with a grant from the Wellcome Trust. These interviews are largely with former colleagues and pupils of Lewis, and with Lady Lewis. They constitute an invaluable source of first hand information about Lewis and the medical scene at his time, with personal recollections going back as far as 1920. They are designated as 'Audiotapes' in the list of references. The following persons were interviewed and the years to which their recollections refer are given in brackets.

Mr Edward Bridger (1926–1933), Mr Reginald Channel (1932), Sir Alan Drury (1920–1925), Dr William Evans (1935), Dr R Gilchrist (1934–1939), Dr LE Glynn (1940–1945), Dr RT Grant (1920–1935), Sir Harold Himsworth (1933–1945), Dr AJ Honour (1927–1945), Mr Stephen Hortin (1927), Lady Lewis (1914–1945), Sir John McMichael (1934-1943), Dr Arthur Morriss (1914), Sir John Nabarro (1939–1941), Professor EB Perry (1933), Lady Pickering (1929–1945), Sir Edward Pochin (1932–1940), Sir Seewoosagur Ramgoolam (1934–1936), Dr Harold Segall (1924), Dr E Joan Stokes (1937–1945), Dr Hugh Sinclair (1934–1944), Dame Janet Vaughan (1927–1929), Sir Edward Wayne (1932–1934), Dame Albertine Winner (1933–1941).

(c) The Centre has 84 bound volumes entitled 'Cardiovascular Reprints' which are original articles by other workers which Lewis collected for the use of himself and his department.

B. The Medical Research Council, London, has a large archive collection. It contains letters and documents which I have examined in the following files.

a) Personal file of Sir Thomas Lewis, PF136.
b) Cardiographic Department and Department of Clinical Research. 2011.
c) Clinical Research Policy 1929–1932. 1617.
d) Personal file of Sir Walter Morley Fletcher, secretary of the MRC. PF139.

C. Dr A Hollman holds a small collection of letters and papers which he will eventually donate to the Royal College of Physicians of London.

D. The National Institute of Medical Research, London, holds 75 boxes containing notes made by Lewis. They contain clinical and experimental data recorded by Lewis on a day-to-day basis. The collection was annotated in 1980 by Dr Joel Howell and his notes are in the Wellcome CMAC PP/LEW catalogue.

E. Informal oral interviews and correspondence, other than those noted in the list of references. Those of especial value have been with Lady Lewis, with her and Sir Thomas' three children, and with Dr AJ Honour who was Lewis' personal laboratory assistant.

# Appendix 2: The Honours and Degrees of Sir Thomas Lewis

Bachelor of Science with first class honours 1902, Doctor of Science 1904, (Wales); University of Cambridge, ex collegio de Cardiff.

University of London, as an external student: Matriculation 1898; 1st part of MB BS 1899; 2nd part of MB BS 1902, with first class and certificate of honour in anatomy, and first class and gold medal in physiology and histology. Bachelor of medicine and surgery (MB BS) with honours and University Medal July 1905. Doctor of medicine (MD) July 1907.

Royal College of Surgeons of England: primary Fellowship 1902, Member 1904.

Royal College of Physicians of London: Licentiate 1904, Member 1907, Fellow (FRCP) 1913.

The Royal Society of London: Croonian Lecturer 1917; Fellow 1918; Royal Medal 1927; Copley Medal 1941; Conway Evans Prize 1945 (jointly with the RCP London).

University College London: Tuke silver medal in pathology 1903, Fellowes silver medal in medicine 1904, silver medal in surgery 1904, Fellow of UCL 1907.

1914 Honorary member Harvey Society of New York; physician in chief pro tempore Peter Bent Brigham Hospital Boston: 1918 Fellow of the Royal Society of London: 1920 Commander of the British Empire (CBE): 1921 Knight Bachelor: 1922 Honorary Doctor of Science (D Sc) Michigan: 1924 Corresponding member of the Society of Internal Medicine of Vienna; honorary fellow Royal Academy of Medicine of Rome: 1926 Honorary member Society of Czech Physicians: 1927 Corresponding member Association of American Physicians; corresponding member Interstate Postgraduate Medical Association of North America; corresponding member Czech Medical Society, Prague: 1928 Honorary DSc Sheffield; honorary Doctor of Law (LL.D) Wales: 1929 Fothergillian Medal of Medical Society of London: 1930 Honorary fellow of New York Academy of Medicine; honorary LL.D Birmingham; corresponding member of Royal Medical Society of Budapest; foreign corresponding member of Royal Academy of Medicine Brussels: 1931 Foreign member of Royal Academy of Belgium; honorary FRCP Edinburgh: 1932 Honorary member of British Society of Dermatology: 1933 Charles Mickle Fellowship University of Toronto; member of Royal Society of Science Uppsala: 1935 Honorary DSc Liverpool; corresponding member

Lombardy Society of Medicine: 1937 Honorary member of Czech Cardiological Society; honorary foreign member of Society of Cardiology of Argentina: 1938 Corresponding member of the French Society of Cardiology; honorary Fellow of the Royal Society of Edinburgh: 1939 Foreign member of the Medical Society of Norway: 1941 Foreign member of Swedish Academy of Science; honorary Fellow of the Royal Society of Medicine.

# Appendix 3: The scientific papers and books of Sir Thomas Lewis

There is a nearly complete list of all Lewis' literary work in the Obituary Notice written in 1945 by Sir Alan Drury and Dr Ronald T Grant (Obituary Notices of Fellows of the Royal Society of London 5: 179–202) and this will not be reproduced here. A few items were missed out of their list and they are appended below.

Lewis ALT, Lewis T (1920) The starling in the woodpeckers nest. Country Life 47: 582–584

Lewis T (1909) Auricular fibrillation. Lancet II: 1820

Lewis T (1912) Meeting of the clinical section of the Royal Society of Medicine, March 20 1912. Proc R Soc Med 4: 183–192

Lewis T (1913) A lecture on the evidences of auricular fibrillation treated historically. BMJ I: 57–60

Lewis T (1914) Walter Holbrook Gaskell BMJ II: 559–560

Lewis T (1914) Research in medicine; its position and needs. The Morning Post April 25. A letter signed Junior.

1917. Lewis T (1917) Croonian Lecture. Upon the motion of the mammalian heart. Proc R Soc Lond B 89: 560–573

1919. Lewis T (1919) The Dogs' Bill. Our dependence on experiment. The Times April 9

1922. Lewis T (1922) Augustus D Waller BMJ I: 459

1925. Lewis T (1925) Sir James Mackenzie. BMJ I: 243

1934 Lewis T (1934) T Swale Vincent. BMJ I: 83–84

1937 Lewis T (1937) 'Relapse' following sympathectomy. Lancet II: 938

1937 Lewis T (1938) The nocifensor system of nerves and its reactions. BMJ I: 431–435 and 491–494

Lewis T (1938) The pathological changes in the arteries supplying the fingers in warm-handed people and in cases of so-called Raynaud's disease. Clin Sci 3: 287–320

Lewis T (1938) Raynaud's disease and preganglionic sympathectomy. Clin Sci 3: 321–336

Lewis T (1939) Professor Thomas Renton Elliott. Univ Coll Hosp Mag Lond 24: 83–86

Lewis T (1939) Editorial preface. Br Heart J 1: 1–2

Lewis T (1940) Visceral pain. Lancet II: 503

Lewis T (1940) The Tourniquet. BMJ I: 457

Lewis T (1941) Professor KF Wenckebach. BMJ I: 219

Lewis T (1942) History of diseases of the heart, by JB Herrick, (book review). Nature 150: 561–562

# Appendix 4: Letter to *The Morning Post* on April 25 1914

**This important letter on research in medicine which Lewis wrote under the pseudonym 'Junior' is here reproduced in full.**

## RESEARCH IN MEDICINE

### Its Position and Needs

During the past twelve months we have heard much of the reorganisation of medical teaching in this country, and especially in the University of London; we have heard less, but a good deal, of the need of medical research. It seems eminently desirable that someone should speak from a different standpoint: the present position and needs of the research *worker*. A simple and clear story is required, and this story, if it is to be told at all, must be told by a unit in the ranks of workers.

Such a unit I count myself; for ten years engaged in medical research work, for six years it has been my chief object in life. At the end of this time I have come fully to recognise the position in which I and those of my fellow-workers in this country who are similarly situated, stand. It is this: we give the best years of our lives, we give the best work of our brains, under conditions which the workers of no sister branch of science would accept; we work for a return which, if offered to a man of business, he would regard as an offence, and which, accepted by us, must stamp us in his eyes as extravagant philanthropists or reckless gamblers. Yet often we are neither the one nor the other, but we are aspirants, who, while we see the extent of the fallow, yearn to turn the few sods we can and enrich the harvest of English medicine, hoping that the day may come when, more properly equipped and more fully trained, we may leave behind us well-ploughed furrows, or gather in the ripe corn in plenty. It is of this fallow, of its enclosure, of the tilling with hoe, of the harvesting in inclement weather, of the wasted endeavour and the heavy rents, that I desire to speak briefly in this article.

And let it not be said that I speak to benefit the farmer: I speak also that hungry mouths may be fed; not only the honest research workers should meet their due, but that their energies may be compressed and fully utilised, that they may be multiplied and that their work may increase in abundance and fruitfulness; that English medicine may progress not in the faltering and fitful steps of the past, but with sure and steady tread.

## FUNCTION OF THE RESEARCH WORKER

I speak especially of research from the standpoint of *Medicine*, work directed to elucidate the cause, to help the recognition, to unravel the course, and to direct the treatment of such disease as comes within the province of the physician. Much of what I say will apply equally to disease with which the surgeon deals; it will apply to a lesser extent to pure pathology. My responsibility is with the first not with the last two.

The primary function of the research worker in medicine, and I shall use this term henceforth in its restricted sense, is to supply the practising hygienist and physician with new knowledge of disease; to advance the science of prevention and the art of practice by the whole means in his power. This end is ultimately utilitarian: he is to seek knowledge; he is to place such knowledge in the hands of those who may apply it. His own function is not to apply, except in so far as preliminary investigation is concerned. We know that success in research comes to few; we know that fruitful research workers are men of peculiar temperaments and abilities.

The researcher seeks, and, finding, he teaches; he teaches the facts he finds; he shows how his new facts link with other knowledge. There ends his task. He may teach by speaking or by writing; he chooses this method or that as circumstances direct him; he selects the quickest and most certain means of thought transference, and resumes his search.

Such, in my view, are the functions of the research worker. What, then, his needs? They are twofold; firstly, to be free and untrammelled in his work; to have broad acres to plough, the best seed to sow, the pick of harrows and reapers, and full control of his farming; secondly, the quickest access to a hungry market.

## PRESENT SYSTEM AND ITS CONSEQUENCES

It does not follow that a man qualified for research also possesses the temperament or type of ability needful to the practising physician. Very often the reverse is true. How imperative in research is hesitancy, that careful and prolonged questioning, which alone avoids the pitfalls of more speedy conclusions. The physician, his duties urging speed, often bids on chance; the research worker, with less thought of time, takes no step till the last if felt secure. Carry the temperament of research to medical practice, and such practice is half paralysed.

At the moment, research work in medicine in this country can be conducted only by those who are not engaged in the practice of medicine, or by those who ultimately aim at so practising. This is unquestionably the chief underlying fault of our present system. For under it, research work is for the most part relegated to the earliest years of the medical career. It comes to occupy a subordinate position, and it is regarded as a fitting preliminary to the practice and teaching of general medicine. It is thought to be a suitable apprenticeship for the junior members of the profession, to be relaxed or abandoned at a later date; and such abandonment is almost universal under present conditions. That is wrong; research at its best should be an introduction to further research and to special teaching; and by special teaching I mean the diffusion of the results of research along the proper channels, and especially the conveyance of new knowledge to those engaged in teaching general medicine.

To be fruitful, research in medicine requires special training and intensive study; witness the recent successes of parasitology. It requires an intimate knowledge of special technique; it calls for exhaustive study of the relevant facts gathered by the allied sciences, be they physiological, morphological, physical, or chemical. Such knowledge is in great measure superfluous to the general physicians, such study is not his real province. The young physician who researches works with the full consciousness that his energies are directed into channels where they must not stray too far, he is acquiring methods and knowledge of facts which will stand him in no stead in practice, the one career open to him. As a consequence such methods of technical skill and such wider knowledge are too often neglected.

The original articles of our medical publications teem with statements which contradict or pervert settled physiological or physical teaching. They are the writings of amateurs, who lack familiarity with the means at the disposal of their science. They are full of constructed hypotheses, which are immediately capable of proof or disproof; yet such proof, or disproof suffers neglect*.

Fruitful and ripe work is attained by continuous study in a limited field of medicine, for the worker in a small field may become conversant with all that he should know to forward his investigation. He saturates himself with all phases of his subject, and becomes a master in his own domain. When a branch of knowledge is complete, so far as it can be taken by methods at his command, he knows it. He does not rest satisfied in publicly propounding hypotheses, he searches for proofs or disproofs.

Research work and guidance of research work is the natural work of long-trained specialists. Yet it largely falls to the lot of the young physician. It falls to his lot because thorough research work seriously inconveniences active practice; the more senior men fall away from research as practice accumulates, and often just at the time when they are becoming most fitted for the former. The younger man takes it, though unpaid, because research work is widely used as a means of advertisement, and is exploited by those who desire practice.

The work is done therefore largely by the junior members of a teaching hospital staff, or by those desiring these appointments. It is undertaken under the most disadvantageous conditions. These men are entering upon their career, not of research, but of hospital and consulting practice. They have the care of patients, not in the wards, but as a medley in crowded in-patient and teaching departments; many have no patients under their care at all; some have a few beds, but the number is always small; the prospect of charge of wards is a prospect of five, ten or fifteen years ahead. They are overburdened with the teaching, not only of general medicine, but of many subsidiary subjects. This work is almost entirely unremunerated. In brief, they have not the material nor the time for serious investigation. To all research supply of material for study is a first essential. In no science is the worker so starved as in medicine. The material is in the hands of the senior who, with a few notable exceptions, fails to utilise it for research. He holds it that he may teach the hospital student, the practitioner in the making, and everything is subordinated to this object. The harvest of the research worker is culled from the fields of others; they leave him stubble, and here and there, by favour or by oversight, a small patch of standing corn. He gathers what he may under disheartening conditions, and too often as he stores his gleanings are sifted, and, if he has gathered too freely, he is charged with pilfering. Let him walk ever so warily, sooner or later he is in danger of arrest for trespass.

Can he discover acres of his own? He can if he is of independent means. He can find them in the wards of hospitals to which no students are attached. But here, too, he must wait serving a long period of apprenticeship before he comes to full control of patients. Moreover, when he moves from the teaching hospital, laboratory accommodation becomes scanty. He works again at a great disadvantage. If he has no means, work in such institutes is well-nigh impossible. Research, he knows, will not in itself support him. It will place him out of pocket; he must assiduously cultivate practice in order to pay his way. It is surprising that under such conditions interest flags and enthusiasm wanes, and that, with the endless irritation of inaccessible material and heavy bills on the one hand and increasing demands for his paid services on the other, the young researcher deserts the vocation for which his capabilities are most suited in order to plunge into practice? He may , it is true, by chance or by rare insight happen upon fact of immediate monetary value. Relying upon such discovery, he gambles with fortune. He *must* find; his finds are his sole merchandise; the seeking is unrewarded. And finding, he must cry his wares, not once, but many times; he must cry them here and cry them there; for his goods sound or base, he is urged to find a purchaser; the inventor becomes a street vendor. Let him fail to cry his goods, they will be cried and sold for him, but not to his advantage.

Such then, are the present circumstances of research in medicine. Physiology and pure pathology, its sister sciences, are eminently productive, the former especially so; their devotees, free and paid, are engaged upon life work. Clinical and experimental medicine are notoriously barren by comparison. Yet how rich is the field of organised research. A worker of a little more than average talent could devote himself under favourable conditions, to no single branch without gathering in a few years a rich store.

## NEEDS OF THE WORKER

It must be acknowledged that no man can successfully engage in the five-fold task; he cannot be at one and the same time (1) an active research worker (unpaid); (2) a teacher of special workers (unpaid); (3) a teacher of general medicine (very limited payments); (4) a hospital physician (unpaid); and (5) a practising physician (fully paid). A division of labour is imperative. The clear duties of the research worker are the first and second, but he must also live. If he is to lead a fruitful existence he must be remunerated; during the years of work he must be independent of practice and of thoughts of practice in the future. If he is not his research is crippled or biased.

His second need is opportunity. He must be equipped with laboratory accommodation; he must be equipped with hospital accommodation. Teaching hospital wards are not the wards in which organised research can be most profitably undertaken, either under present conditions or under proposed conditions. That research is imperative in a teaching institute is granted; it is granted for the sake of teaching, not so much for the sake of research; and research under these conditions is necessarily limited. The same patience cannot be used for demonstration to students and also for observation. Teaching at the bedside, observation at the bedside, one or other, the sick man will willingly tolerate – each is beneficial to the care of the patient; but no sick man should be asked to tolerate both. Neither can observation be successfully practised amidst a crowd of inquiring students or in hospitals where the wards, day after day, become closed class-rooms during the visits of the teaching staff. If research is to have its chance wards must be set apart for research at teaching hospitals or the research work must be conducted at distinct institutes.

In the Poor Law infirmaries of London alone are thousands of patients upon whom no observations are made. A wealth of material goes to waste; it could be utilised without great expense; it could be utilised to the great and immediate benefit of the inmates of these institutes.

Lastly, but by no means least, the research worker should be free within bounds to pursue his studies along his own lines. Successful research directs itself; it follows the path of least resistance. No man can say where it leads; no man can set the course beforehand; he can give at most a general bearing.

Choose the workers rather than select their work; give them a fair competence; engage them half time or full time, as you will; supply their requests for equipment, material, and assistance. They will do the rest.

JUNIOR

*Addendum to Thomas Lewis' letter:*

* A large class of medical writers have long acquired and still maintain the habit of stating hypotheses, making no effort to confirm or disprove them by study. Records of new facts are infrequent, the statement of new hypotheses is universal. A new function is ascribed to an organ by physiologists. There is a hasty effort to explain disease as the perversion of this function; the facts are not analysed. The propounder of a hypothesis defends it through thick and thin: too often, not fact, but every conceivable trick of controversy is brought into the arena. Thoughtful discussion is degraded to the level of partisan debate. It is an almost universal custom of publishers in the sister sciences to restrain hypothesis and render it compatible with the advance of real knowledge. In medicine hypothesis runs riot. A common failing is theorising from the facts which others gather; the teaching ranks of the profession are a curious mixture of workers and philosophers. The philosophers to not appreciate the degree of equality of their trespass, nor do they recognise that the collector of facts is in the long run alone capable of correctly weighing them.

# *References*


1. Adams EB (1990) In search of truth. A portrait of Don Craib. Royal Society of Medicine Services, London, New York
2. Aitken R (1981) A historical dispute. Clin Sci 61: 360–362
3. Anonymous (1920) The mechanism and graphic registration of the heart beat. Thomas Lewis. 2nd edn. (book review). Lancet II: 130
4. Anonymous (1925) The mechanism and graphic registration of the heart beat. Thomas Lewis. 3rd edn. (book review). Lancet II: 605
5. Anonymous (1928) The Harvey celebration. BMJ I: 819–820, 870
6. Anonymous (1930) Research physicians. BMJ I: 503–504
7. Anonymous (1930) Recent advances in cardiology. East CFT, Bain CWC. (book review) JAMA 94: 211
8. Anonymous (1930) Clinical research and experimental medicine. Lancet I: 579–580
9. Anonymous (1931) Sir Thomas Lewis in Boston. New Eng J Med 205: 928–929
10. Anonymous (1933) Progress in cardiology. BMJ I: 791–792
11. Anonymous (1933) The new cardiology. Lancet I: 918
12. Anonymous (1938) Clinical studies of the heart. Nature 141: 533–534
13. Anonymous (1955) Sir Walter Morley Fletcher. In: Brown GH (ed) Lives of the Fellows of the Royal College of Physicians of London 1826–1925. Royal College of Physicians, London, pp 558–559
14. Barron SL (1950) The development of the electrocardiograph in Great Britain. BMJ I: 720–725
15. Barron SL (1952) The development of the electrocardiograph. Cambridge Monograph No 5. Cambridge Instrument Company, London
16. Bedford DE (1939) Left ventricular failure. Lancet I: 1303–1309
17. Bedford DE (1966) Samuel Albert Levine (1891–1966). Br Heart J 28: 853–854
18. Besterman E, Creece R (1979) Waller – pioneer of electrocardiography. Br Heart J 42: 61–64
19. Bickford RG (1937) Experiments relating to the itch sensation, its peripheral mechanism and central pathways. Clin Sci 3: 377–386
20. Booth CC (1979) The development of clinical science in Britain. BMJ I: 1469–1473
21. Booth CC (1986) Clinical research and the MRC. Q J Med 59: 435–447
22. Booth CC (1989) Clinical research. In: Austoker J, Bryder L (eds) Historical perspectives on the role of the MRC. Oxford University Press, Oxford, pp 205–241
23. Bull L (1911) On the simultaneous record of the phono and electrocardiograms. Q J Exp Physiol 4: 289–92
24. Bunker CB (1993) Neuropeptides and Raynaud's phenomenon. Rheumatology 12: 87–89
25. Burch GE, de Pasquale NP (1964) A history of electrocardiography. Year Book Medical Publishers Inc, Chicago
26. Burchell HB (1981) Sir Thomas Lewis: his impact on American cardiology. Br Heart J 46: 1–4
27. Burchell HB (1987) Waller and the first human electrocardiogram. Am J Cardiol 59: 979–983
28. Burchell HB (1987) Did Einthoven invent a string galvanometer? Br Heart J 57: 190–193

29. Burnett J (1985) The origins of the electrocardiograph as a clinical instrument. In: Bynum WF, Lawrence C, Nutton V (eds) The emergence of modern cardiology. Medical History, Supplement 5 pp 53–76
30. Campbell M (1962) The British Cardiac Society and the Cardiac Club: 1922 to 1961. Br Heart J 24: 673–695
31. Cawadias AP (1930) Research in medicine. BMJ I: 667
32. Christian HA (1919) Digitalis therapy: satisfactory effects in cardiac cases with regular pulse rate. Am J Med Sci 157: 593–601
33. Cohn AE (1913) The post-mortem examination of horse's hearts from cases of auricular fibrillation. Heart 4: 221–224
34. Cohn AE (1919) The cardiac phase of the war neuroses. Am J Med Sci 158: 453–470
35. Cotton TF (1920) Observations on subacute infective endocarditis. BMJ II: 851–854
36. Cotton TF (1922) Clubbed fingers as a sign of subacute infective endocarditis. Heart 9: 347–364
37. Cotton TF, Lewis T, Thiele FH (1915) A note on the 'irritable heart' of soldiers. BMJ II: 722
38. Cotton TF, Slade JG, Lewis T (1917) Observations upon dermatographism with special reference to the contractile power of capillaries. Heart 6: 227–248
39. Cournand A (1975) Cardiac catheterization. Development of the technique, its contributions to experimental medicine, and its initial applications in man. Acta Med Scand supplement 579: 7–32
40. Cowan J and others (1939) Some notes on the cardiac club. Br Heart J 1: 97–104
41. Craib WH (1930) The electrocardiogram. MRC Special Report Series 147, HMSO, London
42. Cushny AR (1925) The action and uses in medicine of digitalis and its allies. Longmans Green and Co, London, p 213
43. Cushny AR, Edmunds CW (1907) Paroxysmal irregularity of the heart and auricular fibrillation. Am J Med Sci 133: 66–77
44. Dale HH (1927) The responses of the blood vessels of the human skin. BMJ II: 309–310
45. Dale HH (1933) Sir Walter Fletcher. Lancet I: 1320–1321
46. Dale HH (1945) Sir Thomas Lewis. BMJ I: 461–462
47. Dargie HJ (1989) Heart Failure, management prevention and drug treatment. In: Julian DG, Camm AJ, Fox KM, Hall RJC (eds) Diseases of the heart. Balliere Tindall, London Philadelphia Toronto Sydney Tokyo, pp 58-79
48. Douglas CG (1952) Leonard Erskine Hill 1866–1952. Obit Not Fell Roy Soc Lond 8: 431–443
49. Drury AN (1955) Sir Thomas Lewis. Univ Coll Hosp Mag Lond 40: 70–71
50. Drury AN, Grant RT (1945) Thomas Lewis 1881–1945. Obit Not Fell Roy Soc Lond 5: 179–202
51. Einthoven W (1906) Le télécardiogramme. Arch Int de Physiol 4: 132–163
52. Einthoven W (1912) The different forms of the electrocardiogram and their significance. Lancet I: 853–861
53. Elliott TR (1941) Wilfred Batten Lewis Trotter 1872–1939. Obit Not Fell Roy Soc Lond 3: 325–344
54. Elliott TR (1942) The Copley Medal. Univ Coll Hosp Mag Lond 27: 3–5
55. Feldberg WS (1970) Henry Hallett Dale 1875–1968. Biog Mem Fell Roy Soc Lond 16: 77–174
56. Fletcher MF (1957) The bright countenance. A personal biography of Walter Morley Fletcher. Hodder and Stoughton, London
57. Fraser FR (1940) Effort syndrome in the present war. Edin Med J 47: 451–465
58. Fye WB (1985) Ventricular fibrillation and defibrillation: historical perspectives with emphasis on the contributions of John MacWilliam, Carl Wiggers, and William Kouwenhoven. Circulation 71: 858–865

59. Fye WB (1987) The origin of the heart beat: a tale of frogs, jellyfish, and turtles. Circulation 76: 493–500
60. Fye WB (1987) The development of American physiology. The Johns Hopkins University Press, Baltimore and London, p 221
61. Fye WB (1989) Karel Frederik Wenckebach, 1864–1940. Clin Cardiol 13: 146–148
62. Fye WB (1990) Acute myocardial infarction: a historical summary. In: Gersh BJ, Rahimtoola S (eds) Acute myocardial infarction. Elsevier Science Publishing Co Inc, New York, pp 1–13
63. Fye WB (1994) A history of the origin, evolution, and impact of electrocardiography. Am J Cardiol 73: 937–949
64. Fye WB (1995) Arthur Cushny. Clin Cardiol 18: 360–361
65. Gasser HS, Erlanger J (1927) Role played by sizes of constituent fibres of nerve trunk in determining form of its action potential wave. Am J Physiol 80: 522–547
66. Gavey CJ, Parkinson J (1939) Digitalis in heart failure with normal rhythm. Br Heart J 1: 27–43
67. Grant RT (1926) Observations on the after histories of men suffering from the effort syndrome. Heart 12: 121–142
68. Grant RT (1933) After histories for ten years of a thousand men suffering from heart disease. A study in prognosis. Heart 16: 276–483
69. Grant RT, Iliescu CC (1922) Comparison of the action of quinidine with other cinchona alkaloids in auricular fibrillation. Heart 9: 289–296
70. Guthrie CC (1910) Survival of engrafted tissues III. Blood vessels. Heart 2: 115–126
71. Harper RW, Pitt A (1983) Thomas Lewis – the early years. Br Heart J 49: 403–404
72. Harris I (1930) Research in medicine. BMJ I: 667–668
73. Harris KE, Lewis T, Vaughan J (1929) Haemoglobinuria and urticaria from cold occurring singly or in combination;observations relating especially to the mechanism of urticaria with some remarks upon Raynaud's disease. Heart 14: 305–336
74. Hay J (1930) A lecture on James Mackenzie and his message. BMJ I: 1033–1034
75. Herrick JB (1919) Thrombosis of the coronary arteries. JAMA 72: 387–390
76. Himsworth HP (1945) Thomas Lewis. Univ Coll Hosp Mag Lond 30: 36–37
77. Hoffenberg R (1981) Chairman's remarks. Clin Sci 61: 355–356
78. Hollman A (1945) Thomas Lewis. Univ Coll Hosp Mag Lond 30: 64–66
79. Hollman A (1963) Coronary vasodilators. Med World 99: 217–222
80. Hollman A (1981) Thomas Lewis – the early years. Br Heart J 46: 233–244
81. Hollman A (1985) The history of bundle branch block. In: Bynum WF, Lawrence C, Nutton V (eds) The emergence of modern cardiology. Medical History; Supplement 5, pp 82–102
82. Hollman A (1985) Thomas Lewis: physiologist, cardiologist and clinical scientist. Clin Cardiol 8: 555–559
83. Hollman A (1990) Bernard A Robinson 1888–1979: an unknown pioneer of electrocardiography. Br Heart J 63: 200–204
84. Hollman A (1990) Ronald Thomson Grant 1892–1989. Br Heart J 64: 349
85. Hollman A (1992) Plants in cardiology. BMJ Publishing Group, London, p 21
86. Hollman A (1993) How John Parkinson did the post mortem on Sir James Mackenzie. Br Heart J 70: 587–588
87. Hollman A (1994) Sir Thomas Lewis: clinical scientist and cardiologist, 1881–1945. J Med Biog 2: 6370
88. Hollman A (1996) Heart and the British Heart Journal. Heart 75: 3–5
89. Hume WE (1918) A study of the cardiac disabilities of soldiers in France (V.D.H. and D.A.H.). Lancet I: 529–534
90. Hutchison R (1930) Research in medicine. BMJ I: 565
91. Kekwick RA (1981) Alan Nigel Drury 1889–1980. Biogr Mem Fell Roy Soc Lond 27: 173–197

92. Kellgren JH (1938) A preliminary account of referred pains arising from muscle. BMJ I: 325–327
93. Kellgren JH (1938) Observations on referred pain arising from muscle. Clin Sci 3: 175–190
94. Kellgren JH (1939) On the distribution of pain arising from deep somatic structures with charts of segmental pain areas. Clin Sci 4: 35–46
95. Krikler DM (1969) Alfred Goodman Levy – Bulawayo's first doctor. Centr Afr J Med 15: 97–99
96. Krikler DM (1985) The development of the understanding of arrhythmias during the last 100 years. In: Bynum WF, Lawrence C, Nutton V (eds) The emergence of modern cardiology.Medical history; Supplement 5, pp 77–81
97. Krikler DM (1987) Electrocardiography then and now: where next? Br Heart J 57: 113–117
98. Krikler DM (1987) The search for Samojloff: A Russian physiologist in times of change. BMJ 295: 1624–1627
99. Krikler DM (1987) Historical aspects of electrocardiography. Cardiol Clin 5: 349–355
100. Krikler DM (1987) The roots of british cardiology. Br Heart J 62: 230–234
101. Krikler DM (1990) Paul Rothschild. Br Heart J 63: 369
102. Krikler DM, Hollman A (1990) The last portrait of Willem Einthoven: newly discovered links between Sir Thomas Lewis and Alexander Samojloff. Br Heart J 64: 223–226
103. Krogh SAS (1922) The anatomy and physiology of capillaries. Harvard University Press, New Haven
104. Lawrence C (1985) Moderns and ancients: the 'new' cardiology in Britain 1880–1930. In: Bynum WF, Lawrence C, Nutton V (eds) The emergence of modern cardiology. Medical history; Supplement 5, pp 1–33
105. Lawrence C (1990) Cinema Verité. The image of William Harvey's experiments in 1928. In: Rupke NA (ed) Vivisection in historical perspective. Croom Helm, London pp 295–313
106. Lembeck F (1983) Mediators of vasodilatation in the skin. Br J Derm 109: supplement 25, pp 1–9
107. Levine SA (1929) Coronary thrombosis. Its various clinical features. Medicine 8: 245–418
108. Levy AG, Lewis T (1911) Heart irregularities, resulting from the inhalation of low percentages of chloroform vapour, and their relationship to ventricular fibrillation. Heart 3: 100–110
109. Lewis ALT , Lewis T (1920) The starling in the woodpeckers nest. Country Life 47: 582–584
110. Lewis T (1902) The structure and function of the haemolymph glands and spleen. Int Mschr Anat Physiol 20: 101–155
111. Lewis T (1904) Note on a case of defective development of the lateral cerebellar lobes in a dog. Brain 105: 84–88
112. Lewis T (1906) The pulse in aortic disease: the relation of pulse curves to blood pressure. Lancet II: 714–717
113. Lewis T (1906) The factors influencing the prominence of the dicrotic wave. J Physiol 34: 414–429
114. Lewis T (1908) A lecture on the 'Occurrence of heart-block in man and its causation'. BMJ II: 1798–1802
115. Lewis T (1908) Studies of the relationship between respiration and blood pressure. J Physiol 37: 213–255
116. Lewis T (1909) Single and successive extra-systoles. Lancet I: 382–385
117. Lewis T (1909) Irregular action of the heart in mitral stenosis: the inception of ventricular rhythm, etc. Q J Med 2: 356–367
118. Lewis T (1909) Auricular fibrillation: a common clinical condition. BMJ II: 1528

119. Lewis T (1909) The experimental production of paroxysmal tachycardia and the effects of ligation of the coronary arteries. Heart 1: 98–137
120. Lewis T (1909) Pulse records in relation to their events of the human cardiac cycle. In: Hill LE (ed) Further advances in physiology. Edward Arnold, London, pp 72–111
121. Lewis T (1910) Auricular fibrillation and its relationship to clinical irregularity of the heart. Heart I: 306–372
122. Lewis T (1910) Galvanometric curves yielded by cardiac beats generated in various areas of the auricular musculature. The pacemaker of the heart. Heart 2: 23–46
123. Lewis T (1910) Fibrillation des oreillettes et extrasystoles ventriculaires. Arch Mal Coeur 3: 664–667
124. Lewis T (1910) Die Pathologie de vollstandigen Unregelmassigkeit des Herzens. Verh Dtsch Path Ges 16: 112–116
125. Lewis T (1911) Bad Nauheim. Univ Coll Hosp Mag Lond 2: 44–55
126. Lewis T (1911) Modern English cardiovascular teaching: a rejoinder. Q J Med 4: 301–316
127. Lewis T (1911) Irregularity of the heart's action in horses and its relationship to fibrillation of the auricles in experiment and to complete irregularity of the human heart. Heart 3: 161–172
128. Lewis T (1911) The mechanism of the heart beat. Shaw and Sons, London
129. Lewis T (1912) Electrocardiography and its importance in the clinical examination of heart affections. BMJ I: 1421–1423, I: 1479–1482; II: 65–67
130. Lewis T (1912) A lecture on the evidences of auricular fibrillation treated historically. BMJ: 57–60
131. Lewis T (1912) Observations upon a curious and not uncommon form of extreme acceleration of the auricle. 'Auricular flutter.' Heart 4: 171–220
132. Lewis T (1912) Meeting of clinical section of the Royal Society of Medicine, March 20. Proc Roy Soc Med 4: 183–192
133. Lewis T (1912) Clinical disorders of the heart beat. Shaw and Sons, London
134. Lewis T (1913) The time relations of heart sounds and murmurs with special reference to the acoustic signs in mitral stenosis. Heart 4: 241–258
135. Lewis T (1913) Illustrations of heart-sound records. Q J Med 6: 441–452
136. Lewis T (1913) Clinical electrocardiography. Shaw and Sons, London
137. Lewis T (1913) The pacemaker of the mammalian heart. In: 17th International Congress of Medicine. Oxford University Press, London, section III, pp 107–117
138. Lewis T (1913) An address on the pathology of heart function. Lancet II: 883–888
139. Lewis T (1914) Walter Holbrook Gaskell. BMJ II: 559–560
140. Lewis T (1914) Research in medicine. Its position and its needs. The Morning Post: April 25
141. Lewis T (1914) Observations upon ventricular hypertrophy with especial reference to preponderance of one or other chamber. Heart 5: 367–402
142. Lewis T (1915) A first step in the analysis of the dog's ventricular electrocardiogram. J Physiol 49: xx–xxi P
143. Lewis T (1915) Lectures on the heart. Paul B Hoeber, New York
144. Lewis T (1916) The spread of the excitatory process in the vertebrate heart. Phil Trans Roy Soc Lond 207: 221–310
145. Lewis T (1917) Croonian Lecture. Upon the motion of the mammalian heart. Proc Roy Soc Lond B 89: 560–573
146. Lewis T (1917) Report upon soldiers returned as cases of 'Disordered action of the heart' (D.A.H.) or 'Valvular disease of the heart' (V.D.H.). MRC Special Report Series 8, HMSO, London
147. Lewis T (1917) Osservazioni sopra soldati rinviati all'Ospedale soffernti di sintomi comunemente riferiti al sistema cardio-vasculare. La sindrome della sforzo. Le Mal del Cuore: 421–435
148. Lewis T (1918) The tolerance of physical exertion, as shown by soldiers suffering from so-called 'irritable heart'. BMJ I: 363–365

149. Lewis T (1918) The soldier's heart and the effort syndrome. Shaw and Sons, London
150. Lewis T (1919) The Dogs Bill. Our dependence on experiment. The Times April 9
151. Lewis T (1919) On cardinal principles in cardiological practice. BMJ II: 621–635
152. Lewis T (1920) Notes on the breeding habits of the little tern. British Birds 14: 74–82
153. Lewis T (1920) An address on the relation of physiology to medicine. BMJ II: 459–462
154. Lewis T (1920) The mechanism and graphic registration of the heart beat, 2nd edn. Shaw and Sons, London
155. Lewis T (1920) The mechanism and graphic registration of the heart beat, 2nd edn. Shaw and Sons, London p vii
156. Lewis T (1921) The Linacre lecture. The law of cardiac muscle with special reference to conduction in the mammalian heart. Q J Med 14: 339–351
157. Lewis T (1921) The Oliver-Sharpey lectures on the nature of flutter and fibrillation of the auricle. BMJ I: 551–555 and 590–593
158. Lewis T (1921) Observations upon flutter and fibrillation. Part 9. 'The nature of auricular fibrillation as it occurs in patients.' Heart 8: 193–228
159. Lewis T (1922) The Mellon lecture. Interpretations of the initial phases of the electrocardiogram with special reference to the theory of 'limited potential differences'. Arch Intern Med 30: 269–285
160. Lewis T (1922) The value of quinidine in cases of auricular fibrillation and methods of studying the clinical reaction. Am J Med Sci 163: 781–795
161. Lewis T (1922) The actions of atropine and quinidine in fibrillation of the auricles; clinical and experimental studies. Am J Med Sci 164: 1–13
162. Lewis T (1922) The action of digitalis in cases of auricular fibrillation and flutter. Am J Med Sci 164: 157–173
163. Lewis T (1922) Augustus D Waller. BMJ I: 459
164. Lewis T (1923) Movement of the heart's axis with respiration. Heart 10: 257–270
165. Lewis T (1924) Studies of capillary pulsation, with special reference to vasodilatation in aortic regurgitation and including observations on the effect of heating the human skin. (With appended notes on skin temperature, in collaboration with Dr EP Wolf of Chicago). Heart 11: 151–194
166. Lewis T (1925) Sir James Mackenzie. BMJ I: 243
167. Lewis T (1925) In Memoriam. Sir James Mackenzie. Heart 12: i–vii
168. Lewis T (1925) The mechanism and graphic registration of the heart beat. 3rd edn. Shaw and Sons, London
169. Lewis T (1925) The mechanism and graphic registration of the heart beat, 3rd edn. Shaw and Sons, London, p 340
170. Lewis T (1925) The mechanism and graphic registration of the heart beat, 3rd edn. Shaw and Sons, London, p 366
171. Lewis T (1926) Sayings of the Great. Univ Coll Hosp Mag Lond 11: 172
172. Lewis T (1927) The blood vessels of the human skin and their responses. Shaw and Sons, London
173. Lewis T (1927) In Memoriam. Willem Einthoven. Heart 14: iv–viii
174. Lewis T (1928) A bedstead for use in treating cardiac patients suffering from congestive failure. BMJ II: 997–999
175. Lewis T (1929) Standard colours for use in the study of vascular reactions of the human skin. Heart 15: 1–6
176. Lewis T (1930) Observations on research in medicine: its position and its needs. BMJ I: 479–493
177. Lewis T (1930) Remarks on early signs of cardiac failure of the congestive type. BMJ I: 849–861
178. Lewis T (1931) Muscular pain in intermittent claudication. Bull N Y Acad Med 7: 871–878
179. Lewis T (1932) Pain in muscular ischemia. Arch Intern Med 49: 713–727

180. Lewis T (1932) Raynaud's disease, with special reference to the nature of the malady. BMJ II: 136–138
181. Lewis T (1932) A lecture on vasovagal syncope and the carotid sinus mechanism with comments on Gowers's and Nothnagel's syndrome. BMJ I: 873–895
182. Lewis T (1932) The relation of clinical medicine to physiology from the standpoint of research. BMJ II: 1046–1049
183. Lewis T (1933) The Harveian oration on 'Clinical Science'. BMJ II: 717–722
184. Lewis T (1933) Material relating to coarctation of the aorta of the adult type. Heart 16: 205–261
185. Lewis T (1933) Final editorial note. Heart:16, no page number
186. Lewis T (1933) Clinical observations and experiments relating to burning pain in the extremities, and to so-called 'erythromelalgia' in particular. Clin Sci 1: 175–211
187. Lewis T (1933) Clinical disorders of the heart beat, 6th edn. Shaw and Sons, London
188. Lewis T (1933) Diseases of the heart. Macmillan and Co, London
189. Lewis T (1934) T Swale Vincent. BMJ I: 83–84
190. Lewis T (1934) Clinical science, illustrated by personal experiences. Shaw and Sons, London
191. Lewis T (1934) Clinical science, illustrated by personal experiences. Shaw and Sons, London, preface iv and v
192. Lewis T (1934) Clinical science, illustrated by personal experiences. Shaw and Sons, London, p 3
193. Lewis T (1934) Clinical science, illustrated by personal experiences. Shaw and Sons, London, p 15
194. Lewis T (1934) Clinical science, illustrated by personal experiences. Shaw and Sons, London, p 21
195. Lewis T (1934) Clinical science, illustrated by personal experiences. Shaw and Sons, London, pp 22–23
196. Lewis T (1934) Clinical science, illustrated by personal experiences. Shaw and Sons, London, pp 23–24
197. Lewis T (1934) Clinical science, illustrated by personal experiences. Shaw and Sons, London, p 42
198. Lewis T (1934) Clinical science, illustrated by personal experiences. Shaw and Sons, London, p 81
199. Lewis T (1934) Clinical science, illustrated by personal experiences. Shaw and Sons, London, pp 107–116
200. Lewis T (1934) Clinical science, illustrated by personal experiences. Shaw and Sons, London, p 122
201. Lewis T (1934) Clinical science, illustrated by personal experiences. Shaw and Sons, London, p 165
202. Lewis T (1934) Clinical science, illustrated by personal experiences. Shaw and Sons, London, pp 183–186
203. Lewis T (1935) The Huxley lecture on clinical science within the university. BMJ I: 631–636
204. Lewis T (1935) Experiments relating to cutaneous hyperalgesia and its spread through somatic nerves. Clin Sci 2: 373–417
205. Lewis T (1936) Vascular disorders of the limbs. Macmillan and Co, London
206. Lewis T (1937) Auricular flutter continuing for twenty-four years. BMJ I: 1248
207. Lewis T (1937) Clinical electrocardiography, 6th edn. Shaw and Sons, London
208. Lewis T (1937) Diseases of the heart, 2nd edn. Macmillan and Co, London
209. Lewis T (1937) 'Relapse' following sympathectomy. Lancet 2: 938
210. Lewis T (1937) The nocifensor system of nerves and its reactions. BMJ I: 431–435
211. Lewis T (1938) Suggestions relating to the study of somatic pain. BMJ I: 321–323
212. Lewis T (1938) Research in medicine and other addresses. HK Lewis, London, p 13
213. Lewis T (1938) The pathological changes in the arteries supplying the fingers in warm handed people and in cases of so-called Raynaud's disease. Clin Sci 3: 287–319

214. Lewis T (1939) Editorial Preface. Br Heart J 1: 1–2
215. Lewis T (1939) Professor Thomas Renton Elliott. Univ Coll Hosp Mag Lond 24: 83–86
216. Lewis T (1940) The Soldier's Heart and the Effort Syndrome, 2nd edn. Shaw and Sons, London
217. Lewis T (1940) A note on pulsating manubrial tumor. Brit Heart J II: 260–262
218. Lewis T (1940) The tourniquet. BMJ I: 457
219. Lewis T (1940) Visceral pain. Lancet II: 503
220. Lewis T (1940) Venous pulsation in the orbit. Clin Sci 4: 243–244
221. Lewis T (1941) Professor K F Wenckebach. BMJ I: 219
222. Lewis T (1941) Observations on some normal and injurious effects of cold upon the skin and underlying tissues. BMJ II: 795–797, 837–839, 869–871
223. Lewis T (1941) Personal record of a fellow of the Royal Society. Library of the Royal Society London
224. Lewis T (1941) Caleb Hillier Parry, MD, FRS. (1755–1822). A great Welsh physician and scientist. Proc Cardiff Med Soc, session 1941–1942: 71–90
225. Lewis T (1942) Swelling of the human limbs in response to immersion in cold water. Clin Sci 4: 349–360
226. Lewis T (1942) Trousseau's phenomenon in tetany. Clin Sci 4: 361–364
227. Lewis T (1942) Observations upon the vascular axon reflex in human skin, as exhibited by a case of urticaria with remarks upon the nocifensor nerve hypothesis. Clin Sci 4: 365–384
228. Lewis T (1942) History of diseases of the heart. J.B. Herrick. (book review). Nature 150: 561–562
229. Lewis T (1942) Diseases of the heart, 3rd edn. Macmillan and Co, London
230. Lewis T(1942) Pain. The Macmillan Company, New York
231. Lewis T (1942) Pain. The Macmillan Company, New York, p 51
232. Lewis T (1942) Pain. The Macmillan Company, New York, p 83
233. Lewis T (1944) Reflections on reform in medical education. Lancet 1: 619–621, 649–651, 685–687
234. Lewis T (1945) Congenital tricuspid stenosis. Clin Sci 5: 261–273
235. Lewis T (1945) Exercises in human physiology. Macmillan and Co, London
236. Lewis T (1945) Exercises in human physiology. Macmillan and Co, London, p v
237. Lewis T (1946) Diseases of the heart, 4th edn. Macmillan and Co, London
238. Lewis T (1949) Electrocardiography and clinical disorders of the heart beat. Shaw and Sons, London
239. Lewis T, Allen HW (1913) An instance of premature beats arising in the auriculoventricular bundle of a young child. Am J Med Sci 145: 667–671
240. Lewis T, Barcroft J (1915) Notes of further observations upon dyspnoea and its relation to blood reaction. Q J Med 8: 97–113
241. Lewis T, Embleton D (1908) Split-hand and split-foot deformities, their types, origin and transmission. Biometrika 6: 327–387
242. Lewis T, Grant RT (1923) Observations relating to subacute infective endocarditis. Heart 10: 21–97
243. Lewis T, Kellgren JH (1939) Observations relating to referred pain, viscero-motor reflexes and other associated phenomena. Clin Sci 4: 47–71
244. Lewis T, Landis EM (1930) Observations upon the vascular mechanism in acrocyanosis. Heart 15: 229–246
245. Lewis T, Macnalty AS (1908) A note on the simultaneous occurrence of sinus and ventricular rhythm in man. J Physiol 37: 445–458
246. Lewis T, Marvin HM (1927) Observations relating to vasodilatation arising from antidromic impulses to herpes zoster and trophic effects. Heart 14: 27–47
247. Lewis T, Master AM (1924) Supernormal recovery phase, illustrated by two clinical cases of heart-block. Heart 11: 371–388

248. Lewis T, Mathison GC (1910) Auriculo-ventricular heart-block as a result of asphyxia. Heart 2: 47–53
249. Lewis T, Pickering GW (1933) Observations upon maladies in which the blood supply to digits ceases intermittently or permanently, and upon bilateral gangrene of digits; observations relevant to so-called 'Raynaud's disease'. Clin Sci 1: 327–366
250. Lewis T, Pickering GW (1935) Circulatory changes in the fingers in some diseases of the nervous system, with special reference to the digital atrophy of peripheral nerve lesions. Clin Sci 2: 149–184
251. Lewis T, Rothschild MA (1915) The excitatory process in the dog's heart. Part 2. The ventricles. Phil Trans Roy Soc Lond B 206: 181–226
252. Lewis T, Silberberg MD (1911) Paroxysmal tachycardia accompanied by the ventricular form of the venous pulse. Q J Med 5: 5–10
253. Lewis T, Stokes J (1942) A curious syndrome, with signs suggesting cervical arteriovenous fistula and the pulses of neck and arms lost. Brit Heart J 4: 57–65
254. Lewis T, White PD (1914) The effects of premature contractions in vagotimized dogs, with special reference to atrio-ventricular rhythm. Heart 5: 335–366
255. Lewis T, Oppenheimer A, Oppenheimer BS (1910) The site of origin of the mammalian heart-beat; the pacemaker in the dog. Heart 2: 147–169
256. Lewis T, Ryffel JH, Wolf CGL, Cotton T, Barcroft J (1913) Observations relating to dyspnoea in cardiac and renal patients. Heart 5: 45–92
257. Lewis T, Meakins J, White PD (1914) The excitatory process in the dog's heart. Part 1. The auricles. Phil Trans Roy Soc Lond B 205: 375–426
258. Lewis T, White PD, Meakins J (1914) The susceptible region in A-V conduction. Heart 5: 289–298
259. Lewis T, Cotton TF, Barcroft J, Milroy TR, Dufton D, Parsons TR (1916) Breathlessness in soldiers suffering from irritable heart. BMJ II: 517–519
260. Lewis T, Pickering GW, Rothschild P (1931) Observations upon muscular pain in intermittent claudication. Heart 15: 359–383
261. Lewis T, Pickering GW, Rothschild P (1933) Centripetal paralysis arising out of arrested bloodflow to the limb, including notes on a form of tingling. Heart 16: 1–32
262. Lewis THC (1995) Some recollections of my father, Sir Thomas Lewis, and of my family life. Manuscript in the library of the Royal College of Physicians of London
263. Mackay HMM (1930) Research in medicine. BMJ I: 616–617
264. Mackenzie J (1902) The study of the pulse. Arterial, venous and hepatic and the movements of the heart. Young J Pentland, Edinburgh and London
265. Mackenzie J (1908) The ink polygraph. BMJ I: 1411
266. Mackenzie J (1908) Diseases of the heart. Oxford University Press, London
267. Mackenzie J (1909) Symptoms and their interpretation. Shaw and Sons, London p 85
268. Mackenzie J (1911) Digitalis. Heart 2: 273–386
269. Mackenzie J (1916) The soldier's heart. BMJ I: 117–119
270. Mackenzie J (1925) Diseases of the heart, 4th edn. Oxford University Press, London, p 313
271. Mackenzie J (1925) Diseases of the heart, 4th edn. Oxford University Press, London, p 362
272. Mair A (1973) Sir James Mackenzie, MD 1853–1925, General Practitioner. Churchill Livingstone, Edinburgh
273. Marvin HM (1927) Digitalis and diuretics in heart failure with regular rhythm with especial reference to the importance of etiological classification of heart disease. J Clin Invest 3: 521–539
274. McMichael J (1937) Postural changes in cardiac output and respiration in man. Q J Exp Physiol 27: 55–72
275. McMichael J (1969) Foreword. In: Verel D, Grainger J (eds) Cardiac catheterization. Churchill Livingstone, Edinburgh, pp v–viii
276. McMichael J (1976) A transition in cardiology: the Mackenzie Lewis era. Royal College of Physicians, London

277. McMichael J (1981) Sir James Mackenzie and atrial fibrillation – a new perspective. J Roy Coll Gen Pract 31: 402–406
278. McMichael J, Sharpey-Schafer EP (1944) Cardiac output in man by a direct Fick method. Br Heart J 6: 33–40
279. McMichael J, Sharpey-Schafer EP (1944) The action of intra-venous digoxin in man. Q J Med 13: 123–135
280. McMichael J, Peart WS (1982) George White Pickering 1904–1980. Biog Mem Fell Roy Soc Lond 28: 431–449
281. Meakins JC (1945) Sir Thomas Lewis. Canad Med Ass J 52: 626–627
282. Meakins JC, Parkinson J, Gunson EB, Cotton TF, Slade JG, Drury AN, Lewis T (1916) A memorandum upon heart affections in soldiers with special reference to the prognosis of 'irritable heart'. BMJ II: 418–420
283. Medical Research Committee (1915) Report for the year 1914–1915. HMSO, London
284. Medical Research Council (1933) Report for the year 1931–1932. HMSO, London
285. Medical Research Council (1934) Report for the year 1932–1933. HMSO, London
286. Medical Research Council (1937) Report for the year 1935–1936. HMSO, London
287. Medical Research Council (1947) Medical research in war. Report for the years 1939–1945. HMSO, London
288. Mendlowitz M (1938) Some observations on clubbed fingers. Clin Sci 3: 387–401
289. Merrington WR (1976) University College Hospital and its Medical School: a history. Heinemann, London
290. Morison A (1917) The Lumleian Lectures and medical research. Lancet I: 927–929
291. Nixon PGF (1995) An appraisal of Thomas Lewis's effort syndrome. Q J Med 88: 741–749
292. Paget J (1870) Address by the president. Trans Clin Soc Lond 3: xxxi–xxxix
293. Paget S (1919) Sir Victor Horsley. A study of his life and work. Constable and Co, London, p 190
294. Parkinson J, Bedford DE (1929) Successive changes in the electrocardiogram after cardiac infarction (coronary thrombosis). Heart 14: 195–240
295. Paul O (1986) Take heart. The life and prescription for living of Dr Paul Dudley White. Harvard University Press, Boston, pp 34–35
296. Pickering GW (1934) The cerebro-spinal fluid pressure in arterial hypertension. Clin Sci 1: 397–408
297. Pickering GW (1939) The problem of high blood pressure in man. BMJ I: 1–3
298. Pickering GW (1939) Experimental observations on headache. BMJ I: 907–912
299. Pickering GW (1946) In memoriam. Clin Sci 6: 3–11
300. Pickering GW (1955) Thomas Lewis. Univ Coll Hosp Mag Lond 40: 68–70
301. Pickering GW, Wayne EJ (1934) Observations on angina pectoris and intermittent claudication in anaemia. Clin Sci 1: 305–326
302. Pierach CA, Wangensteen SD, Burchell HB (1993) Spa therapy for heart disease. Bad Nauheim (circa 1900). Am J Cardiol 72: 336–342
303. Pilcher, RS (1973) Wilfred Trotter FRS FRCS. Ann Roy Coll Surg Eng 53: 71–83
304. Pochin EE (1938) Delay of pain perception in tabes dorsalis. Clin Sci 3: 191–196
305. Pochin EE (1955) A journal and a department. Univ Coll Hosp Mag Lond 40: 72–74
306. Pochin EE (1980) Early days of the Medical Research Society. Clin Sci 61: 357–360
307. Pruitt R (1976) Doublets, dipoles and the negativity hypothesis: an historical note on W H Craib and his relationship with F N Wilson and Thomas Lewis. Johns Hopkins Med J 138: 279–288
308. Robinson BA (1914) The science of electrocardiography. The Electrician 63: 485–487
309. Rosenbaum M (1981) Sir Thomas Lewis: a view from the south. Br Heart J 46: 349–350
310. Rothberger CJ, Winterberg H (1909) Vorhofflimmern und arhythmia perpetua. Wiener klin Wochschr 22: 839–844
311. Ryle JA (1930) Research in medicine. BMJ I: 566
312. Sargant W (1940) The hyperventilation syndrome. Lancet I: 314–316

313. Shaw P (1936) Appointments in clinical science. Lancet II: 404
314. Smith TW, Braunwald E, Kelly RA (1992) The management of heart failure. In: Braunwald E (ed) Heart Disease, 4th edn. WB Saunders, Philadelphia London Toronto Montreal Sydney Tokyo
315. Snellen HA (1977) Selected papers on electrocardiography of Willem Einthoven. Leiden University Press, Leiden
316. Snellen HA (1981) Thomas Lewis (1881–1945) and cardiology in Europe. Br Heart J 46: 121–125
317. Snellen HA (1983) Two pioneers of electrocardiography. The correspondence between Einthoven and Lewis from 1908–1926. Donker Academic Publications, Rotterdam
318. Snellen HA (1983) Two pioneers of electrocardiography. The correspondence between Einthoven and Lewis from 1908–1926. Donker Academic Publications, Rotterdam, pp 98–99
319. Snellen HA (1995) Willem Einthoven (1860–1927). Father of electrocardiography.Life and work, ancestors and contemporaries. Kluwer Academic Publishers, Dordrecht Boston London
320. Thomson AL (1975) Half a century of medical research. HMSO, London, p 293
321. Treasure T, Hollman A (1995) The surgery of mitral stenosis 1898–1948: why did it take 50 years to establish mitral valvotomy? Ann Roy Coll Surg Engl 77: 145–151
322. Vincent TS, Lewis T (1901) The proteids of unstriped muscle. J Physiol 26: xix P
323. Vincent TS, Lewis T (1901) Observations upon the chemistry and heat rigor curves of vertebrate muscle, involuntary and voluntary. J Physiol 26: 445
324. Walshe FMR (1942) The anatomy and physiology of cutaneous sensibility: a critical review. Brain 65: 48–112
325. Waterston D (1939) Sir James Mackenzie's heart. Br Heart J 1: 237–240
326. Wayne EJ (1933) Clinical observations on two pure glucosides of digitalis, digoxin and digitalinum verum. Clin Sci 1: 63–76
327. Wayne EJ, Laplace LB (1933) Observations on angina of effort. Clin Sci 1: 103–129
328. Wayne EJ, Pickering GW (1934) Observations on angina pectoris and intermittent claudication in anaemia. Clin Sci 1: 305–325
329. Weber KT (1995) Heart failure: lessons learned over the past 25 years. Clin Cardiol 18: 123–130
330. Weiss S, Baker JP (1933) The carotid sinus reflex in health and disease. Medicine 12: 297–354
331. White PD (1971) My life and medicine, an autobiographical memoir. Gambit Inc, Boston, pp 16–17
332. White PD (1931) Heart Disease. The Macmillan Company, New York, p 487
333. Wilson FN, Jamieson RA (1920) Musical diastolic murmurs in aortic insufficiency. Heart 7: 71–80
334. Wilson FN (1940) Thomas Lewis. Michigan Alum Quart Rev 47: 12–21
335. Wood PH (1941) Da Costa's syndrome (or effort syndrome). BMJ I: 767–772; 805–811; 845–851
336. Wood PH, (1940) The action of digitalis in heart failure with normal rhythm. Br Heart J 2: 132–140
337. Wooley CF (1987) From irritable heart to mitral valve prolapse: World War 1, the US experience and the origin of neurocirculatory asthenia. Am J Cardiol 59: 1183–1186
338. Wooley CF, Stang JM (1988) Samuel A Levine and his world war 1 experience. Am J Cardiol 62: 952–956
339. Zottermann Y (1969 ) Touch, tickle and pain. Pergamon Press, Oxford London Edinburgh New York, pp 234–235.

**Material in the Contemporary Medical Archives Centre (PP/LEW) at The Wellcome Institute for the History of Medicine, London**


340. Abbott ME (1922–1936) Letters to TL A.1/1–27
341. Adrian ED (1941) Letter to TL A.1/777–861
342. Allen HW (1913) Letter to TL A.1/777–861
343. Barcroft J (1918) Letter to TL A.1/553–596
344. Barlow T (1906) Testimonial for TL B.6
345. Bedford DE (1932) Letter to TL A.1/102–151
346. Blalock A (1940) Letter to TL A.1/28–101
347. Bradford JR (1928) Letter to TL E.3/1
348. Bridger, E (1975) Audio-tape
349. Buckle JGT (1910) Letter to TL A.1/777–861
350. Chavez I (1944) Letter to TL A.1/102–151
351. Chromow A (1939) Letter to TL A.1/102–151
352. Cohn AE (1911) Letters to TL A.1/777–861
353. Dale HH (1928) Letter to TL E.3/1
354. Dale HH (1932) Letter to TL B.6
355. Dale HH (1944) Letter to TL B.7/5
356. Elliott TR (1918) Letter to TL A.1/771–861
357. Elliott TR (1933) Letter to TL D.3/2
358. Elliott TR (1941) Letter to TL A.1/777–861
359. Elliott TR (1941) Letter to TL A.1/28–101
360. Elliott TR (1941) Letter to TL A./771–861
361. Elliott TR (1944) Letter to TL D.6/1
362. Elliott TR (1946) Letter to Sir Alan Drury B.9
363. Evans, W (1984) Audio-tape
364. Fletcher WM (1930) Letter to TL D.8/3
365. Fulton J (1930) Letter to TL A.1/205–230
366. Grant RT (1974) Audio-tape
367. Herrick JB (1943) Letter to TL A.1/777–861
368. Hill AV (1941) Letter to TL A.1/777–861
369. Horner G (1930) Letter to TL D.1/3
370. Horsley V (1906) Testimonial for TL B.6
371. Kerr W (1929) Letter to TL A.1/364–389
372. Landis E (1930) Letter to TL A.1/390–459
373. Levine SA (1918) Letter to TL C.1/3
374. Lewis H (1908–1913) Letters to TL B.3
375. Lewis KHD (1909) Letter to TL B.3
376. Lewis KHD (1914) Letter to TL B.3
377. Lewis, Lady (1981) Audio-tape
378. Lewis T (1902) Letters to his mother B.3
379. Lewis T (1904) Letter to his mother B.3
380. Lewis T (1909–1933) Notes and letters about the founding of 'Heart'. E.1
381. Lewis T (1910) Letter to his mother B.3
382. Lewis T (1913) Letter to Dr A Crehore A.1/777–861
383. Lewis T (1918) Correspondence about American officers C.1/4
384. Lewis T (1918) Letter to War Office C.1/2
385. Lewis T (1918) Draft article about sparrowhawks F.21/3
386. Lewis T (1920) Letter to various cardiac consultants C.2/4
387. Lewis T (1921) Letter to Sir James Mackenzie A.1/460–517
388. Lewis T (1924) Letter to Dr Maude Abbott A.1/1–27
389. Lewis T (1927) Letter to Sir John Rose Bradford E.3/1
390. Lewis T (1927) Memorandum on the after care of patients at UCH D.3/10–11

391. Lewis T (1927) Letter to Dr Carl J Wiggers E.1
392. Lewis T (1929) Testimonial for W H Craib D.3/2
393. Lewis T (1929) Memorandum on the Cambridge Scheme D.1/1
394. Lewis T (1930) Draft reply (unpublished) to correspondence in the BMJ D.2/3
395. Lewis T (1930) Testimonial for Dr Janet Vaughan D.3/2
396. Lewis T (1931) Letter to Dr G Horner A.1/28–101
397. Lewis T (1931) Formation of the Medical Research Society D.8/3
398. Lewis T (1931) Letter to editor of *The Lancet* A.1/389–459
399. Lewis T (1932) Letter to Mr S L Barron D.1/3
400. Lewis T (1932) Letter to Dr DE Bedford A.1/102–151
401. Lewis T (1932) Letter to Dr FN Wilson E.2
402. Lewis T (1933) MRC Clinical Committee D.4/3
403. Lewis T (1933) Notes and letters regarding the Harveian Oration D.2/3
404. Lewis T (1935) Letter to Sir William Hume A.1/284–355
405. Lewis T (1936) Letter to Sir Richard Gregory A.1/518–541
406. Lewis T (1936) Letter to Sir Hector Hetherington A.1/234–283
407. Lewis T (1936) Letter to Dr E Landis A.1/389–459
408. Lewis T (1936) Letter to Dr Drew Luten A.1/389–459
409. Lewis T (1936) Letter to BS Oppenheimer B.8
410. Lewis T (1936) Letter to Sir Robert Robinson A.1/597–656
411. Lewis T (1936) Letter to Mr R Sloley A1/695–698
412. Lewis T (1937) Letter to Lord Dawson A1/152–187
413. Lewis T (1937) Letter to Sir Hector Hetherington A.1/234–283
414. Lewis T (1937) Letter to Dr Hugh Maclean A.1/460–517
415. Lewis T (1937) Letter to Dr Wilder Penfield A.1/518–541
416. Lewis T (1937) Letter to Dr WAH Rushton A.1/597–656
417. Lewis T (1938) Letter to Burroughs Wellcome Ltd A.1/28–101
418. Lewis T (1938) Letter to Dr John Parkinson A.1/102–151
419. Lewis T (1938) Movie film on 'The Signs of Venous Congestion'
420. Lewis T (1939) Letter to Dr A Chromow A.1/28–101
421. Lewis T (1939) Letter to Professor FR Fraser C.3/1
422. Lewis T (1939) A note on the Samway tourniquet C.3/2
423. Lewis T (1939) Duties of the house physician D.3/1
424. Lewis T (1940) Letter to Professor A Blalock A.1/28–101
425. Lewis T (1940) Letter to Dr F Boys A.1/28–101
426. Lewis T (1940) Letter to Dr EA Carmichael A.1/102–151
427. Lewis T (1940) Letter to Dr Duckett Jones A.1/357–363
428. Lewis T (1940) Letter to Ministry of Home Security A.1/460–517
429. Lewis T (1940) Letter to the editor of The Lancet A.1/390–459
430. Lewis T (1941) Letter to the British Council A1./28–101
431. Lewis T (1941) Letter to Dr E Landis A.1/390–459
432. Lewis T (1942) Letter to Dr Harold Davies A.1/28–101
433. Lewis T (1942) Letter to Prof JBS Haldane A.1/284–355
434. Lewis T (1942) Letter to Dr E Landis A.1/390–459
435. Lewis T (1942) Letter to Dr Myron Prinzmetal A.1/553–596
436. Lewis T (1942) Letter to Dr FMR Walshe A.1/707–771
437. Lewis T (1942) Letter to Dr FMR Walshe A.1/707–771
438. Lewis T (1942) Letter to Dr PD White A.1/707–771
439. Lewis T (1943) Letter to Mr G Hesling A.2
440. Lewis T (1943) Letter to Dr EP Sharpey-Schafer A.2
441. Lewis T (1943) Letters to Dr FMR Walshe A.1/707–771
442. Lewis T (1944) Letter to Sir Henry Dale B.7/5
443. Lewis T (1944) Letter to TR Elliott D.8/3
444. Lewis T (1944) Letter to Dr EP Sharpey-Schafer A.2
445. Mackenzie J (1918) Letter to TL A.1/460–517

446. Mackenzie J (1920) Letter to TL A.1/460–517
447. Mackenzie J (1921) Letter to TL February 5 A.1/460–517
448. Mackenzie J (1921) Letter to TL March 10 A.1/460–517
449. Mackenzie J (1921) Letter to TL September 2 A.1/460–517
450. Mackenzie J (1923) Letter to TL A.1/460–517
451. Mackenzie J (1924) Letter to TL A.1/460–517
452. Marvin HM (1927) Letter to TL B.6
453. Marvin HM (1928) Letter to TL B.6
454. Marvin HM (1930) Letter to TL B.6
455. Marvin HM (1931) Letter to TL B.6
456. McMichael, Sir John (1974) Audio-tape
457. Medical Research Council (1933) MRC Clinical Committee D.4/3
458. Ministry of Health (1922) Conference of cardiac consultants February 3 C.2/4
459. Moran, Lord (1945) Letter to TL B.7/5
460. Oppenheimer BS (1918) Letter to TL C.1/8
461. Penfield W (1937) Letter to TL A.1/553–596
462. Perry CB (1990) Audio-tape
463. Pickering, Lady (1986) Audio-tape
464. Rothberger CJ (1936) Letter to TL A.1/597–656
465. Rothschild P (1936) Letter to TL A.1/597–656
466. Segall H (1978) Audio-tape
467. Sharpey-Schafer EP (1943) Letter to TL A.2
468. Sharpey-Schafer EP (1943) Letter to TL A.2
469. Sherrington CS (1941) Letter to TL A.1/777–861
470. Sinclair H (1988) Audio-tape
471. Stokes J (1974) Audio-tape
472. Stroud W (1920) Letter to TL A.1/683b
473. Trotter W (1929) Letter to TL B.6
474. Walker MB (1935) Letter to TL A.1/707–771
475. Walshe FMR (1942) Letter to TL June 11 A.1/707–771
476. Walshe FMR (1942) Letter to TL June 15 A.1/707–771
477. Walshe FMR (1942) Letter to TL June 17 A.1/707–771
478. Walshe FMR (1944) Letter to TL D.3/5
479. Wayne Sir Edward (1978) Audio-tape
480. Weiss S (1927) Letter to TL A.1/707–771
481. Welch WH (1914) Letter to TL A.1/777–861
482. White PD (1913) Letter to TL A.1/777–861
483. Wilson FN (1925–1933) Letters to TL A.1/707–771
484. Wright W (1912) Letter to TL A.1/777–861.

### Material in the archives of the Medical Research Council, London

485. Fletcher WM (1915) Letter to TL PF 136
486. Fletcher WM (1918) Letter to Dr George Blacker PF 136
487. Fletcher WM (1927) Letter to TL PF 136
488. Fletcher WM (1930) Letter to Professor TR Elliott PF 136
489. Lewis T (1915) Letter, August 19, to WM Fletcher PF 136
490. Lewis T (1915) Letter, December 8, to WM Fletcher PF 136
491. Lewis T (1916) Letter to WM Fletcher PF 136
492. Lewis T (1919) Letter to WM Fletcher PF 136
493. Lewis T (1920) Letter to WM Fletcher PF 136
494. Lewis T (1921) Letter to Colonel Smallman PF 136
495. Lewis T (1924) Letter to Dr Landsborough Thomson
496. Lewis T (1927) Letter to WM Fletcher PF 136
497. Lewis T (1928) Letter to WM Fletcher File 2011

498. Lewis T (1929) Letter, May 31, to WM Fletcher File 2011
499. Lewis T (1929) Letter, December 2, to WM Fletcher File 2011
500. Lewis T (1932) Letter, June 10, to WM Fletcher PF 116
501. Lewis T (1932) Letter, June 24, to WM Fletcher PF 116
502. Lewis T (1936) Letter, September 4, to E Mellanby File 2011
503. Lewis T (1939) Letter, November 10, to E Mellanby File 2011
504. Lewis T (1942) Letter and memorandum to E Mellanby File 445.

**Material held by Dr A Hollman**

505. Bedford DE (1975) Letter to AH
506. Bland EF (1980) Letter to AH
507. Burchell HB (1990) Letter to AH
508. Clarke CA (1981) Letter to AH
509. Craib WH (1982) Letter to AH
510. Craib WH (1975) Letter to Dr DM Krikler
511. Elliott TR (1945) Letter to Sir Alan Drury
512. Epstein F (1992) Letter to AH
513. Evans W (1981) Letter to AH
514. Fowler A (1987) Letter to AH
515. Himsworth HP (1990) Personal communication to AH
516. Honour AJ (1993) Personal communication to AH
517. Howarth SM (1990) Letter to AH
518. Kellgren JH (1993) Personal communication to AH
519. Kelsall AR (1990) Letter to AH
520. Lewis T (1902 to 1910) Letters to and from his parents
521. Lewis T (1903) Reprints on Ductless Glands, chiefly histological
522. Lewis T (1927) The practitioner's debt to research
523. Lewis T (1935) Manuscript of Vascular Disorders of the Limbs
524. Lewis T (1935) File of letters to him regarding discovery of remedies
525. Lewis T (1935 to 1944) Letters to Dr Eluned Woodford-Williams and Dr E Joan Stokes
526. Lewis T (1944) Pocket diaries, and a scrapbook containing reviews of his books, and his letters to journals
527. Mackenzie J (1910) Letter to Dr William Hume
528. McNee J (1925) Personal communication and his article, The clinical syndrome of thrombosis of the coronary arteries. Q J Med 19: 44–49
529. Morris AD (1965) Letter to AH
530. Morris JM (1995) Personal communication to AH
531. Phillips W (1975) Letter to AH
532. Philps, R (1977) Letter to AH
533. Royal College of Physicians (1928) Letters to TL
534. Savory M (1978) Letter to AH
535. Stern ES (1975) Letter to AH
536. Williams DA (1985) Letter to AH
537. Wolff O (1981) Letter to AH

# Index